Understanding Nursing Research

Using Research in
Evidence-Based Practice

Understanding Nursing Research

Using Research in Evidence-Based Practice

THIRD EDITION

Cherie R. Rebar, PhD, RN, MBA
Associate Professor
Kettering College of Medical Arts
Dayton, Ohio

Carolyn J. Gersch, MSN, RN, CNE
Associate Professor
Kettering College of Medical Arts
Dayton, Ohio

Carol L. Macnee, RN, PhD
Professor
University of Wyoming Fay W. Whitney School of Nursing
Laramie, Wyoming

Susan McCabe, RN, CS, EdD
Associate Professor
University of Wyoming Fay W. Whitney School of Nursing
Laramie, Wyoming

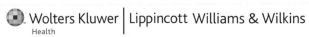 Wolters Kluwer | Lippincott Williams & Wilkins
Health
Philadelphia · Baltimore · New York · London
Buenos Aires · Hong Kong · Sydney · Tokyo

Acquisitions Editor: Hilarie Surrena
Product Manager: Shawn Loht/Eric Van Osten
Director of Nursing Production: Helen Ewan
Design Coordinator: Joan Wendt
Manufacturing Coordinator: Karin Duffield
Prepress Vendor: MPS Limited, a Macmillan Company

3rd edition

9 8 7 6 5 4 3 2 1

Printed in China

Library of Congress Cataloging-in-Publication Data
Understanding nursing research : using research in evidence-based practice /Cherie R. Rebar . . . [et al.].—3rd ed.
   p. ; cm.
   Rev. ed. of: Understanding nursing research/Carol L. Macnee, Susan McCabe. 2nd ed. c2008.
   Includes bibliographical references and index.
   Summary: "This textbook explicitly links understanding of nursing research with evidence-based practice, and focuses on how to read, critique, and utilize research reports. Organized around questions students have when reading reports—how the conclusions were reached, what types of patients the conclusions apply to, how the study was done, and why it was done that way—the text explains the steps of the research process to answer these questions"—Provided by publisher.
   ISBN 978-1-60547-730-5
   1. Nursing—Research. I. Rebar, Cherie R. II. Macnee, Carol L. (Carol Leslie). Understanding nursing research.
   [DNLM: 1. Nursing Research. 2. Evidence-Based Nursing—methods. WY 20.5]
   RT81.5.M235 2012
   610.73072—dc22

                       2010029517

CCS0910

*This book is dedicated to the memory of
Carol L. Macnee and Susan McCabe.*

REVIEWERS

Barbara Celia, EdD, RN
Clinical Assistant Professor
College of Nursing Health Professions
Drexel University
Philadelphia, Pennsylvania

Susan Golden, MSN, RN
Nursing Faculty
Nursing Program Director
Department of Nursing
Eastern New Mexico University—Roswell
Roswell, New Mexico

Joyce P. Griffin-Sobel, PhD, RN, AOCN,
CNE, ANEF
Assistant Dean, Curriculum & Technology
Professor and Director, Undergraduate
Programs
Hunter College, Bellevue School of
Nursing
New York, New York

Vincent P. Hall, PhD, RN
Director
School of Nursing
Western Carolina University
Cullowhee, North Carolina

Cheryl Johnson-Joy, PhD, RN
Professor and Associate Dean
Baptist College of Health Sciences
Memphis, Tennessee

Kimberly Lacey, DNSc, MSN, CNS, RN
Assistant Professor
Department of Nursing
Southern Connecticut State University
New Haven, CT

Kathleen M. Lamaute, EdD, FNP, BC,
CNAA, CNE
Associate Professor
Molloy College
Rockville Centre, New York

Patricia Z. Lund, EdD, RN
Professor Emerita
Western Connecticut State University
Danbury, Connecticut
Adjunct Faculty
Virginia Commonwealth University,
School of Nursing
Richmond, Virginia

Tammie McCoy, RN, PhD
Associate Professor and Chair
Baccalaureate Nursing Program
Mississippi University for Women
Columbus, Mississippi

Barbara Patterson, PhD, RN
Professor
Widener University, School of Nursing
Chester, Pennsylvania

Mary Carol G. Pomatto, EdD, ARNP-CNS
Professor and Chair
Department of Nursing
Pittsburg State University
Pittsburg, Kansas

Kandyce M. Richards, PhD, MSc, BN
Assistant Professor
University of Miami School of Nursing
and Health Studies
Coral Gables, Florida

Beth Rodgers, PhD, RN, FAAN
Professor
University of Wisconsin-Milwaukee,
College of Nursing
Milwaukee, Wisconsin

Cheryl K. Schmidt, PhD, RN, CNE, ANEF
Associate Professor
University of Arkansas for Medical
Sciences, College of Nursing
Little Rock, Arkansas

Shirley Powe Smith, PhD, RN, CRNP
Assistant Professor
Coordinator, Continuing Education
  Program
Duquesne University
Pittsburgh, Pennsylvania

Kathleen F. Tennant, PhD, APRN, BC
Associate Professor
Nursing
Ohio University
St. Clairsville, Ohio

Barbara S. Turner, RN, DNSc, FAAN
Professor
Duke University School of Nursing
Durham, North Carolina

Roberta Waite, EdD, APRN, CNS-BC
Assistant Professor
Division of Undergraduate Nursing
Drexel University
Philadelphia, Pennsylvania

Molly J. Walker, PhD, RN, CNS, CNE
Associate Professor
Nursing
Angelo State University
San Angelo, Texas

Julia P. Wetmore, RN, PhD
Visiting Assistant Professor
Nursing
Western Carolina University
Morganton, North Carolina

PREFACE

We believe that learning should be fun and that learning happens best when students can relate new knowledge to something relevant to them. We also believe that when students are not expected to be researchers, they can enjoy learning how to read and use research as one important form of evidence on which to base practice. We love research, and we are fundamentally practitioners who find excitement and challenge in tackling new information to fill in the gaps in our knowledge about practice. We hope that some of our enthusiasm is communicated in these pages.

Understanding Nursing Research: Reading and Using Research in Practice differs from existing undergraduate research textbooks in a number of important ways. The first premise of this book is that nursing students need to understand the language of research and the underlying concepts of the research process but do not necessarily need to be prepared to conduct a research study. The second premise is that nursing students and practicing baccalaureate-prepared nurses are motivated to read and use research evidence only as it relates to their practice. Given these two premises, it is logical that many nursing students and nurses read only the abstract and the conclusion sections of research reports. Those two sections usually contain less of the technical language of research and address most directly the clinical meaning of a research study, so they are viewed as both understandable and useful for practice. Following that reasoning, we organized this book around the sections of a research report rather than the steps of the research process. It starts with what most practicing RNs are interested in—the conclusions—and then moves forward to the beginning of a research report. We believe that this will help the student recognize the relevance of each section of a typical research report in understanding and using research in evidence-based practice. In addition, five questions that a nurse might ask when reading research are used to further organize the text, and throughout the chapters, the emphasis is on reading, understanding, and using research in practice. In keeping with this, each chapter of the book begins with a clinical case that identifies what information the nurse is seeking from research literature to answer a clinical question. One or two published research articles that directly relate to the clinical case are discussed throughout the chapter to provide specific examples of the concepts addressed; they are reprinted in full in Appendices A.1 through A.9.

It is a challenge to represent the breadth and depth of nursing practice and nursing research in a single textbook. A real effort has been made to include clinical cases that reflect nursing practice in a variety of settings, ranging from acute care to public health, and across a range of specialties. This text also differs from other undergraduate research texts in that we use the research articles as exemplars to discuss both qualitative and quantitative research methods. As nursing science evolves, we recognize the need to use a variety of methods from both the positivist and naturalist viewpoints to develop knowledge that reflects nursing's holistic perspective. Both qualitative and quantitative methods are used to build knowledge in nursing, and rather than artificially separating the discussion of these two approaches, we contrast the approaches while identifying the broader conceptual base that is common to both. However, because combining quantitative and qualitative methods in each chapter may be confusing at times, icons are used to identify the method being described within a paragraph.

Learners learn best by doing, so each chapter of this book ends with a specific learning activity that prepares students for the concepts addressed in the following chapter. The learning activity is directly related to the examples and the clinical case in the chapter. To provide an opportunity for students to be active learners, an in-class questionnaire that can be used as a mini-research study is included in Appendix C, and Appendix B is a fictional article that could have been based on the results from the in-class questionnaire. It intentionally contains flaws that are slightly more glaring than any likely to be found in a published, peer-reviewed research report. The fictional article is used throughout the text as an example, along with the authentic research reports.

The goal of this text is to enable students to read and comprehend published research, so that they can make professional decisions regarding the use of research reports in evidence-based practice. Associated with this goal is the hope that students will develop their interest and confidence in reading research, rather than avoiding it. Our text is designed to be user-friendly, taking a more casual tone than some research texts do, to minimize the intimidating nature of the language and concepts of research. For easy reference, each term in the glossary includes its chapter and page number in the text.

The sign of a successful textbook is that students decide to keep it to use in the future, rather than sell it after they complete their course. We hope ours will be one they keep. We believe that learning to understand and use published research can be fun, interesting, and useful for students if they can see its direct relevance to their practice. The organization of this book is unconventional and the tone conversational, addressing the subject from the perspective of a reader and user of research, rather than from a creator of it. Students tell us this is a helpful perspective and one that they enjoy. As nurse researchers, our greatest goal is to foster appreciation and enthusiasm for the process that we find so challenging and so clinically meaningful. We hope this text contributes to accomplish that goal. And we hope you have some fun!

Cherie R. Rebar

Carolyn J. Gersch

Carol L. Macnee

Susan McCabe

ACKNOWLEDGMENTS

With gratitude and appreciation to our wonderful families, both at home and in the nursing profession, who have supported our endeavors, encouraged our creativity, and challenged us to lend our voices to the continuing evolution of evidence-based nursing.

Cherie R. Rebar

Carolyn J. Gersch

CONTENTS

1

Evidence-Based Nursing: Using Research in Practice

LEARNING OBJECTIVE

The student will relate nursing research to the development of the professional practice of nursing.

KEY TERMS

Abstract
Electronic databases
Evidence-based nursing (EBN)
Key words
Knowledge
Outcomes research

Printed indexes
Research process
Research utilization
Systematic review

Clinical Case • M.D. is a 17-year-old adolescent who is a senior at a local public high school. She has had weight issues for the last 6 years and is considered to be medically obese. She has become concerned about the inability to lose weight, health problems related to obesity, and her self-esteem. She has discussed her concerns with the school nurse and is anxious to take action. The school nurse recognizes that M.D. needs both education and support in achieving her ideal weight. The RN completes a literature search and finds two articles that appear to relate to M.D. and her weight. The first is titled "Sleep, Hunger, Satiety, Food Cravings, & Caloric Intake in Adolescents" (Landis, Parker, & Dunbar, 2009) and the second is titled "The Relationships Among Self-Esteem, Stress, Coping, Eating Behavior, and Depressive Mood in Adolescents" (Martyn-Nemeth, Penckofer, Gulanick, Velsor-Friedrich, & Bryant, 2009). You can find these articles in Appendices A.1 and A.2 of this text.

■ INTRODUCTION

Understanding Nursing Research discusses how you can use nursing research in your nursing practice. Its goal is to teach you, a practicing nurse, to find answers to clinical questions you may have by using nursing research. Another way to phrase this goal is that this book is about practice based on research evidence or evidence-based practice. To base your practice on research evidence, however, you must be able to understand the research language as well as the research process.

Because answering clinical questions is important for a practicing nurse, this book begins at the end of the research process, with the conclusions, and moves forward through the process. While this may seem unusual, research study conclusions often lead to further questions. You may wonder, for example, why the author(s) reached these conclusions. That question may lead to the results section of the study, where specific numbers and measurements are described. You also may wonder to what types of patients these research results apply. That question may lead you to the description of the study sample. If you wonder why a certain patient was studied, or how the author(s) measured some aspect studied (e.g., pain), you must read and understand the methods section of the research study. Finally, the methods section may direct you to review what has been done before and what nursing theory and other theories may suggest about this clinical question. That information is in the beginning or background section of the research report.

Therefore, this book begins at the end and moves forward through a research report to understand both the research language and the process underlying it. The five general questions that are described in the paragraph below are used to organize the end-to-beginning approach. Each chapter discusses a different component of the research report and how that component can help to answer the five questions. These questions also can be used to organize your own reading and understanding of research. They are as follows:

- What is the answer to my practice question—what did the study conclude?
- Why did the author(s) reach these conclusions—what did they actually find?
- To what types of patients do these research conclusions apply—who was in the study?
- How were those people studied—why was the study performed that way?
- Why ask that question—what do we already know?

This book focuses on assisting you to read and understand research reports and to use them intelligently as evidence to guide your clinical practice. Therefore, each chapter begins with a clinical case that raises a clinical question that can be addressed by nursing research. A published research report that is related to the clinical case is part of the required reading for the chapter, and each chapter focuses on what can be decided about practice based on an understanding of the article. To help bring the language and process of research to a practical level, you and your classmates also may participate in a small practice "study" that will be used in the text as a concrete example of different aspects of the research process.

When you finish reading this book, you will be prepared to read nursing research critically and use it intelligently. Critically reading research means reading it with a questioning mind: knowing what information should be presented in a report, understanding what is reported, and asking yourself whether the research is good enough for you to accept and use in your practice. You will not be prepared to be a researcher yourself, but you will understand some of the processes of nursing research and how that research can help you in your practice.

■ ROLE OF RESEARCH IN THE EVOLUTION OF NURSING AS A PROFESSION

This text focuses on the baccalaureate-prepared nurse's role in understanding and using research in evidence-based nursing (EBN) practice: a process used by nurses to make clinical decisions and to answer clinical questions. It also has suggested some other ways that research may be part of the role of the baccalaureate nurse. For example, nurses may be asked to use research as the basis for decisions about the development of clinical programs. They may be asked to participate in some step of the research process, particularly in acquiring informed consent and in collecting data. Equally important, as the nursing profession recognizes the need for clinically relevant and informed research, baccalaureate nurses may be asked to participate in all phases of a research study, from development and refinement of the purpose to interpretation of the results. For example, one of the hallmarks of hospitals that have the highest retention of nurses and quality of patient care—that is, hospitals that have received the American Nurses Credentialing Center (ANCC) Magnet Recognition Program status—is the inclusion of nursing research development and application in the clinical setting.

We begin this book by saying that it is not the goal of this text to give you the tools to implement research independently. Doctoral-level nurses are expected to be the experts in the research process. Nurses prepared at the master's level are expected to be sophisticated consumers of research, who are able to critically evaluate and actively participate in research. Nevertheless, baccalaureate-level nurses often are the foundation from which research is developed and are absolutely the focus for research utilization. Research utilization means the use of research in practice. Your understanding of the language and the process of research, coupled with your clinical experience, will allow you to be a contributor to a research team, should the opportunity arise. One hospital that perhaps best epitomizes the full extent of the potential role of the baccalaureate-prepared nurse in research is housed on the grounds of the National Institutes of Health. Every patient there participates in at least one research study, and the hospital employs only baccalaureate-prepared nurses. The nurses there not only participate in research but also can develop their own cooperative research projects, with support from researchers with advanced preparation. Baccalaureate-level nurses can be members of Institutional Review Boards as well, bringing their knowledge of patients and patient care to assist in assuring that the rights of patients are protected.

Nursing not only has a role in research that directly addresses questions generated within the profession, but it also addresses larger questions in health care. Nursing has moved increasingly to interprofessional teams to address research problems. Nurses also are being sought increasingly to participate in research teams led by researchers from other disciplines. Nursing's unique understanding of health as it affects the whole person, family, and community is a perspective that often contributes important ideas to research studies. Nurses are good at working with people. Thus, researchers from other disciplines often find that nurses can implement sampling plans effectively, with little subject loss.

Beyond generating and participating in research, nursing has an important role in formulating the national research agendas regarding health. The research supported and generated through the National Institute of Nursing Research at the National Institutes of Health has earned the respect of other, more established research disciplines. That development has contributed to ensuring that health concerns particularly focused on nursing have become part of national agendas for health-related research. Nursing research has made great progress since the days of Florence Nightingale, and we can be proud not only of our heritage of research but also of our current and future contributions to meaningful research that improves the care of our patients.

■ HISTORY OF NURSING RESEARCH

History helps us to understand the past and its continuing influence on the future. Nursing research started slowly, but it has evolved at an ever-increasing and progressive rate.

It is widely accepted that the history of nursing research begins with Florence Nightingale and her studies of environmental factors that affected the health of soldiers in the Crimean War. During the last half of the 19th century, nurses, particularly in public health, continued to refine Nightingale's findings published in *Notes on Nursing* (1860). Little is known, however, of any nursing research during that time.

Between 1900 and 1940, nurses conducted research, but the larger focus was the preparation of nurses. During those years, the *American Journal of Nursing* began publication, baccalaureate nursing programs increased, and the first doctoral program in nursing opened at Teacher's College, Columbia University. Each of these developments helped to promote an increase in nursing research.

In the infancy of nursing research, we tended to study ourselves. In the 1940s and 1950s, it primarily focused on studying characteristics of nurses and nursing education. This occurred probably because nursing was relatively new to the university system, and most doctoral-prepared nurses had education degrees. Despite this focus, nursing research made significant progress during this time, as evidenced by the publication of the journal *Nursing Research*.

During the 1960s, nursing began to recognize the need for theoretical foundations to its practice and research. Research also shifted away from the study of nurses toward the study of the clinical care provided by nurses. Within nursing education, nursing faculty began to teach the research process in baccalaureate nursing programs.

By 1970s, nursing research examining clinical practice had increased significantly, as evidenced by the publication of three additional journals to disseminate research: *Research in Nursing & Health*, *Advances in Nursing Science*, and *Western Journal of Nursing Research*. Doctoral nursing programs continued to emerge, leading to steady growth in nurses who were specifically prepared to be researchers. The emphasis in nursing research during this time was traditional quantitative methods, often testing theories borrowed from other fields. Despite this emphasis, nursing theory also was growing during this period, and qualitative methods were increasingly used.

The steady increase in both research itself and nurses prepared to do research reached a critical level in the 1980s, culminating in the establishment in 1986 of the National Center of Nursing Research at the National Institutes of Health. The national recognition of nursing as a science, warranting funding for its own research agenda and center, was a major milestone. Nursing was now acknowledged as an important player among other "big" players, such as the National Institute for Medicine and the National Institute of Mental Health. In 1993, 7 years after its establishment, the National Center for Nursing Research became the National Institute of Nursing Research. This change placed nurses on equal footing with colleagues in medicine and other health-related fields. In addition, during the 1980s and 1990s, five more major nursing research journals were published, and priorities for nursing research were developed. Nursing research had come of age.

At the beginning of the 21st century, nursing research continues to grow exponentially. Nurses preparing at the doctoral level, sources and opportunities for funding of nursing research, and diversity of topics examined in nursing research all have increased steadily. Since the 1990s, when qualitative approaches became recognized and respected as appropriate methods of scientific inquiry, nursing has been implementing mixtures of quantitative and qualitative methods for study design and analysis that fit the unique research problems of the field.

Probably most important, as nursing research has grown, the body of nursing knowledge also has developed, as nurses, we have expanded our horizons to consider outcomes research, international research, and traditional laboratory research. We have replicated and expanded on previous findings. Our researchers have completed multiple studies all related to the same problems, allowing us to truly build knowledge and to find real answers to complex questions. As a result, we now have Centers for Research housed in various universities, where groups of nurses with research expertise in specific areas (such as health-promoting behaviors) can work and build their research together to achieve a better-connected and deeper knowledge. Nurses also have recognized their limits as well as their strengths, moving increasingly toward the creation of and participation in interprofessional teams of researchers, capitalizing on the strengths inherent in the blending of many different disciplines.

■ QUESTIONS FOR PATIENT CARE

In the clinical case at the beginning of this chapter, the nurse has a clinical question and needs answers. The nurse questions how to best meet the complex needs of an adolescent who is medically obese and has health and self-image/esteem issues related to obesity. The nurse knows that educational and supportive interventions will need to be implemented to help M.D. achieve an ideal weight while addressing her health and self-image concerns. The nurse wonders if M.D.'s stress of knowing she is obese, and/or the stress of school and life issues, will in any way alter her coping with becoming a healthy adult. The nurse also knows to consider other complex issues, including psychosocial issues, physiologic issues, health promotion issues, and referral procedures for specialized care if needed for this adolescent. The nurse wonders which factor to focus on first and whether there might be a way to plan nursing care that would promote M.D.'s self-esteem and also focus on several different issues at the same time, given the nurse's busy workload.

This nurse's question is just one example of the kinds of practice-related questions nurses face each day. Any nursing student knows that not all nurses do everything the same way. Therefore, the questions arise, and you may already have had many questions yourself, such as which is the best way to flush a percutaneous endogastric (PEG) tube, maintain an indwelling urinary catheter, or prepare a patient for surgery? And then there are questions about the differences in patients. Why do male patients have a quicker postoperative recovery from coronary artery bypass grafts than do female patients? Why do some patients quit smoking when they are pregnant and others do not? Why do some patients with AIDS keep recovering from infections, when others seem to weaken and die as soon as the first severe complications occur? Which is more helpful to patients with major depression—to urge them to get up and moving each day or to urge them to listen to themselves and follow their own natural schedules? Although nursing knowledge has grown steadily and we know a great deal about providing optimal health care, there are still more questions than there are answers about how to promote health.

■ WHERE TO FIND EVIDENCE FOR PRACTICE

How do you, as a nurse, find answers to clinical questions such as those listed in the previous section? Traditionally, four approaches have been taken, including:

1. Consulting an authority or trusted individual.
2. Using intuition and subjective judgment.

3. Turning to experience.
4. Reading textbooks and other authoritative material.

As you might guess, using these four traditional approaches to answering clinical questions can produce a wide range of answers, some useful and some not so useful. Relying too much on experience or on intuition may prevent new knowledge or understanding from being applied to clinical problems. Consulting with just one trusted person may not bring a range of thoughts and may result in a biased sense of perspective. Because of these concerns, a newer approach is being developed to standardize a nurse's clinical decision-making process and to provide a framework for planning care that answers the kinds of clinical questions nurses may have. This approach is called evidence-based nursing.

EBN practice is the term used to describe the process that nurses use to make clinical decisions and to answer clinical questions. Like traditional approaches, EBN also has four approaches to answer questions. But unlike the traditional approach in which you could choose to use an expert opinion or you could use a textbook, EBN uses ALL of the approaches all of the time for every clinical question. The approaches include:

1. Reviewing the best available evidence, most often the results of research.
2. Using the nurse's clinical expertise.
3. Determining the values and cultural needs of the individual.
4. Determining the preferences of the individual, family, and community.

To answer clinical questions using EBN strategies, the nurse must know how to access the latest research, be able to correctly interpret the research findings, be able to apply the findings to the clinical problem using his or her nursing judgment and experience, and take into account the cultural and personal values and preferences of the patient (STTI, 2005). As more nursing research is conducted, there is more and more evidence that practicing nurses can turn to in order to answer clinical questions. Using EBN allows a nurse to determine the meaningfulness of the available evidence for the patient he or she is caring for and assists the nurse to make decisions about nursing interventions, based on research evidence, that are justified as part of clinical practice.

EBN implies that one of the roles of a professional RN will be to frequently seek out the available evidence in order to plan and implement the best nursing care possible. While the bulk of this book will focus on assisting you to know where to find research evidence and how to interpret it in order to have the research evidence influence your care, it is worth taking a minute to discuss when you should seek evidence. It is ideal to say that you will seek evidence for every patient care situation, but that may be unrealistic. Routine care is often based on protocols or procedures that apply evidence. But there will be moments in your clinical practice when you should actively and independently seek out evidence to inform your care.

Situations in which you should actively seek out research evidence on which to base your care include such times as when something in your clinical practice is out of the ordinary. It may be out of the ordinary because you are caring for a patient with a disease or health need you have not encountered before. An example of this would be if you were caring for an adolescent who has obesity-related physical and psychosocial complications, and although you had cared for adults with these health concerns, you had never cared for an adolescent. Or it may be a situation in which a patient has a characteristic that you have never encountered before, such as a cultural or religious characteristic. An example of this would be if you were working on a step-down unit for postrenal transplant patients and were assigned to care for a Hasidic Jewish patient who has just emigrated from Russia. If you were unfamiliar with the patient care situation, this would be an ideal time to seek research-based evidence in order to improve care.

Another time that you should seek evidence is when the outcomes of the care you are delivering seem to differ in one or more patients without clear reasons. An example of this is given in the clinical case in Chapter 3. It describes a postsurgical patient whose rate of recovery is different from the typical patient the nurse deals with in a specific health care setting. In this case, a search for research-based evidence may well provide increased knowledge, allowing the nurse to provide the best care possible. Another time when an RN should seek out evidence is when there is a need to develop policy or plan standards for care. An example of this may be a nurse who is a unit manager in an ambulatory care unit. The hospital has decided to initiate universal assessment for domestic violence for every patient, male and female, who presents for care. In deciding how to best initiate this change in routine care, the nurse will find that a search of the available literature is very helpful.

While there are four approaches used in EBN, it starts with the ability to locate and then interpret evidence, most often the results of research. This book focuses on how to review the best available evidence. The other pieces of EBN—using the nurse's clinical expertise; determining the values and cultural needs of the individual; and determining the preferences of the individual, family, and community—also are very important and should always be considered (STTI, 2002).

■ DEVELOPING CLINICAL QUESTIONS FOR REAL WORLD PRACTICE

We have been talking about EBN and the professional responsibility of RNs to identify and understand research-based evidence. We have used a clinical case as an example of the common nature of clinical questions that can be answered by examining research. But not every question can be answered by examining research evidence. Sometimes no researcher has studied anything similar to your question, or sometimes even though the health problem has been researched, the aspect of the clinical problem you are most interested in has not been studied. So it is important to be able to state your clinical question effectively and know when you can expect research-based evidence to be of help to you. An effective clinical question for EBN is one that has been asked before by someone else and, at least in part, has been explored by a researcher. In addition, a good clinical question has to focus on a health care issue that can be measured or described in some consistent manner. Finally, a good clinical question that may be answered by examining research-based evidence has to provide information about what nurses want or need to do.

An example of an effective clinical question would be "What is the best patient teaching method for newly diagnosed adolescent diabetic patients treated in ambulatory care clinics?" This question is effective because it clearly focuses on what nurses need to do. Diabetes in adolescents is an area that has been researched, and it can be described or measured. We can use blood sugar levels to measure someone's diabetes. We can interview patients to describe how they learned to cope with their diabetes. A clinical question that is less effective would be "How can I help my young diabetic patient feel better?" While this question is nursing-related, it is less effective because it asks how a nurse can make someone "feel better." Feeling better may mean different things to different people, and it is not easily measured. Another example would be the question "Which insulin pump delivers the most consistent and accurate level of drug to adolescent diabetic patients?" While this is a much more specific and measurable question, it is less effective because it is not directly nursing-related. This type of question is most likely physician-related or pharmacist-related; it does not directly relate to nursing actions.

CORE CONCEPT 1.1

An effective clinical question for evidence-based nursing includes a concern that someone else has studied, focuses on a concern that can be measured or described, and is a concern that is relevant to nursing. The question also addresses Who, Where, What, and When in terms of the clinical concern.

In addition to being related to an area of nursing that has been researched and can be either described or measured, an effective clinical question includes a few other things. It identifies *Who* you are interested in. In our example, the *Who* are adolescent diabetic patients. An effective clinical question also identifies the *Where*. In our example, the nurse identifies his or her interest in adolescent diabetic patients treated in ambulatory care clinics. In addition to *Who* and *Where*, the effective question will identify the *What* and the *When*. The *What* is the health problem of interest or the desired outcome of nursing care. In our example, the *What* is patient teaching. The *When* is often the least identified element of a clinical question, but an important one. The *When* identifies where in the course of the clinical problem the question arises. In our example, we asked, "What is the best patient teaching method for newly diagnosed adolescent diabetic patients treated in ambulatory care clinics?" Our *When* is "newly diagnosed." We are focusing our clinical question on patients who have just been diagnosed. As you can imagine, the patient teaching needs of individuals who have had diabetes for many years are different from those of patients who have just been diagnosed. We could have asked in our example, "What is the best patient teaching method for diabetic patients experiencing neuropathic pain treated in an ambulatory setting?" In this case, our *When* focus is on a time in the course of diabetes that a person has begun to experience the complications of the chronic illness; therefore, the health needs of this person are different from what they were at the start of the illness. Using the *Who*, *What*, *When*, and *Where* approach to forming your clinical question will do a great deal to help you search for the best available evidence to answer your question. For each clinical question in this text, we will identify the *Who*, *What*, *When*, and *Where* in a table following each clinical vignette.

Determining the Best Available Evidence

Practicing EBN implies that nurses use evidence to answer clinical questions. But what is evidence, and is all evidence equally useful for guiding a nurse's decision making? Evidence should be thought of as information that provides a point of view or contributes to finding the solution to a clinical question. But all information is not always equally useful. Some information is from informal sources and is collected under less than rigorous conditions. Other information is obtained from very rigorous procedures, through formal methods. While both kinds of information may be useful, the more formally and rigorously the information is collected, the stronger it is considered as evidence on which to make EBN clinical decisions.

In considering what the best available evidence is, a nurse needs to look at how the information that makes up the evidence was collected, how rigorous the method used to develop the evidence was, and what source was used to share the evidence. In this sense, evidence can be placed into two categories: research-based and nonresearch-based. Figure 1.1 shows examples of both. We will discuss nonresearch evidence first.

Let us say that you have a clinical question regarding the transmission of the H1N1 flu virus. In order to plan how best to prevent the transmission of the flu, you could directly ask people who have had the flu recently how they think they got it. As you ask several people, you may notice some common answers that provide you with information (evidence). But it may not be the strongest evidence on which to base clinical interventions. You could consult a textbook. As a nursing student, you will often use authorities, a type of nonresearch evidence, to answer your patient care questions. As a student nurse, you will regularly seek answers to questions from authoritative sources such as reference books, practice journals, other members of the health care team (such as the pharmacist), and patients. Notice that all these sources of evidence reflect the traditional approaches discussed earlier.

Another approach to answering clinical questions is to use your intuition or subjective judgment. This type of evidence is based on your own experience. Nursing is both a science

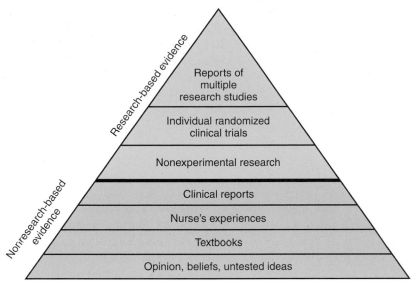

FIGURE 1.1   Sources of evidence.

and an art, and intuition or subjective judgment can be an important way of knowing what to do in clinical situations. Intuition can be a source of indirect evidence that is not explicit and articulated fully. Intuition can be thought of as a form of nonresearch evidence. It differs from common sense or arbitrary choice because it is knowledge—but knowledge that we cannot explicate in detail. Intuition may tell you that a particular day is not the day to push a depressed patient to get out of bed. Intuition may tell you that one patient with AIDS has given up and will not survive hospitalization, whereas another who is equally ill is determined to live. Such intuition will guide your care for each of these patients, perhaps leading to a focus on social support and spiritual care for the first patient and a focus on independence for the second patient. In this sense, intuition is evidence to consider in clinical decision making.

Other approaches to answering questions about nursing care depend on your own experience as evidence. Experience may indicate that patients who had their indwelling urinary catheters changed every 72 hours had fewer urinary tract infections (UTIs) than did those who had theirs changed every 48 hours. Experience may also indicate that depressed patients who were strongly encouraged to get out of bed and follow a daily morning routine were discharged sooner than those who were not encouraged. Personal experience with a health problem may also provide answers to clinical questions. You may know what worked for you or your family, so that is what you will offer or do for your patient.

Clinical reports are another source of nonresearch-based evidence for clinical decision making. This type of evidence is less personal, representing instead the formal experience of someone else. You may find a published article in a practice journal that discusses another nurse's experience with a clinical issue. Or you may find an article that discusses the outcome of a particular approach to patient care. These case reports can provide a rich source of evidence, but the evidence is limited because it may pertain only to that one case and not reflect the unique needs of your patient or the factors that are present in your clinical question.

Each of these sources of nonresearch evidence can assist in answering clinical questions and can be helpful and appropriate. However, sometimes you cannot get the answer from an authority, and you have no intuitive or experiential basis on which to answer the question. Or there may not be a case report on the clinical problem you face. Sometimes the answers from these diverse sources of evidence may differ and lead to a more confusing picture. Take the question about how the RN at the high school can best assist M.D. to control her weight, given that she has not succeeded on her own. The nurse in the clinical case could talk to a peer who works in a larger high school and see if they have any protocols for this type of care. The nurse could also check the standardized care plan for patients diagnosed with obesity to see if health needs are addressed and if they seem helpful to such patients. The nurse's experience with her 15-year-old niece who is overweight might tell the nurse that adolescents who are overweight do not respond well to interventions such as "lecturing," but sharing concerns and ideas may work. However, all of these sources of evidence are biased, reflecting subjectively held beliefs or opinions. Despite using these forms of evidence, the question of how to best implement care for M.D. remains.

Finding Answers Through Research

Research-based evidence, in the form of nursing research, may provide the nurse with an answer to a clinical question that avoids the subjective concerns or the informal nature of nonresearch evidence. Often it is exactly the types of questions that are not answered in textbooks, and that everyone has a different idea about or experience with, that are the questions studied in nursing research. However, while very useful, reading and analyzing research is not necessarily the easiest way of gathering evidence for answering clinical questions.

Just as there are several sources of nonresearch-based evidence, there are several kinds of research-based evidence. Research-based evidence is considered to be stronger evidence on which to base decisions about nursing care. It is the result of carefully designed and implemented research that has been thoughtfully and precisely conducted to answer a specific question. The research process, as you will learn in this book, involves a set of systematic processes that formalize the development of evidence, which is why this type of evidence is stronger than nonresearch evidence.

The sources of research-based evidence are discussed in depth in later chapters. They include nonexperimental research and randomized clinical trials. The strongest forms of research-based evidence are reports that combine multiple research studies such as metasynthesis, meta-analysis, and systematic reviews. We will discuss these further in this chapter as well as in later chapters.

In our clinical example, the nurse asks the clinical question of how to best implement care for M.D. The nurse can look to research to find answers. To look for answers in research, the nurse must

1. Identify research in the area of interest.
2. Access the research report(s).
3. Read and understand the research report(s).
4. Decide whether the research is relevant and useful in answering the question.
5. Decide whether to accept and use what is found in the research.

Rather than completing all of these steps, it is easier to ask someone who is an expert or an authority, hoping that he or she has read the research. However, it is not uncommon for the answer to the question to be "I do not know," or for the answer to differ among sources. As a professional nurse, you will be an authority from whom others will be seeking answers. This book gives you the skills needed to use research intelligently in your practice, whether for answering direct clinical care questions based on systematic reviews or individual research reports, or for developing and evaluating quality of care standards. However, to read and understand research, you first must know more clearly what research is.

Identifying Applicable Research Reports

Finding research reports is the first step in using research in clinical practice. Identifying research has become easier with the widespread use of the Internet and the increasing numbers of journals that are published electronically. In the clinical case for this chapter, the nurse used the high school's Internet to search for research about planning care for an adolescent who has obesity-related health issues. Not every article about a health condition is a research article. In fact, most information one can access through journals, texts, and the World Wide Web is not research. So, what is nursing research?

CORE CONCEPT **1.2**

Nursing research is the systematic gathering of information to gain, expand, or validate knowledge about health and responses to health problems. Evidence-based nursing uses research-based evidence to plan and implement quality care.

The definition of nursing research includes two key components. First, for a written report or a Web site to be considered research, it must describe the systematic gathering of information to answer some questions. Systematic means that a set of actions was planned and organized. The information-gathering actions may include interviews, observations, questionnaires, or laboratory tests, but they must have been guided by a plan and administered methodically or systematically.

Second, the information must have been gathered to answer a question that addresses a gap in our knowledge about nursing. **Knowledge** is what is understood and recognized about a subject. Information can be gathered for many other purposes, including evaluation, reporting, or accounting for resources. Research seeks to gather information so that we can understand or learn something about which we do not yet have knowledge. Research begins with a question—an unknown—and develops new knowledge. In contrast, evaluation, reporting, and accounting usually describe or validate something that is already known or occurring.

What if an article, found by our nurse working with M.D., describes, for example, the prevention and treatment of childhood obesity and mentions that adolescent obesity has increased? While this is of interest, it would not be considered a research report. Even if the article-provided statistics or numbers about characteristics of adolescent obesity, it still would not be a report of research. A research report about the complications in children of all ages who are obese would formulate a question about those complications and then describe the process and results of a systematic effort to answer that question. Therefore, facts and numbers alone do not make a source of information a report of research. A research report provides a description of the systematic gathering of information to gain, expand, or validate knowledge.

Not only is it important to differentiate research reports from those that are not research, but also it is important to identify and find primary sources of research. A primary source is a report of the research written by the original author(s). Professional newsletters and journals often include summaries of research that have been presented at a conference or published elsewhere. Although these summaries are a quick source of information, they do not allow you to fully understand and evaluate the actual research because they are another individual's summary of that research. These summaries are helpful, however, for identifying research studies that may be potentially interesting and important in your practice. To use research intelligently, you must find and read the original research.

As you read more research, the difference between reports of research and other scholarly and informative work becomes clearer. In fact, many of the computer sources used to find research reports have an option that allows you to select only reports that are research, eliminating the need to even decide if an article is a research report. But it is important to understand that what you find when you read a research report is not just a description of facts, ideas, theories, or procedures but is also a question and a systematic effort to gain information to address that question.

Accessing Research Reports

Once you know what you are looking for, the next step in finding research reports is knowing where to look. As a nursing student, you are probably already aware of numerous nursing research reports. One of the obvious sources is a journal that includes the words "nursing research" in its title (i.e., *Research in Nursing and Health* or *Nursing Research*). Most professional nursing journals, even those whose primary purpose is not publishing research, often do include research articles, usually specifically labeled as research in the table of contents. However, simply picking up and scanning journals at the library or at a hospital is a somewhat hit-or-miss approach if you are interested in a specific clinical question. Three primary sources that allow you to search for research on a specific question or topic are (1) printed indexes, (2) the Internet, and (3) electronic databases. Table 1.1 lists examples of these three primary sources.

Printed Indexes.   **Printed indexes** are written lists of professional articles that are organized and categorized by topic and author, and they cover articles written from 1956 to today. They usually can only be found in formal academic libraries and are being used more infrequently since the development of computerized electronic databases. Printed indexes are, however, the only source that lists and categorizes research that was done before 1982. Because indexes are tedious to use, are not as available as other sources for finding research, and provide a catalog of studies that are older and thus not current, they should be considered a last resort for research. However, indexes can be helpful in providing ideas for key words to use in a computer search on a topic as well as indicating the kinds of research that have generally been done in your area of interest.

The Internet.   Programs called *search engines* can be used to search the Internet; they often come already loaded on the hard drive of a new personal computer. Because the Internet is a source of information from computers throughout the world, a tremendous and potentially overwhelming amount of information can be found on it. However, because almost anyone can put information on the Internet, the accuracy, completeness, and even honesty of information found there must be considered carefully.

When you use the Internet to look for research, it may help to use the word "research" in the search in addition to words that describe your question. Initially, you will probably get thousands of results, or "hits." These vary from connections to large databases, specific journals or newsletters, and organizations, to connections to individuals' Web pages. You then narrow the search to specific links that will give you research reports. Examples of sites that may provide links that could be helpful in answering clinical questions are those of the CDC and the National Institute for Nursing Research (visit thepoint.lww.com/Rebar3e for the direct links). Links to large and well-established health-related organizations such as these can assure you high-quality information, and many of these sites provide selected research reports. Links to little-known organizations or sites, however, should be used cautiously because the information may be incorrect or incomplete.

When the RN in our clinical case used the Internet to search for ideas about helping M.D. resolve her health concerns, the search led to a link with a site that discussed resources associated with childhood obesity (visit thepoint.lww.com/Rebar3e for the direct link). Another site provided the nurse with a practical overview of strategies for preventing and

Table 1.1

Sources to Search for Nursing Research About a Specific Clinical Topic

TYPE OF SOURCE	LEVEL OF EVIDENCE FOR PRACTICE IMPLICATIONS	ADVANTAGES AND DISADVANTAGES	SPECIFIC EXAMPLES
Print			
Indexes: provide lists of articles that are organized by topic and author from a range of journals; include all types of articles, including research articles published as early as 1956	No evidence to support practice	Not available via computer/Internet Studies that are older may not address research of clinical questions relevant to current health care Tedious to use Can provide key words for use in searching for specific research articles	Printed *CINAHL (Cumulative Index to Nursing and Allied Health Literature)*, also known as Red books *Index Medicus* *International Nursing Index*
Card catalogs: list all materials held by the library, including books, audiovisuals, theses, and dissertations organized by topic and author	No evidence to support practice	Provides lists of sources available	
Abstract reviews: summaries of research studies and prepared bibliographies	Low level of evidence to support practice	Provides summaries of research and prepared bibliographies to assist in finding relevant research articles	*Dissertation Abstracts International* *Psychological Abstracts* *Sociological Abstracts*
Electronic			
World Wide Web (WWW)	No evidence to support practice	May not be reliable Can assist in finding relevant research articles Can assist in developing key words	Popular search engines include: www.yahoo.com www.go.com www.altavista.com www.dogpile.com www.google.com
	Low to moderate level of evidence to support practice	Provides basic health information for consumers and health care professionals May or may not provide research articles Provides current information	Health/Medical search engines include: www.fealth.com www.healthfinders.gov www.medscape.com www.scirus.com
		Current and reliable sources in locating research articles and standards of practice based on research	Relevant nursing-related Web sites include www.ana.org/American Association of Nursing www.nih.gov/ninr/ National Institute of Nursing Research

(continued)

Table 1.1

Sources to Search for Nursing Research About a Specific Clinical Topic *(continued)*

TYPE OF SOURCE	LEVEL OF EVIDENCE FOR PRACTICE IMPLICATIONS	ADVANTAGES AND DISADVANTAGES	SPECIFIC EXAMPLES
			www.cdc.gov/Centers for Disease Control and Prevention hwww.dhhs.gov/ Department of Health and Human Services www.nursingsociety.org/ Sigma Theta Tau International Nursing Honor Society www.cna-nurses.ca/ Canadian Nurses Association
Electronic databases: categorized lists of articles from a range of journals, organized by topic, author, and source			CINAHL—includes articles from 1982 to the present MEDLINE (medical literature analysis and retrieval system) PsycInfo (psychology information) PubMed (database provided by the National Library of Medicine)
Systematic reviews	Strongest level of evidence for practice	Provides a review of multiple research articles May not be relevant for specific cases that have unusual or uncommon characteristics not addressed in articles	Cochrane Reviews Joanna Briggs Collection

managing adolescent obesity–related complications (visit thepoint.lww.com/Rebar3e for the direct link) and provided ideas for planning care to help M.D.

Electronic Databases.   Besides using search engines on the Internet, you also can use the Internet to make a connection with academic libraries through most university Web sites. Once you make that connection, you can usually access the large electronic databases available at these libraries. Electronic databases, the most commonly used source to find research reports, provide categorized lists and complete bibliographic citations of sources of information in a broad field of knowledge. Examples of computer databases include the Cumulative Index to Nursing and Allied Health Literature (CINAHL), which categorizes information that relates to the practice of nursing and allied health professions, and PubMed, which is a database provided by the National Library of Medicine that provides access to more than 11 million health-related and medicine-related citations. Electronic databases can be found in CD-ROM format as well as online. Most are organized similarly so that you can initiate a search for information using key words, terms that describe the information you are interested in getting. In the case of the clinical example, the nurse might have used key words such as "adolescent," "obesity," and "self-esteem." Sometimes the most difficult part of using an electronic database is determining which key words to use to narrow your search. As mentioned, a quick look at printed indexes may help identify appropriate key words.

Electronic databases also allow you to search for information written by a specific author, or for a specific article using its title. Searches can be limited by date of publication or type of information sought, such as research only. The results of an electronic search include a list of references with bibliographic citations and, usually, an abstract or summary of the article. Again, remember that not all articles found in a search will be research articles unless you have specified that you only want research articles. Although occasionally the title of an article alone may clearly tell you that it is relevant to the question you are asking, you may also need to read the abstract to decide whether it is relevant. Abstracts are discussed in detail later in this chapter.

After finding a citation for a possibly relevant research report, the next challenge may be to acquire a copy of it. Copies of research reports may be acquired in several ways. One way is to subscribe to those journals that usually print the types of research articles that are of interest to you. This allows the article you are interested in reading to be available in your home. A second way is to join one or more professional organizations that provide subscriptions to their journals as a membership benefit. For example, membership in Sigma Theta Tau International includes a subscription to *The Journal of Nursing Scholarship*, which includes many research reports. Another option for acquiring research reports is by obtaining them from your place of practice, as most health care organizations subscribe to several professional journals.

Because numerous journals are now published online as well as in print format, a third way to acquire a research report is to get it online. Although most online journals provide full-text articles only to subscribers, many academic libraries have subscriptions to both print and online journals. As a nursing student, you may be able to get articles online. You also may be able to request an interlibrary loan of an article from a journal to which your library does not subscribe. If you do so, be sure to find out whether there is a charge for the article. Finally, you can acquire articles by visiting the closest academic library that subscribes to the journal that you need.

Reading and Understanding Research Abstracts

The nurse in our clinical case will read the published online abstract to decide whether to take the time and trouble to acquire the entire text of the research article. However, reading and understanding the abstract to decide whether the report is potentially useful may be a challenge. Because the abstract for a research report is frequently available when a nurse uses one of the different sources to find research, let us examine what usually is included in an abstract of a research report.

An abstract is a summary or condensed version of a research report. Although one meaning of *abstract* is "to summarize," another is "to take away." Because an abstract is a condensed summary, it does "take away" from the total picture or information about a research study and gives only limited information about the study itself. Therefore, the abstract should not be depended on for understanding a research study or making decisions about clinical care. However, if you are trying to decide whether to acquire the full report of a research study, the abstract can certainly be useful. Abstracts vary from journal to journal in format and length. They also vary depending on the type of research performed. Abstracts may be organized by headings, such as Background, Problem, or Results, or they may be written as a single paragraph. However, they are organized, almost every abstract identifies the general problem or research question and the general approach taken to implement that research. Most abstracts also briefly describe the people included in the study (called the *subjects* or *participants*) and one or two of the most important findings. Abstracts vary in length from 100 to 500 or more words; those that are more limited in the number of words obviously provide less information. Even longer abstracts, however, provide only a "skeleton" of the key ideas from the research report.

Despite the abstracts' limitations, they still can be useful in determining whether the research study reported is one that you want to acquire and read. The abstract usually provides a clear idea about two important factors: (1) whether the research addressed the clinical question of interest and (2) whether it studied patients or situations that are similar to your clinical case, so that the research is relevant.

Often you can determine from reading an abstract whether the study addressed is the topic you are interested in exploring. For example, a search of the CINAHL database using the key words "adolescent" and "obesity" might return a citation for an article titled "Prediction of acceptance of self in obese adolescents using the Rosenberg Self Esteem instrument"—a fictional title simply used as an example. This title suggests that the research might be relevant to caring for adolescents who are obese. The abstract for this article, however, might indicate that the purpose of the study was "to describe the relationship between how an adolescent accepts self and obesity." Because the nurse in our clinical case is sure that the high school health clinic does not use this instrument for students, a review of the abstract would allow the nurse to conclude that this article is not worth acquiring at this time. It is also possible that although the purpose of this study does not fit with the clinical question, the RN may choose to acquire this research report anyway because of its general clinical interest. Besides giving you information about the purpose of a study, most abstracts include information about who was included in the study. Regarding the question about obesity-related care, if an abstract tells you that the people (subjects) in the study were all boys who were involved with sports, you may decide that this study will probably not be helpful for your specific purpose. But if it said the people (subjects) in the study were all girls in high school, it might be very helpful. Be careful, because searching for research on a topic of interest can be a bit like eating peanuts—each one leads to yet another. It is easy to become distracted from the clinical question of interest by related studies. Because you may have limited time and resources, it is important to have as clear an idea as possible regarding the clinical question of interest before you begin searching and reading abstracts of research reports.

■ PUBLISHED ABSTRACT: WHAT WOULD YOU CONCLUDE?

To better understand the usefulness of reading and understanding research report abstracts, read the abstract of the article found by the nurse in our clinical case: "The relationships among self-esteem, stress, coping, eating behaviors, and depressive mood in adolescents" (Martyn-Nemeth et al., 2009). You can find this article in Appendix A.2. Remember that the nurse in the clinical case is trying to plan care to assist her adolescent patient who is medically obese. Consider the following questions as you read the abstract:

1. What do you understand or not understand in the abstract?
2. Do you believe that reading the entire report will be helpful in deciding what nursing care would be necessary to assist M.D.? Why or why not?
3. Based on the abstract alone and what you know about the clinical question, can you make a decision about what would go into a care plan for M.D.? Why or why not?

It is likely that you will not understand all the language in the abstract; do not be discouraged. The goal of this book is to help you learn to understand that language, and the next chapter directly addresses that topic. However, it is likely that you will understand some of the abstract, and reading even limited information about the research will add to your knowledge about adolescents and obesity. Some abstracts are organized by major headings (such as *Methods* or *Subjects*) that can be helpful to your understanding, such as this example. The abstract indicates that overweight adolescents are prevalent. It states the researchers were looking for relationships between self-esteem, stress, coping behaviors, and support systems among 102 high school students. It tells you that the study found low self-esteem and avoidant coping were related to unhealthy eating behaviors. The results indicated that "teaching adolescents skills to reduce stress, build self esteem, and use more positive approaches to coping may prevent unhealthy eating behaviors and subsequent obesity" (Martyn-Nemeth et al., 2009, p. 96). So even if you did not understand the entire abstract, you can see that this research report is relevant to planning for the patient in our clinical case.

CORE CONCEPT 1.3

Abstracts from research reports are an important source of evidence and can be helpful in narrowing down or focusing on the appropriate research to acquire and read. They cannot, and should not, be depended on to provide a level of understanding of the research that would support clinical decision making.

Good, solid, practice-related decisions cannot, however, be based on information gleaned only from the abstract of a research report. Specifically, the research abstract does not give enough information for you to:

1. Understand all the results of the study.
2. Identify who was in the study.
3. Recognize how the results fit or do not fit with existing knowledge.
4. Decide intelligently whether the study was performed in a way that makes the results realistic for clinical practice.

For example, the abstract from the Martyn-Nemeth et al. (2009) does not tell you that most of the research participants were in public high schools in suburban areas within the Midwest and that they had to be able to complete a 45-minute questionnaire written in English. The abstract also does not tell you how the subjects were assessed. Because the RN in the clinical case is interested in how to implement care to assist the patient in the complex work of achieving ideal weight and health status, it is important to determine what assessment techniques were included in the study. The RN must read the entire research report to find the answer to these questions and to decide if the study's findings can be helpful in planning care for M.D.

■ SYSTEMATIC REVIEWS IN EVIDENCE-BASED NURSING

This book treats EBN in the broadest sense by including all types of research, as well as other sources of knowledge, as evidence. Currently, however, there is a particular emphasis in nursing on a process of evidence-based practice that addresses clinical questions by searching the literature, evaluating evidence, and choosing an intervention. The product of this process is a *systematic review* of the research regarding a particular clinical question and is considered by many as one of the strongest forms of evidence for EBN. Thus, there is a *process* that is often referred to as implementing a systematic review as a basis for evidence-based practice, and there is a *product* that also is often referred to as a systematic review. Although it might be easier to refer to the process of implementing a systematic review as the process of evidence-based practice, doing so significantly limits the breadth of evidence that may be used in nursing. Therefore, throughout this text whenever the term *systematic review* is used, the specific usage of the word will be made explicit to avoid confusion.

Like individual research reports, a systematic review includes an abstract and a statement of the problem. However, rather than developing a systematic plan to directly gather information from patients about that question, a systematic review gathers reports of research studies, which have already been completed that, address the problem. The review summarizes these studies, considering aspects of the research process (such as designs and samples) and then draws conclusions about what is known about the clinical question based on the entire group of studies. Here, as with abstracts of individual studies, a nurse can review the abstract to decide whether the review is directly related to the question of interest. Again, even reviewing the abstract requires a basic understanding of the research language.

Dr. Archie Cochrane, a physician and epidemiologist, was the developer of the "Cochrane Reviews," an electronic database similar to CINAHL, which consists of systematic reviews in various health care fields. If you search for topics in this database, you will find a short, focused systematic review, along with a list of relevant primary sources (visit thepoint.lww.com/Rebar3e for the direct link).

Another source for systematic reviews that is focused on the health professions is the Joanna Briggs Collaboration (visit thepoint.lww.com/Rebar3e for the direct link). This collaboration is a coordinated effort by a group of centers from around the world to promote evidence-based health care, education and training, conduct of systematic reviews, development of Best Practice Information Sheets, implementation of EBP, and conduct of evaluation cycles and primary research arising out of systematic reviews. There are currently more than 20 collaborating centers covering the disciplines of nursing, midwifery, physiotherapy, nutrition and dietetics, podiatry, occupational therapy, aged care, and medical radiation. Other databases are now incorporating systematic reviews as an option when searching for evidence-based literature.

The Cochrane Reviews, the Joanna Briggs Collaboration, and other databases all serve an important function in improving the use of research in practice because they pull together disparate studies into an easily accessible and organized form. This allows the nurse to find multiple studies on the same clinical question already synthesized into a single review that ends with recommendations for practice. Clearly then, systematic reviews address the issues of access to research and, to some extent, applicability of research to practice.

Evidence-Based Nursing Practice: Pros and Cons

Use of systematic reviews for EBN has limits as well as strengths. Just as a researcher implementing a traditional research study must make decisions about methods and sample, the author(s) of a systematic review must make decisions about what research to include. This raises the question of what constitutes the "best" evidence. Often, the standard set for appropriate studies include in a review that they be *empirical*, a term used for studies using quantitative approaches. Although there is no question that studies using a quantitative approach are important and useful for answering some questions in nursing, many problems in nursing do not lend themselves to the level of quantitative study. Therefore, an overdependence on systematic reviews of clinical research may limit both the types of problems that

Table 1.2

Five Research Questions Applied to Systematic Reviews	
GUIDING QUESTIONS	APPLICATION TO SYSTEMATIC REVIEWS
Why ask that questions—what do we already know?	What do we already know that suggests the need for a systematic review?
How were those people studied—why was the study performed that way?	Why was a systematic review used? Why were the studies that were included in the review performed that way?
To what types of patients do these research conclusions apply—who was in the study?	What types of studies were included as evidence in the review? What types of samples were used in the studies reviewed?
Why did the author(s) reach that conclusion—what was found?	Why did the review reach its conclusions? What did the studies find?
What is the answer to the research questions—what did the study conclude?	What is the answer to the clinical question?

practitioners consider appropriate for research utilization and the dissemination of important knowledge acquired using other research methods.

Systematic reviews as a type of research have an important place in EBN. Reading and understanding systematic reviews should be conducted using the same five questions mentioned throughout this book and keeping the same openly questioning, critical mind. The difference in reading and understanding systematic reviews is that you must answer the five questions at two different levels, rather than just at one level. For example, when considering the question "How were those people studied—why was the study performed that way?" you must consider the methods for the different studies included in the review. However, you also must consider the rationale for use of a systematic review approach to this clinical question. Probably the toughest two-layered question will be "To what types of patients do these research conclusions apply—who was in the study?" To answer, you must consider the samples in the different studies in the review as well as the sample of "studies" that comprise the review. The second layer becomes "Why did the reviewer include those studies and not others?" Table 1.2 provides an overview of how one might apply the five questions to a systematic review.

Systematic reviews are an important source of evidence for practice, but they are not the only evidence, and they are not even the only source of research evidence. As an intelligent reader and user of nursing research, you must find how the use of evidence in the form of systematic reviews can be most useful to you in your clinical practice.

■ SUMMARY

In summary, we have examined the history of nursing research and how that has led to today's professional nursing practice. This chapter starts you on the way to critically reading, understanding, and intelligently using research in practice by (1) defining research, (2) describing sources of research reports, and (3) discussing how to use abstracts to select which research to read. You should now have a working sense of what is meant by EBN and how you might format a clinical question that could be answered through EBN strategies. The next chapter discusses the language of nursing research as well as the components of published research reports and how they can guide your understanding and decisions about using the research in clinical practice.

OUT-OF-CLASS EXERCISE

Get Ready for the Next Chapter

To prepare for the next chapter and to give you a concrete example of the components of a research report, read the fictional research report titled "Demographic characteristics as predictors of nursing students' choice of type of clinical practice" in Appendix B. This report describes a fictional study similar to one in which you may participate during your first class period. As you read this report, make two lists: one containing important words or ideas that you understand in the report and one listing important words or ideas that you do not understand. Once you have read the report, you are ready to read the next chapter. Also, make sure you read the "Discussion" and "Conclusion" sections of the two articles that our nurse found in the clinical case (Landis et al., 2009; Martyn-Nemeth et al., 2009).

References

Landis, A., Parker, K., & Dunbar, S. (2009). Sleep, hunger, satiety, food cravings, and caloric intake in adolescents. *Journal of Nursing Scholarship, 41*(2), 115–123.

Martyn-Nemeth, P., Penckofer, S., Gulanick, M., Velsor-Friedrich, B., & Bryant, F. (2009). The relationships among self-esteem. Stress, coping, eating behavior, and depressive mood in adolescents. *Research in Nursing & Health, 32*, 96–109.

Resources: Printed

Agan, R. D. (1987). Intuitive knowing as a dimension of nursing. *Advanced Nursing Science, 10*(1), 63–70.

American Nursing Association (ANA). (1989). *Education for participation in nursing research.* Kansas City, MO: Author.

Burns, N., & Groves, S. K. (2002). *Understanding nursing research* (3rd ed.). Philadelphia, PA: W.B. Saunders.

Carper, B. A. (1978). Fundamental patterns of knowing in nursing. *Advances in Nursing Science, 1*(1), 13–23.

Cronin-Stubbs, D. (1992). Publishing research for staff nurses' use. *Applied Nursing Research, 5*(4), 157.

Heath, H. (1998). Reflection and patterns of knowing in nursing. *Journal of Advanced Nursing, 27*, 1054–1059.

Huycke, L. I. (2001). Evidence-based nursing practice. *Southern Connections, 15*(2), 2.

LoBiondo-Wood, G., Haber, J., & Krainovich-Miller, B. (2002). Overview of the research process. In G. LoBiondo-Wood & J. Haber (Eds.), *Nursing research: Methods, critical appraisal, and utilization* (5th ed.). St. Louis, MO: Mosby.

Nahas, V. L., Chang, A., & Molassiotis, A. (2001). Evidence-based practice: Guidelines for managing peripheral intravascular access devices. *Journal of Nursing Administration, 31*(4), 164–165.

Polit, D. F., & Beck, C.T. (2007). *Nursing research: Principles and methods* (8th ed.). Philadelphia, PA: Lippincott Williams & Wilkins.

Thompson, C., McCaughan, D., Cullum, N., Sheldon, T. A., Mulhall, A., & Thompson, D. R. (2001). Research information in nurses' clinical decision-making: What is useful? *Journal of Advanced Nursing, 36*(3), 376–388.

Resources: Online

www.aacap.org/cs/root/facts_for_families/obesity_in_children_and_teens
www.cdc.gov
www.cochrane.org
www.in.gov/isdh/20064.htm
www.joannabriggs.edu.au
www.ninr.nih.gov
www.nlm.nih.gov

CHAPTER

2

The Research Process: Components and Language of Research Reports

LEARNING OBJECTIVE

The student will differentiate the terminology in and the components of research reports.

KEY TERMS

Conclusions
Data
Data analysis
Descriptive results
Hypothesis
Limitations
Literature review
Measures
Meta-analysis
Metasynthesis
Methods
Multivariate
Problem
Procedures

Process improvement
p value
Qualitative methods
Quality improvement
Quality improvement study
Quantitative methods
Results
Sample
Significance
Statistics
Systematic review
Themes
Theory

Clinical Case • The RN described in the case in Chapter 1 begins to read the two research reports found regarding adolescent obesity, self-esteem, and health problems associated with being overweight. It has been a long time since the nurse has read research reports, and the nurse is struggling with some of the language. But the nurse is reminded of the overall similarity in the organization of research reports. The two articles the RN found are available in Appendices A.1 and A.2. If you have not done so, read through them quickly to make the best use of the examples that are provided in this chapter. Do not worry about fully understanding the articles right now, but do keep a list of words or ideas that you do not understand.

■ INTRODUCTION

This chapter provides an overview of the major components or sections in most research reports as well as some of the unique research language that identifies these different sections. As you probably discovered when reading the articles in Appendices A.1 and A.2, not understanding certain terms in a research report is frustrating and creates barriers to your ability to use evidence-based nursing (EBN) intelligently in practice. This chapter discusses the meanings of some of the language of research and gives an overview of the research process. The remaining chapters will walk you through the individual sections of a research report and will elaborate on definitions of terms used in those sections. Viewing the entire report first will allow you to see the whole "picture" and will help you to understand where each section fits when we begin to review each specific part. Recognizing and understanding nursing research language will make it easier for you to start reading and comprehending the research and to use it in your practice.

The language and style of research reports are unique and, therefore, can be difficult to read. They are generally written in a scientific writing style, the goals of which are to be clear, precise, and succinct. Like health care language, research language is formal, technical, and terse, with many ideas compounded into each sentence. This makes research reports reliable methods of communication for anyone immersed in the language of science, but it also makes them inscrutable to the novice who is just beginning to learn the language of research.

Learning to read research reports is similar to learning to read a patient's chart. The first time that you read a sentence such as "The patient is a 64 yo m w m, presenting c̄ RUQ abd pain, post a MVA yesterday a.m.; denies LOC or pain at time of accident," it probably made little, if any, sense to you. Now, however, you know that this sentence refers to a patient being a 64-year-old married white male who has come to seek health care because he has pain in the upper right quadrant of his abdomen. He was in a motor vehicle accident yesterday morning but says that he did not lose consciousness or have pain at the time of the accident. Notice that it took two sentences and many more words to say the same thing in everyday prose. The language of research is much like the language of health care—it, too, is packed with meaning in every sentence and uses unique terms that communicate clearly to anyone familiar with it. Just as you have mastered or are mastering the language of health care, you can master the basics of the language of research.

Paradigms for Research: What Do You Believe?

Have you ever found yourself thinking: What is research? Do I really believe in research? Is research overrated? What does research do for me, as a nurse? I don't have time to look for research, it is easier to ask someone else or look in a book. If you have thought any of these thoughts, you are not alone.

Has your perception of the value of research in nursing changed since reading Chapter 1? Chapter 1 defines research and its value to nursing practice in general. What about you as an individual nurse? The first question is to ask yourself is "How can research help me provide quality care?" In the past and still today, nurses are using interventions that are scientifically weak. In other words, some nursing actions are based in tradition; what they have learned in nursing school, what more experienced nurses have been doing for decades, and/or what they were taught by others. Currently, research is being used to provide nurses evidence that can be translated to nursing care. This new knowledge assists nurses in developing the most effective, safe, and competent care. Also, the field of nursing education is using research to assist nurses in gaining the knowledge they need to enhance patient care. In the future, research has the potential to provide the nursing profession with the knowledge needed to provide evidence-based care to any patient in any situation. Patients, whether individuals, families, groups, or communities, will benefit from EBN practice.

■ THE LANGUAGE OF RESEARCH

This chapter presents several terms that are unique to research. Each will be defined in this chapter, but do not be discouraged if you are not completely clear about all of them. They are also included and defined in the glossary, and we will revisit these terms as we discuss the different sections of a research report in more detail in the following chapters. The learning outcome for this chapter is that you differentiate the different sections or components of a research report and the language associated with each of those sections, not that you understand each of the terms in depth. Table 2.1 provides a summary of the sections of a research report and their associated language.

You were asked at the end of Chapter 1 to read the fictional article from Appendix B and compile a list of terms that you did and did not understand. Hopefully, this chapter will touch on some of the terms that were not clear to you and, perhaps, add to your understanding of those that you believed you already understood. Again, you can think of reading research as being similar to reading a patient's chart. The first time you read a patient's hospital chart, a great deal of the information in it may not have made sense to you, and you may not have even known which section to look in for different types of information. With time, however, you learned the unique language of the health care field and found your way around a chart with ease. The same thing will happen with research reports. Just as you learned where to look for physicians' orders as well as the unique language used in those orders, you will learn where to look for specific information about a research study and to understand its unique research language. For example, you will learn where to look for information about procedures in a research study and some of the unique language used to describe those procedures so that you will have a good start at reading and better understanding research reports. As you read the different research reports used in this book, keep

Table 2.1

The Sections of a Research Report and Associated Terms

RESEARCH REPORT SECTION	ASSOCIATED TERMS
Problem or Introduction: describes the gap in knowledge that will be addressed in the research study	• Literature review • Theory • Research question • Hypothesis
Methods: describes the process of implementing the research study	• Qualitative • Quantitative • Measures • Sample • Procedures
Results: summarizes the specific information gathered in the research study	• Data • Data analysis • Themes • Descriptive • Significant • Multivariate
Conclusions: describes the decisions or determinations that can be made about the research problem	• Limitations • Implications for practice

adding to your list of words or ideas that you do not understand, then periodically review it and cross out those words you believe you understand. You can use the list to guide your own reading and can share it with your fellow students and your faculty to assure clarification of the words to facilitate your own and fellow students' learning.

■ COMPONENTS OF PUBLISHED RESEARCH REPORTS

In addition to an abstract, almost every research report has at least four major sections:

• Introduction or Problem
• Methods
• Results
• Conclusions or Discussion

Table 2.1 describes each of these sections and lists some of their associated research terms. Because this book discusses research by beginning at the end or the conclusions of a research report and moving to the beginning of the report or introduction, we will look at each of the sections of a report, starting with the end.

Conclusions

The word conclusions is used in research reports much as it is generally used outside of the research setting. Conclusions identify what was found and complete a report by identifying an outcome. They specifically describe or discuss the researcher's final decisions or determinations regarding the research problem.

   In nursing research reports, conclusions usually include a description of implications for nursing practice. That is why practicing nurses often start with the conclusions of a report. That section provides the "so what" by providing the meaning of the research for practice. What distinguishes conclusions in a research report from those in other reports is the expectation that they contain either new knowledge or confirmation of previous knowledge. This is a core concept. The goal of the research process is to generate knowledge that can be used in practice. In the conclusions section of a research report, the findings or results of a study are directly translated into that new knowledge. So, you should expect that the conclusions go beyond simply saying what was found in a study; they present the implications or meaning of those findings for future practice. As such, the conclusions of research reports are powerful because they are the evidence for EBN. They are used as the basis for decisions about direct patient care, whether in program planning, or in one-to-one direct patient care, such as that being planned by the RN.

CORE CONCEPT 2.1

What distinguishes conclusions in a research report from those in other reports is the expectation that they contain either new knowledge or confirmation of previous knowledge.

Because of the power and importance attached to them, the statement or decisions described in the conclusions of a research report are carefully worded and should list any relevant cautions or limitations. This cautious presentation may, however, make the conclusions weak or not helpful to the nurse who is looking for clear and direct answers to clinical questions.

For example, the RN in our clinical case is looking for specific advice about how to provide care for M.D. and finds the conclusions of the two reports described in sections labeled "Discussion" and "Conclusions." From reading these sections, the nurse learns that there is a relationship between daytime sleep and food cravings that may lead to overeating and obesity (Landis, Parker, & Dunbar, 2009). The nurse also learned that "low self esteem and avoidant coping emerged as significant predictors of unhealthy eating behavior, and thus may influence the use of emotional eating to cope with stress among adolescents" (Martyn-Nemeth, Penckofer, Gulanick, Velsor-Friedrich, & Bryant, 2009). This is useful information for the RN, but it does not provide specifics about how to assist M.D. as she goes through her teen years or how to promote self-esteem and healthy behaviors. The discussion in the self-esteem and eating behavior article goes on to state: "A large sample of both normal-weight and above normal-weight adolescents would have been beneficial to more adequately test for associations with body weight" (Martyn-Nemeth et al., 2009, p. 106). The sleep and hunger in adolescents article states: "Several intrinsic limitations to this study are noted. Sleep data were reported subjectively. Self-report sleep diaries are subject to recall biases and missing data" (Landis et al., 2009, p. 121). The authors of each article clearly express their conclusions cautiously and may do so for several reasons. Chapter 3 examines in more detail why conclusions often are constrained or hesitant.

The conclusions section of a research report usually has fewer unique research terms than does the rest of the report. This is probably another reason why the conclusions section is sometimes the first part read by nurses. One term that regularly appears in the conclusions section is *limitations*. Limitations are the aspects of how the study was conducted that create uncertainty concerning the conclusion that can be derived from the study as well as the decisions that can be based on it. These limitations often address the information presented in the beginning sections of the report, such as the study's methods and sample.

Just as the cautious language used in the conclusions section can be frustrating when you are looking for practical answers to clinical questions, the limitations described may make you wonder whether you can use conclusions as evidence on which to practice. That is why the limitations are included in the conclusions: to remind the reader that there are constraints or limits to the knowledge being reported. Limitations do not mean that the results of a study are flawed or meaningless. They do, however, indicate the boundaries of or constraints to the knowledge generated by the research. One might view the limitations as the fence that surrounds and "limits" the new knowledge in the report. To decide whether to use the knowledge described in a research report and how it will be used, you must understand not only the knowledge but also the "fence" that surrounds it. This requires understanding of other aspects of the research process, such as sampling or methods that may fence or boundary the new knowledge.

Finally, the conclusions section of a research report usually contains recommendations for future research regarding the problem of interest. These recommendations often directly address the limitations that have been described and suggest additional studies that are needed to further build on the new knowledge generated and stretch the boundary of that knowledge.

Results

The results section of a research report summarizes the specific findings from the study. Almost no research report can give all of the information that was gathered during a research study, so the results section contains a summary or condensed version of what the authors believe are the most important findings. *Data* is a word that is often used and has specific meaning in research. Data are the information collected in a study. Organizing and compiling data are called *data analysis*. Data analysis pulls elements or information together to present a clear picture of the information collected, but it does not interpret or describe the implications for practice of that picture of the information.

CORE CONCEPT 2.2

The difference between results and conclusions is that results are a summary of the actual findings or information collected in the research study, whereas conclusions summarize the potential meaning, decisions, or determinations that can be made based on the information collected.

Some of the unique language found in this section is a result of how the data were analyzed and what analysis methods were used to summarize the information collected. Results or findings may be reported in the form of numbers, words, or both. Which form is used depends on the type of information or data collected. If the study collected information about people's beliefs and experiences, the results section summarizes the words collected using terms such as *themes*, *categories*, and *concepts*. Themes are abstractions that reflect phrases, words, or ideas that appear repeatedly when a researcher analyzes what people have said about a particular experience, feeling, or situation. A theme summarizes and synthesizes discrete ideas or phrases to create a picture from the words collected in the research study. For example, in the fictional research report in Appendix B about nursing students' choices of type of clinical practice, the results section mentions "three distinct themes that represent the meaning of life experiences related to choice of field of nursing." The authors of this article do not list the answers given by 30 different nursing students; rather, they have looked for recurring ideas or words in those answers and have categorized them into themes or findings.

In contrast, the research study on sleep and hunger in adolescents is primarily collected in the form of numbers, such as scores on the body mass index (BMI) and the Self-Rating Scale for Pubertal Development. Again, the authors do not list all the responses/results from the 85 different adolescents who completed assessment measures; rather, they summarize

Box 2.1

Descriptive Results of the Depressive Mood, Self-esteem, Coping, and Eating Study

"Eating behavior scores ranged from 13 to 35 ($M = 23.1$). Several unhealthy eating behaviors were reported. Breakfast was the least frequently eaten meal, with only 13% of the students reporting eating breakfast every day over the past week. Only 36% reported eating lunch every day, despite having a scheduled lunch period in school. Dinner was the most frequently eaten meal (59%), yet only 16% of students reported eating daily meals with most of the family; and 51% indicated that they were too busy to eat dinner with the family over the past week" (Martyn-Nemeth et al., 2009, p. 103).

the numbers in different forms, such as means. The language that describes data analysis of information in numbers is called **statistics**, and the language of statistics is often some of the most intimidating language to readers of research. We do not have to be statistical experts to develop a greater understanding of that language, and we will focus on the language of statistics in Chapters 4 and 5. However, a few key terms are worth highlighting here to help us get started.

Almost all research reports, even those that are mostly reporting results of interviews in the form of words, include descriptive results. **Descriptive results** summarize information without comparing it with other information. For example, descriptive results may state how many people were in a study, the average age of those studied, or the percentage who responded in a specific manner. In the depressive mood, self-esteem, coping, and eating study, almost all of the results presented are descriptive. In Box 2.1, the paragraph describing eating behavior from the article is repeated. Here, the authors describe the percentage of adolescents who ate at specific meals.

Thus far, we have talked about descriptive results, but the authors of the depressive mood, self-esteem, coping, and eating study also provide some correlation statistics in the paragraph headed "Coping" (Martyn-Nemeth et al., 2009). Here, the authors are doing more than just describing the findings because they are looking for connections between the variables in their study. Specifically, the authors are looking for a connection between the adolescents who use food to cope and BMI. The computation of a correlation statistic to look for connections between variables requires consideration of two important statistical concepts: significance and p values.

Let us look at what *significance* means first. The last sentence in the Coping section of the depressive mood, self-esteem, coping, and eating study indicates that: "Using food to cope was positively correlated with a higher BMI percentile ($r = -.26, p = .009$)" (Martyn-Nemeth et al., 2009, p. 104). **Significance** is a statistical term indicating a low likelihood that any differences or relationships found in a study happened by chance. In research, we often try to make decisions about clinical care for a large group of patients based on what we have found in a small group of patients. Statistical significance is important because we need to be sure that what was found in the small group of patients studied is not something that happened by chance rather than because of some factor we are studying. The correlation described as $r = -.26$, which the authors of the depressive mood, self-esteem, coping, and eating study tell us is significant, indicates that the connection between using food to cope and BMI did not occur by chance alone. Thus, we could expect that in another group of adolescents, we would find some relationship between using food to cope and BMI. This significant relationship has a p value equal to .009, which leads us to the second important statistical concept.

So if significance is indicated by p values, what is a p value? P values indicate what percentage of the time the results reported would have happened by chance alone. For example, a p value of .05 means that in only 5 out of 100 times would one expect to get the results by chance alone. If it is unlikely that the results happened by chance, then we can summarize the findings by saying that the results are statistically significant. In order to consider if the results of a study help to answer your clinical question, and in order to practice EBN, you will need to look for these p values. For example, the p value given for the correlation between using food to cope and the BMI percentile is "$p = .009$" (Martyn-Nemeth et al., 2009). This tells us that the connection found between these two scores would happen by chance alone in less than 1% of samples. What that connection means and how it affects our clinical planning are not discussed until the conclusions section of the report. However, summarizing and reporting the finding of a connection that is not likely to happen by chance alone are important so that the reader knows why the researchers reached their conclusion.

Another term that is often found in the results section of a research report is *multivariate*. If you think about this term, it is easy to figure out that multivariate indicates that the study reports findings for three (multi) or more factors (variate) and includes the relationships among those different factors. The fictional article in Appendix B, the sleep and hunger in adolescents article, and the depressive mood, self-esteem, coping, and eating article all report multivariate results because it looks at relationships and differences between more than two factors. For example, the fictional article does not use the word *multivariate*, but it does describe results of a statistical procedure called a *logistic regression*, which included the three factors of age, rating of health, and choice of field of nursing. Now that you know what the word means, you can count the number of factors analyzed and identify that this study is, indeed, multivariate. Logistic regression is a statistical procedure that allows us to look at relationships between more than two factors and test whether those relationships are likely to occur by chance. Statistical language such as this is discussed further in Chapters 4 and 5.

The information summarized in the results section of a report depends on who was studied, how the study was conducted, what the research question asked, and how the researcher(s) analyzed the information. To understand more completely what was implemented in a study and who was studied, we must look at the methods section of the research report.

Methods

The methods section of a research report describes the overall process of how the researchers went about implementing the research study, including who was included in the study, how information was collected, and what interventions, if any, were tested. Remember from Chapter 1 that one of the things that distinguishes research from other ways of answering questions is its systematic collection of information. The methods section of a research report should describe those procedures used to collect information. Chapter 8 examines, in detail, the variety of research methods, along with the many names used for them. For now, remember that research methods can be broadly categorized under two major headings: qualitative and quantitative methods. Because qualitative and quantitative methods are used both separately and together in nursing research, both methods are discussed throughout this text. To assist you in understanding the differences between them and how the differences may affect your use of the research in practice, the following eight chapters will be organized so that general information relating to both approaches is described first, followed by specific information related to qualitative and then to quantitative methods. These sections will be identified by use of an icon, just as the two following paragraphs are identified. Be sure to read carefully and note the icons, as it is easy to get the two approaches confused. At this point, we will briefly differentiate qualitative and quantitative methods.

FIGURE 2.1 The differences between qualitative and quantitative methods.

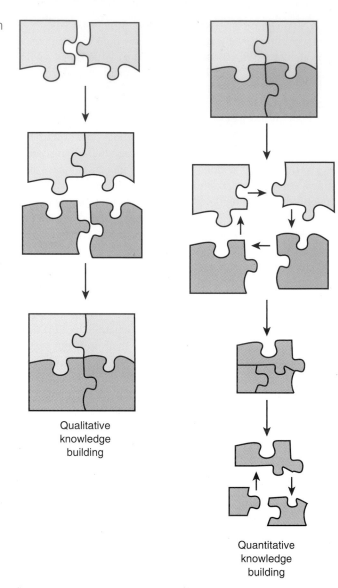

Qualitative
knowledge
building

Quantitative
knowledge
building

Qualitative methods focus on understanding the complexity of humans within the context of their lives. Research that uses qualitative methods attempts to build a complete picture of a phenomenon of interest. Therefore, qualitative methods involve the collection of information as it is expressed by people within the normal context of their lives. Qualitative methods focus on subjective information and never attempt to predict or control the phenomenon of interest.

Quantitative methods focus on understanding and breaking down the phenomenon into parts to see how they do or do not connect. Therefore, quantitative methods involve collecting information that is specific and limited to the particular parts of events or phenomena being studied. Quantitative methods focus on objective information and can yield predictions and control. The sleep and hunger in adolescents study used in Chapters 1 and 2 is a study using quantitative methods.

Figure 2.1 illustrates the differences between knowledge building using qualitative versus quantitative methods: qualitative research assembles the pieces of a puzzle into a whole picture, whereas quantitative research selects pieces of a completed puzzle and breaks them down into their component parts.

Methods sections of research reports, whether they use qualitative or quantitative methods, usually include information about three aspects of the research method: (1) the sample, (2) the data collection procedures, and (3) the data analysis methods.

Sample

A sample is a smaller group, or subset of a group, of interest that is studied in a research. Using the sleep and hunger in adolescents study as an example, you will see that the researchers were interested in gaining knowledge that could help a provider do a better job of caring for adolescents, but they only had the time and resources to study a group of 85 teenagers from one community and high school.

Therefore, in planning care for M.D., the RN must consider whether the 85 adolescents from a community and high school in the research report are similar to the adolescents in their school. The effort to assure that the subgroup or sample and what happens to them is similar to the other patients or people being studied is emphasized in quantitative research methods. However, describing the sample, that is, who was studied, is important for understanding the results of a qualitative study as well as those of a quantitative study.

CORE CONCEPT 2.3

Most research attempts to gather information systematically about a subset, or smaller group of patients or people, to gain knowledge about other similar patients or people. Many of the methods in research are aimed at assuring that what happens in the subgroup or sample studied is as similar as possible to what would happen in other larger groups of patients or people.

The sampling subsection in the methods section of a research report describes how people, or studies in the case of the metasynthesis, were chosen, what was done to find them, and what, if any, limits or restrictions were placed on who or which research could be done in the study. It also usually describes how many patients or people declined to be in the study, withdrew from it, or were not included in it for specific reasons. For example, the fictional article states that the sample was one of convenience, meaning that no special efforts were made to get a particular type of student to participate. The students chose whether or not to participate in the study and did not provide identifying information on the questionnaire. Therefore, no restrictions were placed on who would participate; all the researcher did was approach a class of students and ask them to volunteer. This is an example of a simple sampling procedure.

In contrast, a research report using multiple studies such as a *metasynthesis* contains a more complex sampling method, involving the analysis of information about each individual study's report in order to identify the sample of reports that best met the criteria of the study. Understanding samples and sampling is an important part of making intelligent decisions about the use of research in practice and is discussed in more detail in Chapters 6 and 7.

Procedures

In addition to information about samples, the methods section usually includes information about procedures used in the study. Nurses are familiar with procedures within the context of health care. Research procedures are similar because they are the specific actions taken by researchers to gather information about the problem or phenomena being studied. Research procedures in qualitative and quantitative studies differ because the purposes of the two approaches to research differ.

Because the systematic collection of information in a qualitative study involves looking as much as possible at the whole phenomenon being studied, procedures for qualitative studies are systematically planned activities—such as observations or open and unstructured interviews of people in their natural life situations—to see and hear as much as possible of the complexity of those situations. A qualitative researcher may videotape or audiotape interviews with individuals so that every word, expression, and pause can be carefully considered and studied. In addition, qualitative researchers keep detailed notes of their observations of the environment where the information is collected as well as the expressions and actions of those being studied. This is not a haphazard process but an organized, systematic, and intensive process to collect and then analyze the complexity of experiences.

In contrast, because the methods used in a quantitative study involve identifying specific aspects of a problem, the procedures involve actions to isolate and examine those particular aspects or pieces. The focus of a quantitative study is on clearly defining and examining that which is believed to be relevant to the problem being studied. Therefore, procedures may involve carefully defined repeated observations at set time intervals, such as taking a blood pressure reading immediately before and after a patient is suctioned. Another example may be a specific protocol for teaching each patient, in exactly the same manner, to use visualization to relax before surgery.

In summary, quantitative and qualitative methods lead to different approaches and procedures. Control and objectivity are hallmarks of quantitative methods, whereas naturally occurring conditions and subjectivity characterize qualitative methods.

Often, the procedures in a quantitative study involve taking measurements, sometimes directly, such as taking a blood pressure reading, but often indirectly, such as in a written questionnaire. **Measures** are the specific method(s) used to assign a number or numbers to an aspect or factor being studied. For example, in the article about sleep and hunger in adolescents, the authors used a 28-item self-report to collect information about specific food cravings. They did not do extensive nutritional testing on the adolescents; rather, they depended on the teenager's self-report of how many food cravings he or she experienced in relation to type of craving. The final numbers used in this study are the average or mean scores on this self-report of cravings. Thus, the abstract concept of cravings is converted into a number that can be analyzed.

Another example of the use of measures is found in the fictional article in Appendix B. The study examines factors that cannot be directly observed. The article has a section labeled "Measures," which describes a three-part written questionnaire. This questionnaire was used to assign numbers to aspects that were studied, such as perceived well-being or choice of field of study. So again, abstract concepts are converted into a number that can be analyzed using statistical procedures. Based on the previous discussion of qualitative and quantitative studies, it should make sense that both the depressive mood, self-esteem, coping, and eating study as well as the sleep and hunger in adolescents study used quantitative methods because the goals were to break down and describe aspects of the health of adolescents. It carefully defined the factors to be studied and established a clear, easily reproduced approach to get information. Similarly, the fictional article describes measures used to translate the factors that were studied into numbers, indicating a quantitative approach, but also includes what the author calls a "qualitative question." By using the word *qualitative*, the author indicates that this part of the research attempted to look broadly or holistically at the students' experiences, without selecting specific pieces and asking focused questions. Therefore, the fictional article describes the use of both qualitative and quantitative procedures in its methods section.

An important point to understand is that although this book describes and defines many of the terms used in the research process and found in research reports, the terms can have various meanings and can, at different times, be used broadly or more specifically. This can be frustrating or discouraging because the words or ideas are new, and you are just beginning to understand them. However, the more experience you gain from reading and learning about research, the easier understanding it will be. You will find the same situation with many of the words used in the health care field. For example, "normal" body temperature is defined as 98.8°F. Fever is clearly present when a patient has a temperature of 100.8°F or higher, but a temperature between 99.8°F and 100.8°F is not considered either febrile or "normal," and a patient can feel "feverish" with a "normal" temperature. With practice, nurses learn to recognize these variations in the meaning of the words *fever* and *feverish*. Similarly, with practice, you will learn to recognize and be comfortable with the variations in meanings or use of research terms. Although we have said that quantitative and qualitative methods usually look different, which suggests that an individual research study will use only one of the two broad approaches, at times, researchers use a combination of the two methods to address the same research problem. The fictional article is an example of such a study.

CORE CONCEPT 2.4

Many of the terms used in research have a range of meanings rather than a single, discrete, locked-in meaning.

Data Analysis Plan

In addition to describing the sample and procedures used in a study, the methods section often includes a description of the data analysis. Remember that data are the information collected in a study, and data analysis is a description of what was done with that data to obtain a clearer picture of what the information tells us. Although the results section summarizes the outcome of data analysis, the methods section often describes in detail how the researchers worked with or analyzed the data. In the article depressive mood, self-esteem, coping, and eating, the authors describe some of the procedures they used to analyze reports under heading titled "Data Analysis." In other reports, the authors may not have a specific heading for data analysis, so you may need to look for such headings as "Evaluation of reports" and "Metasummary and Metasynthesis." Similarly, the depressive mood, self-esteem, coping, and eating study includes paragraphs under the heading of "Methods" that describe how data were collected and how they were analyzed. The fictional article has a much shorter "Analysis" subsection, in which the author informs the reader that a specific computer program was used to analyze the data that were numbers, and then describes the analysis procedures for the data that were words. Again, the approaches to analyze quantitative and qualitative data are different and are discussed further in Chapter 4.

Problem

So far, we have reviewed the conclusions, results, and methods sections of research reports: Conclusions discuss the outcomes, decisions, or potential meanings of the study; results summarize what was found; and methods describe how the study was implemented. This brings us to the beginning of a research report, a section often labeled "Problem" or "Introduction." Just as the word suggests, the problem section of a research report describes the gap in knowledge that is addressed by the research study. In this section, the researcher explains why the study was needed, why it was carried out in the manner that it was, and, often, what the researcher is specifically asking or predicting.

The introduction or problem section of a research report usually includes a background or literature review subsection, which is a focused summary of what has already been published regarding the question or problem. The literature review gives us a picture of what is already known or has already been studied in relation to the problem and identifies where

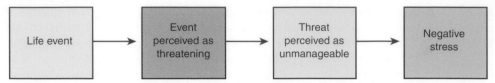

FIGURE 2.2   Proposed relationships among the four factors in Lazarus's theory of stress and coping (1993).

the gaps in knowledge may be. It may report, for example, that studies have only been done with selected types of patients, such as with children but not with adults. Or, it may report that no one has ever tried to ask a particular question before: Perhaps studies have examined occurrence of one or two specific health problems in adolescents, but only a few have examined multiple physical and mental variables associated with obesity.

The literature review does not necessarily only include published *research* studies. It also may include published reports about issues related to practice or a description of a theory. A **theory** is a written description of how several factors may relate to and affect each other. The factors described in a theory are usually abstract, that is, they are ideas or concepts—such as illness, stress, pain, or fatigue—that cannot be readily observed and immediately defined and recognized. Nursing theories such as Roy's theory of adaptation (1984), Neuman's system model (1982), and Watson's theory of human caring (1985) are examples of written descriptions of how the four major components of nursing (persons, health, environment, and nursing) may interrelate.

Lazarus's (1993) theory of stress and coping is another example of a theory that most nurses know and that is somewhat simpler than many nursing theories. It proposes relationships among four abstract factors: life events, perceptions of threat, perceptions of ability to manage a threat, and stress. The relationships proposed in the theory are if a life event occurs that is perceived as threatening, and there are no perceived approaches to manage or mitigate that threat, then stress results. Figure 2.2 illustrates the proposed relationships among these four factors.

When a research report discusses a theory in its introduction or problem section, the study usually tests or further explains the relationships proposed in that theory. Therefore, if a study report discussed Lazarus's theory of stress and coping (1993) in the introduction, we expect that the study will be based on, or will examine, some aspect of how life events and perceptions affect stress as described in that theory. If a research study is based on an existing theory, then the researcher often already has an idea of what relationships are expected to be found. These ideas are stated in the form of a **hypothesis**—a prediction regarding the relationships or effects of selected factors on other factors. Not every study will have a hypothesis. For a study to include a hypothesis, there must be some knowledge about a problem of interest so that we can propose or predict that certain relationships or effects will occur. If you remember from earlier in the chapter, qualitative research does not try to predict outcomes, and therefore, a hypothesis is seldom appropriate. The depressive mood, self-esteem, coping, and eating study was guided by a theoretical framework (theory), purpose, and three research questions. This study also includes descriptions of several factors that may influence the problem of interest and suggests that the knowledge gap results from not knowing the effects or relationships among these factors.

■ THE RESEARCH PROCESS AND THE NURSING PROCESS

We started this book by stating that the goal was not to make you a researcher, but, rather, to give you the knowledge and tools needed to understand and use research intelligently. However, we do not want to continue this chapter with an emphasis on how complex and arduous the research process can be or the many potential barriers there can be to both implementing and publishing research. The research process is a wonderful and exciting challenge. It is like a giant interactive puzzle because as each piece is solved and fit into place and the rest of the pieces change and must be addressed in their new form, given what has already been completed. Fitting each piece into the puzzle can be extremely satisfying, and finishing small sections of the puzzle through completion of a research study can be rewarding.

Part of the reason the research process is fun is because it is a continuous learning experience for those involved. When one is trying to develop new knowledge, the challenges of planning and implementing a valid and meaningful study always require problem solving and creative solutions, so the opportunity to learn and create can be immense. More and more, we are recognizing that most research is best approached by using teams with members from different backgrounds and disciplines. This allows the knowledge brought to bear on a research problem to be wide ranging and to enhance the potential for a high-quality product.

It is the authors' hope that as you read and use research, you will develop an interest in and excitement about the process of research as well as for the problems that it addresses. Although the baccalaureate nurse is not expected to plan and implement research, there are several roles for nurses in the research process, such as participation in planning a study or in subject recruitment and data collection.

As we discussed the research process, you may have noticed some similarities between it and the nursing process. For one thing, both are processes and both have been broken down into steps. In the broadest sense, the nursing and research processes are similar because they are used to solve problems. Both a research problem and a patient care problem (whether the patient is an individual, family, or community) can be viewed as a complicated puzzle, where often only some of the pieces are available at any time point.

Both types of problems are initially addressed through gathering information. In the nursing process, this gathering of information is referred to as assessment, and in the research process, it is referred to as describing and refining the knowledge gap or problem. However, in both cases, we are collecting information to guide us in understanding the problem and formulating a plan.

The second, third, and fourth steps of the nursing and research processes also initially may appear similar, although they differ in some major ways. Although the second step of the nursing process is planning and the second step of the research process is developing a detailed plan, the two processes differ because they have fundamentally different purposes. The purpose of the nursing process is to provide informed, scientifically based nursing care for human responses to potential or actual health problems. The purpose of the research process is to develop or validate knowledge. The goal of the nursing process is action to promote the established outcome of improved health. The goal of the research process is to acquire new knowledge, and the outcomes for that new knowledge cannot be known until the knowledge is established. Therefore, the second and third steps of the nursing process address planning and implementing care, whereas the second and third steps of the research process address planning and implementing acquisition of new information. As a result, the fourth steps of these two processes have different focuses because evaluation in the nursing process is concerned with outcomes, whereas data analysis and interpretation are concerned with understanding. Table 2.2 summarizes the similarities and differences between the two processes. We discuss the roles of nursing in research more in the next chapter.

Although there are some similarities and differences in the processes of nursing and research, it is essential that there be a strong relationship between the two. The research process should provide knowledge that is the basis for the nursing process. This is why this entire book focuses on understanding and intelligently using research in practice. In addition, the nursing process will often be the source of problems that need to be addressed

Table 2.2

Comparison of the Research Process and the Nursing Process		
	RESEARCH PROCESS	NURSING PROCESS
Similarities	A process with steps A form of problem solving Complex "puzzle"	A process with steps A form of problem solving Complex "puzzle"
Differences	Purpose is to develop knowledge	Purpose is to provide scientifically based care
	Plans and implements knowledge acquisition	Plans and implements delivery of care
	Analysis and interpretation concerned with knowing	Evaluation concerned with outcomes

using the research process. As we plan, implement, and evaluate nursing care, we often find problems or face questions about the best ways to achieve our outcome of improved health. The nursing and research processes differ in purpose, but they are closely linked and together ensure the growth and development of nursing as a profession.

CORE CONCEPT 2.5

While different in purpose, the nursing process shares several steps and skills with the research process.

Metasynthesis, Meta-analyses, and Systematic Review Reports as Evidence for Nursing Practice

We have been discussing the sections and language in research reports in general; however, there are several unique types of reports we should recognize. These include reports of a single study, metasynthesis, meta-analysis, systematic reviews, and quality improvement.

Metasynthesis, meta-analysis, and systematic reviews can be used as evidence for nursing practice. The two studies we have been using in this chapter are reports of a single research study. These studies answer specific clinical questions in a specific situation that are often used in nursing practice. Another type of study that may be used as evidence for nursing practice is a metasynthesis, which is a report of a study of a group of single research studies using qualitative methods. A meta-analysis is a quantitative approach to knowledge development that applies statistics to numeric results from different studies that addressed the same research problem to look for combined results that would not happen by chance alone. Both of these methods examine a question or problem about which there have been a number of studies and actually take a sample of studies, rather than a sample of individuals. Metasynthesis and meta-analysis are similar to another special type of research report called a *systematic review*. As you recall from Chapter 1, a systematic review addresses a specific clinical question by summarizing multiple research studies, along with other evidence. Systematic reviews differ from metasynthesis and meta-analysis because they by definition will address a clinical question and they do not generally apply statistical procedures to the information collected from individual studies or develop a systematic metasummary of the content of each study.

The sections of reports of metasynthesis, meta-analyses, and systematic reviews resemble those of single studies but may differ in some important ways. Table 2.3 summarizes

Table 2.3

Components of Reports for Individual Research Studies, Metasynthesis, Meta-analysis, Systematic Reviews, and Quality Improvement Reports

COMPONENTS OF REPORTS	TRADITIONAL RESEARCH STUDY	METASYNTHESIS	META-ANALYSIS	SYSTEMATIC REVIEW	QUALITY IMPROVEMENT STUDY
Problem or introduction	Review of the literature; theory; statement of a knowledge gap; predictions or hypotheses	Identification of a problem that has been addressed in only a few studies with limited findings	Identification of a problem that has been addressed in several studies with inconsistent results	Statement of a practice problem, including a broad overview of the relevant clinical questions related to the problem	Statement of a standard for patient care that is measurable and specific, usually including a summary of the research basis and clinical basis for the standard
Methods	Description of quantitative or qualitative procedures; sampling methods; data analysis methods	Description of the procedures used to find and select the individual research studies; description of the procedures used to analyze the individual studies	Description of the procedures used to find and select the individual research studies; description of procedures used to code and analyze results from the individual studies; usually includes a table of studies	Description of search strategies and criteria used for including a study in the review	Description of the procedures used to identify selected patient care situations and methods used to collect information about the care in those situations
Results	Description of findings; summary of themes or concepts or results of statistical procedures	Summary of findings, concepts, or themes across the sample of studies	Summary of results of statistical tests on groups of results from individual studies	Summary of research findings categorized and synthesized under clinically meaningful topics; usually includes a table of studies	Summary of the patient care practices that were identified
Discussion or conclusions	Summary of key findings; comparison of results to previous studies; speculation about the meaning of results in relation to theory; description of limitations; recommendations for additional research and final conclusions	Summary of key findings and identification of how these might differ from what is generally accepted understanding; identification of needs for additional research and of limitations in existing studies	Summary of key findings and identification of how these might differ from what is generally accepted understanding; identification of needs for additional research and of limitations in existing studies	Specific identification of practice implications derived from the synthesis of the literature; identification of needs for additional research	Summary of key findings; comparison of findings to established standards; speculation about reasons for differences found; recommendations for changes to remedy any deficits found

what you might expect to find in the different sections of reports of a systematic review, metasynthesis, and meta-analysis. All three begin with a section that identifies the problem of interest. In metasynthesis or meta-analysis, the problem identified may be anything that has been addressed in several individual research studies. In contrast, a systematic review addresses a specific patient care or clinical practice question because the intent of the review is to provide evidence for practice.

A systematic review has defined procedures, but they are not always described in the report under a heading titled "Methods." The procedures in a systematic review involve searching and identifying all published reports or primary studies that examine or are related to a particular clinical care problem. The researcher has to define the problem and determine which studies are and are not related to that problem. The researcher also describes the procedures used to search the literature after describing the problem, or perhaps at the end of the report, under a heading such as "Search Strategies."

In contrast, metasynthesis or meta-analysis reports usually have clearly identified methods sections in which the search strategies used, the inclusion and exclusion criteria used for the sample of studies, and the analysis methods applied to the sample of studies are all described. Remember that a metasynthesis or meta-analysis examines a sample of research studies rather than a sample of patients.

The results sections of metasynthesis or meta-analysis and systematic reviews differ because the metasynthesis reports specific integrated concepts extracted from the individual reports, while meta-analysis specifically describes the numeric values from findings of the different studies and the statistical tests used to test those numbers. A systematic review usually summarizes the available studies that address a clinical care question but does not yield new findings in either numerical or written form. A metasynthesis or meta-analysis may summarize the nature of the studies used, but the core of the findings will be new knowledge in either a numeric or conceptual form. Both systematic reviews and meta-analyses usually provide a table identifying the basic characteristics of the individual research studies that were included, which allows the reader to view the individual studies as needed.

Finally, metasynthesis, meta-analyses, and systematic reviews all have a conclusions section in which the potential meaning of the findings is described. As with single research reports, these types of reports may identify limits to what has been reported and usually recommend areas for future research. A systematic review always addresses implications for clinical practice.

Although systematic reviews are an important form of research that can be used in practice, quality improvement is a process that resembles, yet differs from, the research process. Quality improvement is a process of evaluation of health care services to see if they meet specified standards or outcomes of care and to identify how they can be improved. Quality improvement often is based on research, and the process and product resemble the research process. The questions in quality improvement are whether a certain set of actions is occurring and how desirable outcomes can be facilitated. This is a form of a descriptive research question. The standard or outcome itself usually is based on earlier research that indicates the set of actions or outcome that can and should be achieved. Standards of care change as research findings suggest better approaches to and potential outcomes of care.

In addition to asking a descriptive question about the presence or frequency of a set of actions or outcomes, quality improvement studies also often examine relationships among factors that may affect the outcome or actions of interest. Just as we want to know what factors may influence a clinical problem of interest, we want to know what factors influence the consistency of achievement of standards or outcomes.

In such ways, traditional research often serves as the basis for quality improvement standards. Moreover, many of the methods used in research directly apply to the process of evaluating quality. Finally, gaps in quality of care may indicate fresh areas requiring research as well as needs for changes in practice.

Although quality improvement studies are an important form of research that can be used in practice, process improvement is a process that resembles, yet differs from, the quality improvement and research process. Process improvement is a management system in which all participants involved strive to improve customer satisfaction. While meta-analysis, metasynthesis, and systematic reviews seek to find the best practices and development of standards of care to improve patient outcomes, process improvement methods seek to improve the process in which decisions/changes in care delivery are carried out. For example, a traditional research study may seek to answer whether customer satisfaction is improved when a professional translator is assigned to a patient versus the use of a family member for a patient who is Chinese, whereas a process improvement method seeks to improve an approach that increases customer satisfaction for all patients within an organization.

Therefore, process improvement is a management system, whereas quality improvement seeks to find practice-related answers. However, process improvement reports can resemble a quality improvement study by identifying problems using data, planning and implementing a change, and evaluating results. Quality improvement and process improvement systems use the same quality principles. Although we have explained differences between quality improvement studies and process improvement, the terms are often considered synonymous. Process improvement methods are based extensively in the business industry to remove process errors and increase efficiency within an organization leading to overall customer satisfaction. Health care organizations are successfully using these methods to increase patient satisfaction, efficiency, and effectiveness and decrease costs. In other words, these methods focus on meeting and/or exceeding customer requirements, needs, and expectations.

How does quality improvement play a role in health care services? According to the Health Care Improvement (HCI) project, quality improvement can be defined as "all activities that contribute to defining, designing, assessing, monitoring, and improving the quality of healthcare" (HCI Project, n.d.). The HCI project uses quality management principles to develop tools and methods to improve health care services. These principles focus on four areas: patient, systems and processes, measurement, and teamwork. The HCI project has improved health care services in many arenas. Another health care organization known as Agency for Healthcare Research and Quality (AHRQ) uses quality improvement research to improve health care services. The AHRQ focuses on health care outcomes, quality, cost, use, and access. Visit thepoint.lww.com/Rebar3e for the direct link. The Joint Commission (TJC) works to improve the quality of care and safety of patients within the United States. The TJC evaluates and uses accreditation to verify health care organizations and programs provide safe, quality care to individuals and communities. Visit thepoint.lww.com/Rebar3e for the direct link. The TJC Center for Transforming Healthcare uses the Lean Six Sigma process improvement model to help health care entities reduce waste, decrease health care errors, and to improve quality of care (TJC Center for Transforming Healthcare, 2010). These organizations, along with The Institute for Healthcare Improvement, National Association for Healthcare Quality, The Institute for Safe Medication Practices, and American Society for Quality, are committed to using quality/process improvement principles to improve quality in health care services.

Health care organizations using process improvement methods rely on each employee at every level to strive for continuous improvement in health care services. The results could and do have drastically changed how nurses practice. For example, data is collected on a surgical unit in a local hospital regarding the number of surgical wounds that have developed an infection. The nurses identified possible causes of the infection and developed a procedure in caring for surgical wounds based on research indicating actions that decrease the risk of infection. Data was collected for several months after the procedure was initiated and the number of infected surgical wounds decreased. What do you think happened to the patient satisfaction scores after the procedure was followed?

There are several process improvement methods currently being used in health care organizations today. Each method uses quantitative data to assess for process improvement opportunities. Total Quality Management (TQM) is a management system involving all organizational shareholders and requires a change in attitude that allows and encourages the participants to focus on quality and meeting customer's needs. The first priority in TQM is the customer. What can be done to improve customer satisfaction? What do customers want/need/expect? The Deming Cycle, also known as the PDCA model uses four steps in improving quality: plan, do, check, and act. In the planning step, a nurse might identify an issue and plans for a change. The nurse implements the plan/change on a small scale then collects data to determine if the results were significant. If the change had significant results, the change may be broadened to include other areas. Results are then collected and the cycle continues. Continuous Quality Improvement (CQI) is another management system based in the belief that products, processes, and services can always be improved. CQI research focuses on customer satisfaction, scientific approach, and teamwork to develop strategies in improving the health and well-being of individuals.

A written report of a quality improvement study resembles a report of a traditional research study, but there are some differences between the two. The problem addressed in a quality improvement study usually concerns whether certain expected clinical care was completed, so the question involves discovering what is being done or what has happened, rather than trying to understand a phenomenon. As with traditional research, a quality improvement study usually examines only a subset of all the occasions when a specified type of care was given. Methods to collect data for a quality improvement study include questionnaires, direct observation, and chart reviews. The report of a quality improvement study describes how information was collected concerning the clinical care and a summary of what was found. This is similar to the methods and results sections of a research report. The conclusions of this type of report include recommendations for improving the quality of care based on what was found regarding the care currently given. The recommendations are similar to the conclusions that are drawn from a research study. See Table 2.3 for a summary of the sections of quality improvement reports compared with individual research reports, metasynthesis, meta-analyses, and systematic reviews.

The usefulness of a quality improvement study can be understood using the same five questions discussed throughout this book. Table 1.2 outlines how they might be applied. We can consider why the standard or outcome was established—what is the evidence for that standard? We can ask about the manner by which the study was implemented because various methods can be used to implement quality improvement, including chart review, observation, interviews, and questionnaires. Various approaches can be taken to the "sample" for a quality improvement study, including convenience, random selection, and purposive sampling. Similarly, data from a quality improvement study can be handled and analyzed in several ways, making the fourth question about what was actually found appropriate to consider. The last question of what the study concluded is obviously also relevant to quality improvement studies. Just as an accurate and meaningful research study can inform clinical practice, an accurate and meaningful quality assurance study can evaluate and strengthen practice. Findings from a quality improvement study that indicate standards are being met support continuation of existing practices. Findings indicating that standards are not being met should guide revision of existing practices to improve care. As with traditional research, findings from a quality improvement study may lead to the need for another study to further clarify issues that may relate to meeting standards or outcomes.

■ RESEARCH REPORTS AND THE RESEARCH PROCESS

So far, we have discussed the elements of a published research report. However, in doing so, we have had to at least touch on what a researcher does to conduct a research study. Although this book is not intended to teach you how to be a researcher, it is impossible to use research intelligently if you do not understand the basics of the research process. Just as you do not have to be a cardiac surgeon to understand what open heart surgery entails, you do not have to be a researcher to read and use research in EBN. Fortunately, the research report is written in a manner that closely mirrors the actual research process, so as we focus on understanding and intelligently using research, we also can learn the basics of the process. We overview the steps in that process now and then discuss the different steps further in the following chapters.

Steps in the Research Process

Figure 2.3 illustrates the five steps in the research process and the relationship between them and the sections of a research report. The first step is to define and describe a knowledge gap or problem. Frequently, this step begins with a clinical question or problem, such as the one raised by the RN in the clinical case who wants to find evidence to guide her care

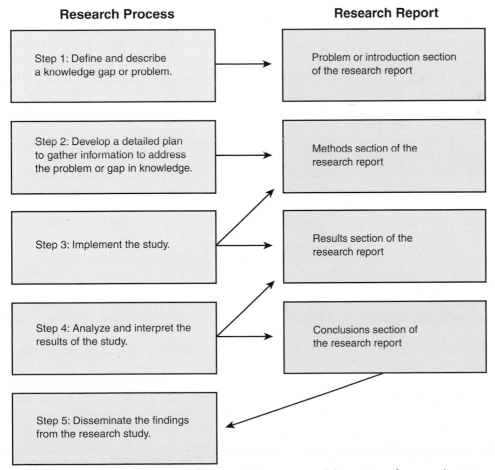

FIGURE 2.3 The relationship between the research process and the sections of a research report.

of M.D. A researcher interested in this type of clinical question then performs a literature review to determine what is already known about the problem. Performing a literature review requires using databases, as discussed in Chapter 1, and the researcher should search for and read as many pertinent published articles on the topic as possible. As part of defining and describing the knowledge gap, the researcher also investigates whether anyone has ever implemented a study addressing the clinical question as well as how other people have studied or described aspects of the problem. Although this process may help the researcher to gain a clearer picture of how to construct a study to address the clinical question, it also may make the problem more complicated and confusing. Often, a researcher's question changes as he or she learns about what has already been studied or described. Therefore, the focus of the first step is to narrow and identify something specific for the study, and its culmination is a statement of a problem or purpose. The problem section of a research report partially reflects this step by providing a description of the relevant literature, possibly a theory, and one or more of the following: a research problem, question, or hypothesis. However, the neatly written problem or introduction section of a research report certainly will not reflect all of the thinking, sorting, and comparing involved in the first step of the research process.

The second step is to develop a detailed plan for gathering information to address the identified knowledge gap. Planning the study depends on the problem or question being asked, and the designs of qualitative and quantitative studies differ, partly because of the type of questions asked and partly because of the researcher's beliefs about how best to gain meaningful knowledge.

Knowledge gaps that lend themselves to studies using qualitative methods are usually related to the experiences, beliefs, feelings, or perceptions of individuals, and often, little is known about the area in question. Because of this limited knowledge, qualitative methods provide a broad picture by describing the whole experience from the patient's viewpoint. In addition, a researcher may approach knowledge gaps by using qualitative methods because he or she believes that we can best learn and understand the phenomenon of interest by examining the phenomenon in its usual context.

In contrast, knowledge gaps that involve a concrete response or action, such as the relationships between depressive mood, self-esteem, coping, and eating, lend themselves to a quantitative approach in which each factor that might contribute to understand a problem is identified, defined, and measured. A researcher who uses a quantitative approach believes that knowledge can best be generated by breaking down a phenomenon into its different pieces and objectively measuring and examining each piece and its relationship to the other pieces.

In this step, the specific methods used to study the problem are planned, including who will participate in the study, what will be done to collect information, and how that information will be analyzed. It requires understanding the various approaches used to systematically gather information, considering what has been done in the past and what kinds of problems have occurred, and planning carefully to maximize the knowledge that will be the product of the study. The methods section of the research report, like the problem section, summarizes the decisions made in this step by specifically describing the sample, procedures, and data analysis used in the study. For example, in the fictional article about nursing students' preferences for first clinical jobs, we are told that the study included junior-year undergraduate nursing students and that, in this program, traditional 4-year, RN-to-BSN and LPN-to-BSN students were included. The report also tells us that a written questionnaire was used to collect the data. The researcher in this study could have decided to study graduating seniors rather than juniors or to conduct in-depth interviews with selected students rather than using a questionnaire. The researcher had reasons for using juniors and having them complete a questionnaire, such as time constraints, student availability, and the researcher's view on meaningful ways to gather knowledge. What we read in the research report usually only reflects the final decisions of the second step of the research process, and the researcher will likely only provide a limited explanation of the methods used.

Because research is a process, a study may not occur as it was designed and planned; therefore, the methods section also may describe any changes made to the study plan as it was implemented. The depressive mood, self-esteem, coping, and eating study reports that only 102 of the 119 high school participants were accepted into the study (Martyn-Nemeth et al., 2009).

The third step in the research process is to implement the study by gathering and analyzing the information in the systematic manner planned in the second step. As mentioned in the discussion of procedures, this may involve numerous different actions, such as tape-recording interviews, performing carefully controlled clinical experiments, or mailing and compiling responses to a questionnaire. In addition to gathering the information, this step involves managing, organizing, and analyzing the information to address the problem being studied. The outcome of this step is reported in the results section of the research report, which is why that section describes the sample and summarizes the answers or outcomes for each measure. Those results may not directly answer the research question, but they do allow the reader to have a better understanding of what happened during the study. For example, the researchers in the depressive mood, self-esteem, coping, and eating collected data from two public high schools whose student population equaled 3531 students. The number of students was narrowed down by the study's criteria of the participant having the ability to read and write English in order to complete a 45-minute questionnaire. The researchers do not indicate how the students who were given the questionnaire were selected, other than the ability to complete the 45-minute questionnaire written in English. It is likely that the researchers did not plan on only having such a small percentage of high school students who agreed to be in the study. We do not know if one type of adolescent was more likely than another to participate. However, the researchers indicate that the ethnic/racial distribution between the community's population and the participants was similar, and they describe the demographic and health information of the adolescents who participated. It is important to remember this when reviewing the conclusions because they may or may not apply equally to all patients.

The fourth step is the detailed analysis and interpretation of the results. In qualitative research methods, this step is woven closely with the third step, with analysis often guiding additional data collection. In quantitative methods, some preliminary analysis and summary of the data usually occur during the implementation step. However, additional analysis and careful interpretation of the meaning of the findings occur only after all the information from the study is gathered. The researchers will analyze the data, compare their findings to those from previous studies, and decide what they can conclude from the study. At this point, the researcher hopes to answer the question posed, confirm or not confirm the prediction made, or create a meaningful understanding of the phenomenon of interest. The actual findings from the study are summarized in the results section of the research report, whereas the implications, or potential meaning of those findings, are included in the conclusions section. As with all the other sections of a report, what is actually included does not reflect everything that the researchers did during this step. They will distill their analysis into a few paragraphs to provide the reader with a succinct summary of what they found and what it may mean for clinical care.

The fifth and final step of the research process is the sharing or dissemination of the findings. Gathering information to gain new knowledge is not a particularly useful activity if no one ever learns about the new knowledge, so an important obligation and commitment of the researcher is to share that research through publications, presentations, posters, and teaching. Research reports, such as the one on depressive mood, self-esteem, coping, and eating, are obviously a major method for disseminating research. However, these reports do not accomplish the goal of disseminating research if the people who need the knowledge cannot understand them. This brings us back to the importance of understanding and intelligently reading and using research in nursing practice.

■ SUMMARY OF THE RESEARCH PROCESS CONTRASTED TO THE RESEARCH REPORT

The first step of the research process—describing and defining the knowledge gap or problem—is summarized in the background and literature review sections of a research report. These sections give us the context for a research problem and tell us about relevant theory and research regarding aspects of it. The information included in the research report is a synopsis of the much more extensive information that was gathered and synthesized during the first step. The research purpose and specific questions or hypotheses that conclude the first sections reflect the final refinement of the research problem into specific variables and a specific type of research question.

The second step of the research process is reflected in the methods section of a research report. This section tells us the study design, sampling plan, methods of measurement, and procedures. Again, all the previous research, practicalities, and experience that enter into the decisions about settings for a study, the sample, and the measurement are distilled into a few paragraphs describing the final decisions that were reached about the study plan.

The third step of the research process—implementing the study—is usually reflected in the results section of a research report because it is there that we learn who actually participated in the study. We also may see part of the implementation reflected in the methods section if what occurred during the implementation process changed the sampling or measurement approaches taken. In either case, the information included in a report rarely reflects all of the details of a study's implementation.

The fourth step of analysis and interpretation of the results of a study is reflected in both the results and conclusions sections of a research report. Of all the steps of the research process, probably this one is the most fully described in the report. However, even with this step, a great deal more goes into the process than is reflected in the results and conclusions sections of most reports.

Finally, the fifth step in the research process is the research report itself. However, developing and publishing a research study report also require more effort than may be obvious when looking at the final product. Publication depends on several factors. These include the fit between the purpose of the study and the emphasis of journals that publish research, the relevance and quality of the research study, and the ability of the researcher to express clearly and succinctly all the pertinent elements that are needed to fully understand and use the research. The first two factors primarily affect those who will use the research because they affect what research is available through journals and online. Some research journals publish all types of research in each issue; others develop themes for different issues, limiting the types of studies they will publish at any particular time. Other journals reflect specialties, such as obstetric nursing, and are only interested in research that is relevant to that specialty. Some journals do not want to publish research that is highly theoretical because they target readers who want practical and practice-focused information. To disseminate the study findings, a researcher first has to find journals that fit with the purpose of the completed study.

Some research is not published because problems with the quality of the research are identified during the review process that decreases the meaningfulness or validity of the study's results. This does not mean that the research was bad but simply that some flaw or aspect of the study creates enough doubt about the findings or meaning of the results to preclude its warranting publication.

Another factor that affects publication is the ability of the researcher to express in writing adequate information to describe accurately the entire research process. Many of the common errors in research reports that we will discuss throughout this book are errors of omission or lack of complete information. The research process requires much more thought and work than can be described in a research report. The challenge for a researcher, then, and for the reviewers and editors who contribute to the final publication, is to describe clearly and completely all the aspects of the research process that were relevant to their particular study. The goal is to provide the readers with enough information to allow them to understand the study fully and to make intelligent decisions about the usefulness and meaning of the research for practice. One way this is accomplished is by using the language of research to limit the need to fully explain each study aspect. Yet, that very language of research may interfere with using research in practice because the practitioner may not be familiar with or understand the language.

Critically Reading Research for Practice

In Chapter 1, you were introduced to five questions that will be used to organize this text. These questions also provide a broad framework for critically reading reports to evaluate their usefulness as evidence for your EBN practice. As a bachelor's-prepared nurse, you are not expected to critique research reports in depth for their scientific soundness; however, it is important that you are able to critically evaluate research reports to decide whether they can serve as evidence related to your clinical practice question. Therefore, at the end of most of the chapters, we will include a section about common errors in research reports and list a set of questions to ask yourself that will allow you to critically evaluate research reports. Figure 2.4 presents six boxes containing the critical reading questions for the five broad questions that organize this text. Each of these sets of questions will be discussed in detail in the later chapters and are included here primarily to introduce you to them.

■ PUBLISHED REPORT—WHAT DID YOU CONCLUDE?

We have discussed briefly all of the sections in the published research studies about adolescents and obesity. The authors of those studies report directly that adolescents with obesity face health-related issues affecting both their experiences as an adolescent and an adult. The studies also report that adolescents need support for their weight concerns. If you were the RN in the clinical case, would you now know how to develop a plan of care for M.D.? Why or why not?

One reason it may be difficult to decide how to develop a care plan for M.D. based on the research report is because the nurse may still have questions about the research. What kinds of questions do you think the RN may have about how to proceed in her care of M.D.? One question might be whether you can believe the results of the study about depressive mood, self-esteem, coping, and eating or whether the results are "strong" enough that you are willing to develop a plan of care around that evidence. A second question might be why the depressive mood, self-esteem, coping, and eating study did not address the issue of health-promoting behaviors in relation to weight. A third question might pertain to what adolescents perceive as important to promote the health of themselves. You can probably think of other questions. With a further understanding of the research language and the research process, it is possible to answer most of the

How to Critically Read the Conclusions Section of a Research Report

Does the report answer the question
"What is the answer to my practice question—what did the study conclude?"

Did the report include a conclusions section?
Did the conclusions section assist me with my clinical problem?
Did the conclusions assist in a general manner or provide specific information about my
clinical problem?
Did the conclusions section include limitations of the study?
Did the limitations diminish my ability to use the conclusions in practice?
Do the conclusions seem reasonable or warranted based on the results of the study?

How to Critically Read the Results Section of a Research Report

Does the report answer the question
"Why did the authors reach these conclusions—what did they actually find?"

Did the report include a clearly identified results section?
Were the results presented appropriately for the information collected?
Were descriptive versus inferential results identifiable if this is a quantitative study?
Were themes or structure and meaning identifiable if this is a qualitative study?
Were the results presented in a clear and logical manner?
Did the results include information about the final sample for the study?

How to Critically Read the Sample Section of a Research Report

Does the report answer the question
"To what types of patients do these research conclusions apply—who was in the study?"

Did the report include a clearly identified section or paragraphs about sampling?
Did the report give me enough information to understand how and why this sample was chosen?
Is there enough information about the sample to tell me if the research is relevant for my clinical
population?
Was enough information given for me to understand how rights of human subjects were protected?
Would my patient population have been placed at risk if they had participated in this study?
Can I identify how information was collected about the sample?   *(continued)*

FIGURE 2.4   Questions for critically reading research reports.

questions posed by reading the published report in more detail. In the next chapter, we look more closely at the conclusions of research reports and what they can tell us about patient care questions.

■ SUMMARY

In this chapter, we have examined all the components of a research report and at least have begun to become familiar with the unique language of research. Specifically, we have learned that conclusions are the last section of most research reports and that they identify what was found and complete a report by identifying an outcome. We now understand that the results section of a report contains a summary or condensed version of what the authors believe are the most important findings and that results may be presented as numbers or as words, depending on the data collected for the study. We understand that the methods section of a research report describes the overall process of how the researchers went about

---

How to Critically Read the Methods Section of a Research Report

Does the report answer the question
"How were those people studied—why was the study performed that way?"

Did the report include a clearly identified section describing methods used in this study?

Do the methods make this a quantitative or a qualitative study?

Do I understand what my patient population would be doing if they were in this study or a study using similar methods?

Do the measures and procedures in this study address my clinical problem?

Do I think that the measures used in this study would provide helpful and useful information when used with my patient population?

Do I think what the researcher collected and the method of collection was the best way to address the clinical question?

Do I think that the researcher(s) should have planned the study differently in order to answer my clinical question?

How to Critically Read the Description of Study Design in a Research Report

Does the report answer the question
"How were those people studied—why was the study performed that way?"

Did the report include a clearly identified section describing the research design?

Does the design make this a quantitative, qualitative, or mixed method study?

Does the report address approaches taken to assure study rigor, internal validity, and/or external validity?

Do I think that the researcher(s) should have designed the study differently in order to answer my clinical question?

How to Critically Read the Background Section of a Research Report

Does the report answer the question
"Why ask that question—what do we know?"

Did the report include a clearly identified background and/or literature review section?

Do I think the background discusses aspects of my clinical question?

Does the literature help me understand why the research question is important to nursing?

Is the majority of the literature cited current (less than 5 years old) or very important to understanding the research question?

If a nursing or other theory was presented, does it connect to my clinical question?

Is the specific research question/problem/hypothesis connected logically to the literature and/or theory presented in the background section?

Is the specific research question/problem/hypothesis relevant or related to my clinical question?

FIGURE 2.4   (*Continued*)

implementing the research study, including who was included in the study, how information was collected, and what interventions, if any, were tested. We learned that there are two broad approaches to research: (1) qualitative methods, which focus on understanding the complexity of humans within the context of their lives and attempt to build a whole or complete picture of a phenomenon of interest and (2) quantitative methods, which focus on understanding and breaking down the different parts of a phenomenon into its parts to see how they do or do not connect as well as involve collecting information that is specific and limited to the particular parts of events or phenomena being studied. Last, we discussed the problem section of a research report, which describes the gap in knowledge addressed by the research study. In this section, the researcher explains why the study was needed, why it was carried out in the manner that it was, and, often, what the researcher is specifically asking or predicting.

Besides examining all the components of a research report, we looked at how those sections relate to the actual steps of the research process, and we considered some special types of research reports such as a metasynthesis, meta-analysis, systematic review, and quality improvement reports. We are now ready to begin looking at each section of a research report in detail in order to assure that you can read and use research as evidence for your professional practice.

OUT-OF-CLASS EXERCISE

Differing Conclusions From the Class Study

The fictional article in Appendix B represents the kind of report that might be written based on a questionnaire that you may have completed in class. In that article, the author suggests that older students may be interested in nonacute settings because they have had more experiences with health care in several settings. In preparation for the next chapter, write a concluding paragraph that could be used to end the fictional article by taking the position that nursing programs must focus on recruiting older students so that more nurses can be obtained for general care and nursing home settings. Then, write a different paragraph taking the opposite position that age should not be considered when recruiting nursing students because it is not clear whether it contributes to choice of nursing practice after graduation. Base your arguments on the findings reported in the fictional article—not solely on your opinions or ideas. Once you complete this exercise, you are ready to read Chapter 3.

References

Landis, A., Parker, K., & Dunbar, S. (2009). Sleep, hunger, satiety, food cravings, and caloric intake in adolescents. *Journal of Nursing Scholarship, 41*(2), 115–123.

Lazarus, R. S. (1993). Coping, theory and research: Past, present and future. *Psychosomatic Medicine, 55,* 234–247.

Martyn-Nemeth, P., Penckofer, S., Gulanick, M., Velsor-Friedrich, B., & Bryant, F. (2009). The relationships among self-esteem, stress, coping, eating behavior, and depressive mood in adolescents. *Research in Nursing & Health, 32,* 96–109.

Neuman, B. (1982). *The Neuman system model: Application to nursing education and practice.* East Norwalk, CT: Appleton-Century-Crofts.

Roy, C. (1984). *Introduction to nursing: An adaptation model* (2nd ed.). Englewood Cliffs, NJ: Prentice-Hall.

Watson, J. (1985). *Human science and human caring: A theory of nursing.* Norwalk, CT: Appleton-Century-Crofts.

Resources: Printed

Locke, L. F., Silverman, S. J., & Spirduso, W. W. (2009). *Reading and understanding research* (3rd ed.). Thousand Oaks, CA: Sage Publications.

Resources: Online

www.ahcpr.gov
www.asq.org
www.hciproject.org
www.jointcommission.org
www.centerfortransforming healthcare.org

3

Discussions and Conclusions
What Is the Answer to My Question—What Did the Study Conclude?

LEARNING OBJECTIVE

The student will interpret the conclusions of research reports for their potential meaning for evidence-based nursing (EBN) practice.

KEY TERMS

Conceptualization
Confirmation
Discussion
Generalization

Replication
Speculation
Study design

Clinical Case • C.T. is a 63-year-old elementary school teacher who has had a mastectomy at her community hospital and has been discharged to home several weeks ago. She is currently undergoing radiation therapy and has been given a favorable prognosis. C.T. has been encouraged to participate in activities of daily living, as much as possible; however, she is doing very little other than daily grooming. During a follow-up visit at the oncology clinic, C.T. states she is very concerned about her level of fatigue; "I'm not getting better! I can't do any baking, or cleaning, or gardening without becoming short of breath and so tired!" She is also concerned that she is becoming depressed and does not enjoy life anymore. The RN working with C.T. has had minimal experience with post–breast cancer care and begins to question if any nursing interventions could improve C.T.'s fatigue and short of breath on exertion. The RN reviews conversations with C.T., as well as her chart. The RN does a quick search in CINAHL using the keywords "breast cancer" and "recovery," which yields numerous hits regarding factors affecting recovery. One appears particularly relevant, since the patient population in the study is patients who have had breast cancer and are undergoing various cancer treatments. The article is titled "Effects of a Supervised Exercise Intervention on Recovery From Treatment Regimens in Breast Cancer Survivors" (Hsieh et al., 2008). You can find this article in Appendix A.3. Reading the conclusion or discussion sections of this article will help you to understand the examples discussed in this chapter. In addition, Table 3.1 summarizes the clinical question and the key search words used by the RN in the clinical case. We will include similar tables after clinical cases in later chapters to help you see how a good question for EBN is formed and how you could search for available evidence.

■ THE END OF A RESEARCH REPORT—DISCUSSIONS AND CONCLUSIONS

In this chapter, we address the first of the five questions that are used to organize this book: What is the answer to my practice question—what did the study conclude? As mentioned in Chapter 1, the major reason a practicing nurse wants to read and understand research is to answer clinical questions, so nurses, such as the one in the clinical case, often go directly to the last section of a research report. That section is sometimes labeled "Discussion," "Conclusions," or both, but its content usually includes both a discussion and conclusions as described here.

When the RN who is interested in finding interventions that decrease fatigue in patients who are undergoing breast cancer treatments reads the discussion section of the report on effects of exercise on recovery study, the RN learns that fatigue is the most prevalent side effect of the cancer itself as well as various treatments and is the most

Table 3.1

Development of a Clinical Question From the Clinical Case

What nursing interventions can decrease fatigue in patients undergoing breast cancer therapies after discharge from a hospital?

The *Who*	Patients with breast cancer
The *What*	Fatigue
The *When*	Undergoing breast cancer therapies
The *Where*	Outpatient setting
Key search terms useful in finding research-based evidence for this practice question	Breast cancer Recovery Exercise

common unmanaged side effect. The RN continues reading the discussion and learns that other studies that were done on decreasing fatigue using exercise programs demonstrated an improvement in cardiopulmonary functioning; however, no studies have determined whether the benefits of supervised exercise are influenced by the type of treatment, for example, surgery, chemotherapy, radiation, and surgery (Hsieh et al., 2008). Additionally, the RN who reads the study finds that individualized exercise programs alleviate cancer treatment–related side effects by improving resting heart rate, blood pressure, oxygen consumption, oxygen saturation, and increasing the length of time on a treadmill. Further, the "Discussion and Conclusion" section of the report on exercise and impact on recovery and fatigue associated with cancer indicates that patients are likely to have adversely affected quality of life and well-being. The RN reads that the study implies that "moderate intensity, individualized, prescriptive exercise maintains or improves cardiopulmonary function with concomitant reductions in fatigue regardless of treatment received for breast cancer" (Hsieh et al., 2008). The RN's likely response to reading the discussion and conclusion sections of this report is "While I now know that exercise should decrease fatigue and improve ability to perform activities of daily living and quality of life, how do I go about setting up a standard plan of care for patients with cancer-related fatigue?"

The discussion and conclusion sections of research reports initially may not be helpful in clinical questions for several reasons, including

- The study may not address the question you are asking.
- The researchers may have had problems implementing the study, resulting in an unclear answer.
- The results of the study may have been unexpected or complex and increase, rather than decrease, possible answers to the question.

Later chapters address why research questions may not directly address clinical questions and the many problems that can occur when carrying out a research study. Although this chapter discusses briefly how unexpected results can affect clinical usefulness, understanding results and the results sections of research reports are discussed more completely in Chapter 4. This chapter focuses on a fourth reason why the conclusion of a report may not answer a clinical question: The nurse having inappropriate or unclear expectations about what information can be found in the conclusion of a research report. Just what should we expect to find from the discussion and conclusion sections of research reports?

■ DISCUSSIONS

This book treats discussions and conclusions as two separate sections, but remember that you often find them combined in published reports. Table 3.2 summarizes the major components of most discussion and conclusion sections. The discussion section of a research report summarizes, compares, and speculates about the results of the study. Let us examine these pieces, starting with summarizing.

Summary

The first part of the discussion section in a research report usually includes a summary of the study's key results. This summary usually addresses the results that directly relate to the major research question posed by the researcher(s). It also includes the unexpected results and those that stood out as being particularly meaningful. However, this summary usually is brief because it follows a detailed description of the results. It is also likely, unless the study had few findings, that it will not include all of the results from the study. What the brief

Table 3.2

General Components of the Discussion and Conclusion Sections of Research Reports	
SECTION OF REPORT	MAJOR COMPONENTS OF THE SECTION
Discussion	• Summary of key findings • Comparison of results with those of previous studies • Description of whether findings confirm results of similar studies or predictions based on theory • Speculation about possible interpretations of results
Conclusion	• Description of the new knowledge that can be accepted based on the study • A conceptualization of the meaning of the results or a generalization of the findings • A description of study limitations

summary does include are the specific results from the study that the researcher believes are particularly important and meaningful.

For example, the discussion section on the effects of exercise on recovery study (Hsieh et al., 2008) tells us that "the exercise intervention resulted in significant reductions in behavioral fatigue, affective fatigue, sensory fatigue, cognitive and mood fatigue, and total fatigue in the surgery and chemotherapy; surgery and radiation therapy; and the surgery, chemotherapy, and radiation therapy groups" (p. 911). It also states that "the breast cancer survivors in the surgery alone group showed significant reduction in fatigue on the behavioral and affective subscales and the total fatigue score but not on sensory and cognitive and mood subscales after exercise training" (p. 911). The author specifically identifies the types of fatigue, but does not explain the meaning of the factors in this section of the report.

Comparison

After a brief summary of key or important results, the discussion section of a research report debates the possible meanings of the study results. Questions addressed in research studies are rarely simple or readily answered completely by only one study; therefore, the results provide information that can be explained or understood in several different ways. Hence, the pros and cons of different explanations for the results may be described, forming a written debate. Further, the meaning of the findings usually must be interpreted within the context of existing knowledge, so the discussion section frequently compares the study's results with those of previous studies. The match or lack of match of results of a study to results from previous studies supports the different explanations offered regarding the results. Another important reason for comparing is to provide confirmation of previous findings. Confirmation is the verification of results from other studies. Rarely are we comfortable deciding that we are completely certain of the answer to a clinical question based on the findings of only one study. One goal of research is to build knowledge, with each research study adding a new piece to our understanding. However, as with the parts of any building that is going to be stable and strong, the pieces of knowledge must overlap and unite to make a cohesive whole. A study that is a duplication of an earlier study is called a replication study, and its major purpose is confirmation. Usually, however, a research study differs from past studies in some ways by, for example, using a different patient group in the study or by using different procedures on the subjects. Whether a study is a replication or a variation of previous studies, the discussion section of the research report describes how the findings do or do not overlap with previous knowledge.

CORE CONCEPT 3.1

The summary of findings in the discussion section of a research report only contains selected results from the study. It does not give the reader a complete picture of the results but does give information about some key or important results.

In addition to discussing how a study's results do or do not confirm those of previous studies, the authors may compare their findings with the predicted results that were based on existing theory. Theory might be considered to be the plans for the knowledge being built about a clinical question: Like the blueprints of a building plan, a theory provides the description of how all the parts of a phenomenon should fit together. Not all research studies are based on a theory or test a prediction from a theory because not enough may be known about a clinical question. However, if the study tests a prediction or hypothesis that was based on a theory and the results show the pieces fitting together as the theory predicted, then the results are considered to confirm that theory. We discuss how theory directs and is built by research in Chapter 10.

Our effects of exercise on recovery article that the RN found did not attempt to specifically test theory. Nor, did the authors tell us whether the studies cited in the discussion section were based on theory. However, the discussion section of the article does cite previous studies demonstrating that exercise improves cardiopulmonary functioning. While in this example the findings of the recovery from article are similar to past studies, it is not uncommon for results from a study to differ from previous studies. This is why we usually need multiple studies to inform our EBN and to make clinical decisions. Results that differ from findings in previous studies require that the author(s) suggest reasons for those differences, which lead us to the third component of most discussion sections.

Speculation

In addition to comparison, the discussion section of a research report speculates about the reasons for the results of the study. Speculation is the process of reflecting on results and offering some explanation of them. The debate, or speculation, in a discussion generally considers several alternative explanations for the results and provides a rationale for the author's judgments about which is the best explanation.

CORE CONCEPT 3.2

The discussion section of a research report contains a debate on how the results of the study fit with existing knowledge and what those results may mean.

As a Core Concept from Chapter 2 stated, the results section provides the findings of the specific study, whereas the discussion and conclusion sections of a report interpret those findings in light of existing knowledge and theory. This interpretation is appropriately called a *discussion* because it is open to debate. It reflects not fact, but thoughtful informed speculation. Although such speculation is thoughtful and informed and considers alternative possibilities, it is based on the author's knowledge and selection of previous research or theory. Another author might know or select a different theory or body of research to use in his or her discussion.

Why are the meanings of results from almost any study open to debate? The answer lies, in part, in the nature of research. We learned in Chapter 2 that research usually examines a question using a subgroup or sample of people. Although great pains often are taken to include diversity in the people, samples cannot possibly reflect all of the variation that exists in humans. What works with or happens to a few subjects is unlikely to always be exactly what happens with many patients or with everyone.

In fact, qualitative methods assume that experiences are subjectively unique and that although we can increase our understanding regarding a particular question, there may always be individual variations. Returning to our analogy of building knowledge piece by piece, the qualitative research perspective is that the picture of the phenomenon, which is the product in knowledge building, is constantly evolving because our world and our individual experiences are always changing.

Conceptualization is a process of creating a picture of an abstract idea; in the case of nursing research, it is a picture of some aspect of health. Discussions and conclusions of qualitative studies conceptualize some phenomenon related to health as opposed to those of quantitative studies that objectify and isolate parts of the phenomenon. For example, a qualitative study might conceptualize patient satisfaction as a person's overall sense of the quality of the care that is received. A quantitative study may examine patient satisfaction as the total score on a survey of the patient's care experience. If theory is the blueprint or plan for a building, we can view a qualitative study as providing results that are an artist's rendition of how the building looks. Similarly, we can view quantitative results as a detailed parts list for constructing the building. The artist's rendition provides a clear sense of how a building might look or even feel and smell, whereas the parts list gives us a sense of how it looks when it is put together and how it might be used, but not of how we will actually experience the building. Figure 3.1 illustrates this concept.

From a qualitative perspective, knowledge is built by creating a "picture album" filled with different "pictures" of a particular aspect of health. Each study result, or picture, gives

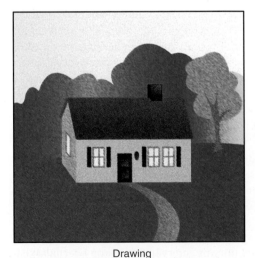

Drawing

Product of qualitative research is like
an artist's rendition.

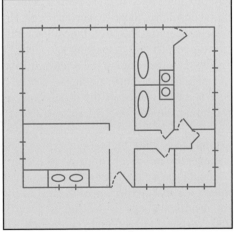

Blueprint

Product of quantitative research is like a
blueprint, showing details and
how parts go together.

FIGURE 3.1 Products of qualitative versus quantitative research.

a sense of the aspect of health at a unique moment in time. As we look at more and more pictures, we get a greater sense of the whole phenomenon. Each qualitative study provides a unique picture that adds to our overall understanding.

Quantitative methods do not assume that knowledge is always changing and evolving; they assume that there are answers to questions and that we can find those answers by reducing, objectifying, and quantifying the components of a phenomenon to understand the relationships among the components. Quantitative methods assume that we get a greater sense of the whole phenomenon by breaking it down to smaller parts, and we get closer and closer to "knowing" the "real" answer to questions when we get the same results in different studies with different groups. The quantitative researcher expects that each study will add more details to the same detailed building plan.

The goal of research is to generalize a study's results. Generalization is the ability to apply a particular study's findings to the broader population represented by the sample. The authors of the effects of exercise on recovery study, for example, conclude that exercise programs can be effective in improving cardiopulmonary function and in decreasing fatigue in breast cancer treatment regardless of type. Both qualitative and quantitative research strives to develop knowledge that can be applied to a broader population. However, the term *generalization* is more commonly applied to quantitative research than qualitative research. Nonetheless, a qualitative researcher will often do several procedures to make sure that the findings can also be applied to the population in the area of interest. The value of being able to generalize study findings is an important concept. If the study is conducted well, whether it is a qualitative or quantitative study, then a nurse who reads the study can make better clinical decisions regarding the value of applying the research findings to work with similar populations.

Implications for Practice

The discussion in a nursing research report often includes a debate on the meaning of the study results for nursing practice. For example, the effects of exercise on recovery article found that a moderately intense exercise program decreased fatigue for patients undergoing treatment for breast cancer. The authors then suggest that nurses can assist patients in improving quality of life by referring patients to exercise-supported therapies and that health care providers need to consider if a higher intensity exercise program would be more beneficial or safe for those cancer survivors. However, it is important to realize that choices are made concerning the best clinical interpretation of results, just as choices are made about how the results add to existing knowledge in general. This means that the discussion section needs to be read critically and with an awareness of the different meanings that could be assigned to the study findings.

The RN who reads the discussions on effects of exercise on recovery in the article is reading the author's interpretations of what is believed to be the key findings. The author clearly states that cardiopulmonary function was increased in all groups after treatment and that total fatigue scores were reduced. The author interpreted the findings that exercise positively impacts all patients undergoing breast cancer treatments. This is a speculation by the author about the meaning of the results and is most likely based on beliefs and past experiences as well as the results of previous research. The author did not specifically test or measure or identify gender or racial differences as the exercise study consisted of a female population. However, the RN caring for C.T. has one possible answer to the clinical question about what nursing intervention to consider in assisting C.T. in decreasing fatigue and improving activity endurance. The RN must read previous sections of the report to decide if the author's practice implications drawn from the results match the nurse's beliefs and experiences. We return to the RN's dilemma later in this chapter.

CONCLUSIONS

The conclusions of a research report describe the knowledge that the researcher believes can be gained from the study, given its "fit" with other studies and theories. As stated in Chapter 2 in the discussion of sections of a research report, conclusions from a research study can be powerful because they are used to guide practice. Conclusions move beyond debate or speculation about the results to a statement of what is now "known" about a question or problem. As a result, they generally are worded carefully. Conclusions also may be statements about what we do not know, particularly if the study results do not fit with theory or replicate previous studies. Therefore, it is possible for a conclusion to state that we now know we cannot get the answer for our question using the methods or measures or sample that was used in the study being reported. More often, conclusions include recommendations for building knowledge about a clinical question or health aspect. In either case, the conclusion section almost always describes the limits that must be placed on the knowledge that has been gained from the study.

The effects of exercise on recovery article does not provide concrete answers to questions that could have been addressed. One reason for this is because when questions are complex, the research results are open to debate and interpretation. Another reason is because almost every study has limitations. A third reason is because researchers will often collect information via investigation, as opposed to constructing research questions to answer during the study. Remember from Chapter 2 that limitations are the aspects of a study that create uncertainty about the meaning or decisions that can be derived from it. We suggested that limitations can be viewed as a fence around the results of a research study that confine or limit what we can conclude.

Several aspects of a study may be viewed as limitations, and Figure 3.2 illustrates some of these. We have already alluded to one factor that often limits a study: the sampling—who was included in the study. Although the effects of exercise of recovery study included a convenience sample of women between the ages of 47.5 and 68.3 and included data on height and weight, the study did not include data on race, health status, or other population characteristics. Additionally, all of the women in the study were identified as being from the same geographical location, patients from the Rocky Mountain Cancer Rehabilitation Institute. This aspect of the sample leaves us with uncertainty about the meaning of the results for male patients, patients with complex health needs, and patients who are of different racial backgrounds than those involved in the study. The study aims to produce findings that can be used in various breast cancer treatments, so the limit on the sample indicates that the picture provided by the study results is a picture of only women between the ages of 47.5 and 68.3 and who live in the same geographical location. As we will see in Chapters 6 and 7, many other sampling-related aspects can create limits to a research study.

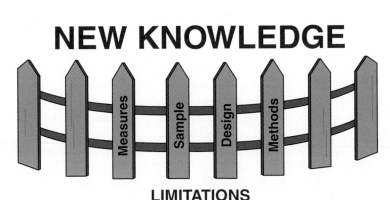

FIGURE 3.2 Some limitations of the research process, represented by the fence posts.

A second factor that may be a limitation is the study design—the overall plan or organization of a study. Some study designs create more uncertainty than do others. For example, if the RN in the clinical case read a study that described the cognitive, behavioral, and psychological factors that affect a patient's self-perception of fatigue, the RN would be uncertain about whether those factors were present before the operative intervention and thus whether they impacted the patient's recovery. However, the effects of exercise on recovery study use a pretest and post-test design, in which measures of cardiopulmonary function and fatigue are taken before and after the exercise intervention, which would remove some of the uncertainty about the clinical use of results because we would know the outcome change that occurred between the beginning and the end of the study. Many factors affect a researcher's decision about a study design, including the type of question being asked, the level of existing knowledge, and the availability of resources. Chapter 9 discusses research designs in more detail.

A third factor that may be a limitation involves the measures used in the study. Several problems can occur with study measures. For example, a study's measures may be inconsistent. If blood sugar is measured by using a glucometer that loses calibration halfway through the study, the resulting measures will be inconsistent. Sometimes paper-and-pencil questionnaires are unclear or confusing, causing people to be inconsistent in their understanding of, and therefore answers to, the questions. Another possible problem is that measures may be inaccurate or incomplete. Returning to the study using a glucometer for measuring blood sugars, if the glucometer had gone out of calibration before the study began, the resulting measures would be consistent but inaccurate throughout the study. That is, the measures would consistently be inaccurate. Accuracy and consistency of measures are referred to as *validity*, *rigor*, and *reliability* in research. The examples given in this paragraph are all reflective of quantitative research, although accuracy and consistency are also a problem in qualitative research. These ideas are the focus of Chapter 8 and will be explored in detail in that chapter.

Finding accurate measures of concepts in quantitative research is a problem in nursing because it is difficult to find ways to quantify some concepts that are important to nurses, such as anger, quality of life, pain, or self-confidence. If measures do not exist, the researcher will either have to make one or not include that factor in the study. Excluding an important factor limits the conclusions that can be drawn. For example, hypothetically, if a limitation was identified where the author did not assess fatigue levels in the participants before the exercise intervention, the researcher might assume that some of the findings are related to exercise. Without baseline measures taken before the exercise intervention, the researcher's finding is just an assumption. This lack of the measurement presents the possibility that fatigue levels as measured after exercise intervention may actually be better than they were before the exercise intervention and therefore are really not factors impacting fatigue associated with breast cancer treatments.

The methods used in a study are a fourth factor that may limit the conclusions. Not only does a measurement need to be consistent and accurate, it also must be used consistently and accurately. An appropriately calibrated glucometer will still provide results that are inconclusive regarding a person's blood sugar if it is used at different times during the day and with different techniques to acquire blood samples. Similarly, a measure of a person's knowledge about HIV will not be conclusive if one group completed the measure immediately after a patient education program and the other group completed it 2 weeks after their education program. Therefore, the methods used to conduct a study also may lead to limitations in the conclusions.

The discussion and conclusions sections of a research report, then, include a summary of key results, a comparison of those results with findings from other studies or to existing theory, speculation and debate about the possible explanations for the results and how they fit with current knowledge, and finally, some carefully worded decisions about new knowledge gained in the study. These sections includes debate, speculation, and cautious language because research questions are complex, each study contributes only one new piece to the puzzle or one more picture to the phenomenon, and almost every study has some limitations.

Can Conclusions Differ?

At the end of Chapter 2, you were asked to write two concluding paragraphs for the fictional article in Appendix B, taking two different positions regarding who should be recruited for nursing programs based on results reported in the article. Reviewing the results reported in that study, we find that age, type of program, and rating of health-affected choice of nursing field. We assume that the goal is to focus recruitment of students on increasing the number of graduates who enter fields that are not considered acute, a goal with which you may not personally agree. One way to interpret the results is to focus on the finding that age was an important factor in choice of field and conclude that older students should be recruited. Therefore, the new knowledge gleaned from the study would be that recruiting older students will increase the numbers of new graduates entering nonacute nursing fields.

However, the finding that health rating was important could mean that the relevant factor is not age and experience, as the author suggests. Rather, the relevant factor may instead be level of health, with students who perceive themselves as less healthy selecting fields of practice that are generally considered less physically strenuous. If this is true, then age is not the relevant factor. Rather, schools of nursing must recruit students who want less physically strenuous positions. This second conclusion would probably be considered relatively implausible, but it illustrates that conclusions can differ based on the interpretation of the results. Because the conclusions drawn from study results can differ as you read discussions and conclusions of research reports, you should carefully consider whether the interpretation provided makes sense to you in terms of your own knowledge and practice.

Do We Change Practice?

We have emphasized that the conclusions of research reports can be powerful because they are used to change practice. We also have pointed out some of the uncertainty that is reflected in most conclusions. Most importantly, we have said that the purpose for nurses to intelligently understand research is for them to use it in practice. Recognizing the limitations of each research study and the complexity of building new knowledge does not imply that research cannot and should not be used in practice. However, it does mean that it is essential to have some understanding of more than just the study conclusions. We must understand why and how much the limitations such as sampling, measures, methods, or design make the results uncertain, and we must look intelligently at the study findings to determine whether the author's interpretation is logical.

Each research study reflects only one piece or picture in the process of knowledge building, which is why nurses and other health professionals emphasize the use of systematic reviews. Systematic reviews include the results from many studies as evidence for practice. They compile the results of multiple studies regarding the same clinical question and organize the findings around key aspects related to practice. A systematic review also addresses differences in research studies, such as design, sample, and methods. The end of a systematic review is usually titled "Practice Implications" and summarizes the practice-related points that are most strongly supported by different research studies.

As with individual studies, however, systematic reviews are open to interpretation because the findings of particular studies can be given more or less attention. For example, the author of a systematic review may place less emphasis on negative findings about a procedure and interpret the positive findings to warrant a change in clinical practice. An author may also believe that any negative finding about a procedure questions its use and interpret any negative research to indicate that a procedure should not be adopted in practice. As in individual studies, the conclusions of systematic reviews include some hesitancy or caution and almost always include recommendations for further research. Systematic reviews as evidence for practice can be helpful, but the nurse still must read the review carefully and intelligently to decide how the findings should be used in practice.

■ COMMON ERRORS IN RESEARCH REPORTS

To be read and used intelligently in practice, the research report must clearly and completely give the reader the needed information. Many nurses assume that if they are not comfortable in their understanding of a research study, it is because they lack knowledge. While this may be the case, it is also possible that part of the problem is a lack of clarity in the research report. While we will summarize below the common ways in which a report can be unclear, we will also discuss common errors that may be found in research reports in later chapters. We do this to help you recognize that sometimes the problem lies not with your knowledge, but with the information provided to you.

As an example of errors in research reports, you may see a failure to include one or more major aspects of a discussion and conclusion. The authors should provide the information discussed in the discussion and conclusions sections. As a research reader, you should expect to find a summary of key findings, a comparison of the findings with previous research, and an interpretation of the meaning of the findings within the context of current knowledge. Also, you should find some discussion of the study limitations. The fictional article in Appendix B provides an example of a report that does not include important aspects because it neither compares its results with previous studies nor includes any discussion of study limitations.

A second common error is presenting a confusing summary of key findings or presenting new results. The summary should use language that is consistent with both the common use of terms and how the terms were used throughout the report. It should not include key findings that were not already described in more detail in the results section. Because we are starting at the end of a report, we might not know that information in the discussion was not addressed in the results, but we can quickly find this out if we read the results section. The summary of key findings is a brief, succinct summation. If a result is only provided at the end of a report in this manner, we will likely not have enough information about it to judge intelligently the usefulness of that finding for practice.

A third common error in research reports is overinterpreting the results. Like nurses in practice, researchers want answers to the questions they study. Therefore, it is tempting to overinterpret results by reading into them, generalizing them beyond what was actually found, or discounting the limitations. It is expected that a researcher will understate or be conservative when interpreting study results. However, occasionally, a report presents an interpretation that makes suggestions that are more than what can reasonably be concluded based on the results of the study. For example, if the author of the effects of exercise on recovery article had concluded that fatigue levels would predict who had a higher quality of life or sense of well-being, the authors would have drawn a conclusion that interpreted the results beyond what was indicated—the authors did not track what factors affected quality of life or well-being, only what affected cardiopulmonary function and fatigue.

Similarly, occasionally, a research report draws conclusions that are not directly related to the question under study. It is important to read the conclusions of a study carefully and remember that conclusions are, in part, the speculation of the author. Part of being an RN who uses EBN effectively is to be a careful reader who thinks discriminately about the conclusions drawn from a study.

■ CRITICALLY READING DISCUSSION AND CONCLUSION SECTIONS OF REPORTS

In Chapter 1, you were introduced to five questions that will be used to organize this text. These questions also provide a broad framework for critically reading reports to evaluate their usefulness as evidence for your EBN practice. Remember, as a bachelor's-prepared nurse, you are not expected to critique research reports in depth for their scientific soundness. However, you are expected to be able to critically evaluate research reports to decide whether they can serve as evidence related to your clinical practice question. Therefore, Box 3.1 presents a set of six questions that you can use to help you in the process of critically reading the discussion and conclusion sections of a report.

The first question to ask yourself is "Did the report include a discussion and/or conclusion section?" While this may seem like a simple question, some reports of research do not present much of a conclusion section, or it is not easy to find and may be buried toward the end of the article. The recovery from surgery article includes a section labeled as "Discussion."

A second question to consider when critically reading the discussion and conclusion sections of a report is "Did the discussion/conclusion section assist me with my clinical problem?" To answer this, one needs to compare the *Who*, *Where*, *What*, and *When* contained in the discussion with that of your clinical question. The RN in our clinical case asks the question "What nursing interventions can decrease fatigue in patients undergoing breast cancer therapies after discharge from hospital? If we look at the discussion section effects of exercise on recovery article, we find that it discusses patients' fatigue, cardiovascular endurance, and pulmonary function, making it a very good match to our RN's clinical question. The RN in our clinical case would learn how exercise could be used in trying to decrease fatigue in patients undergoing breast cancer treatments.

The third question to ask yourself as you critically read the discussion and conclusion sections of a report is "Did the discussion/conclusion assist in a general manner or provide specific information about my clinical problem?" The answer is based on the RN's sense

---

Box 3.1

How to Critically Read the Discussion and Conclusion Sections of a Report

Do the discussion and conclusion sections answer the question "Did the section provide an answer to my practice question—what did the study conclude?"

1. Did the report include a discussion and/or conclusion section?
2. Did the discussion/conclusion section assist me with my clinical problem?
3. Did the discussion/conclusion assist in a general manner or provide specific information about my clinical problem?
4. Did the discussion/conclusion section include limitations of the study?
5. Did the limitations diminish my ability to use the conclusions in practice?
6. Do the discussion/conclusions seem reasonable or warranted based on the results of the study?

of how easily he/she can change their practice after reading the conclusions of the effects of exercise on recovery report. While the report assisted the RN in knowing that fatigue was a common unmanaged symptom of breast cancer and its treatments, the ways in which it was measured may not easily translate into routine clinical practice and may require more thought and evidence searching to identify potential interventions.

A fourth question "Did the discussion/conclusion section include limitations of the study?" is answered by examining the discussion section of the report. The effects of exercise on recovery study had a section labeled "Limitations" within the last few paragraphs of the article. The authors discuss the convenience sampling of the study as a limitation as well as the fact that the participants were from the same geographical area. The importance of these limitations will be discussed in more detail in Chapter 6, which addresses sampling. Such patients may not be typical and may not closely resemble the patients our RN sees in the clinical case.

It is important to stop and think about statements such as made by the researcher in the "Limitations" section, which leads us to the next question we need to ask ourselves when critically reading the discussion and conclusion sections of a report: "Did the limitations diminish my ability to use the conclusions in practice?" What do you think it means that the authors used a convenience sampling? How could it influence the interpretation of the findings that are presented? Does it increase, decrease, or not affect the RN's willingness to use these results in resolving the clinical question? This is the process of critically thinking about the evidence for EBN. As you answer these questions, it is important to remember that all studies will have limitations. It is an unavoidable aspect of studying living patients. The question to answer is whether or not the limits are so limiting that the results cannot be generalized to your patients.

The final question to ask when critically reading the discussion and conclusion sections of a report is "Do discussion/conclusions seem reasonable or warranted based on the results of the study?" To answer this, you need to think about what the conclusions seem to say that a nurse should do, and then see if the results section of the report supports this. In the effects of exercise on recovery article, the author tells us that the results section supported the conclusion that "exercise improved cardiopulmonary function and reduced fatigue in patients undergoing breast cancer treatment, regardless of the type of treatment." To know if this is a logical and clear conclusion, we will need to read the results section carefully. How this should be done is presented in Chapters 4 and 5. We will revisit this question after we learn more about critically reading the results section of research reports.

■ PUBLISHED REPORTS—WHAT WOULD YOU CONCLUDE?

The discussion and conclusion sections of the report found by the RN in the clinical case tell us several different things. It tells us that fatigue is common and is usually left unmanaged for patients undergoing breast cancer treatment. This confirms the RN's impression that there is something that could be done to meet C.T.'s needs. The conclusion also suggests that exercise to address fatigue and cardiovascular endurance in patients undergoing breast cancer treatment is important for all patients, regardless of the nature of the treatment. The discussion did not tell the RN what specific assessments were done to assess fatigue, cardiovascular endurance, or pulmonary function, the RN will have to read the results section to answer that question.

The conclusions from this report may contradict another report found by the RN. This is often one of the most confusing and frustrating aspects of EBN. However, it is most often possible to fit the conclusions of apparently contradictory studies together in a meaningful way. For example, the RN might decide from the effects of exercise on recovery article that he/she must help other staff to recognize and look for cardiovascular intolerance and fatigue in all patients undergoing breast cancer treatments. At the same time, another study may suggest that cardiovascular intolerance and fatigue in patients who have breast cancer is associated with protein deficits. The RN might plan to have his or her staff assess the protein intake of patients.

The discussion and conclusion section of a research report provides useful information for using research in practice, including a summary of key findings from the study, a comparison of the findings with previous research and theory, and an interpretation of the meaning of the findings. However, although the conclusions begin to answer the RN's clinical question, he/she will probably want to know more about the assessments that were used in determining fatigue and activity endurance. This means that the RN must read the preceding section of the research report—the results section.

OUT-OF-CLASS EXERCISE

How Do We Organize a Large Amount of Information to Make Sense of It?

Chapters 4 and 5 discuss the results section of research reports. As we mentioned in Chapter 2, these sections often include some of the most complex and confusing language for those readers who are not advanced researchers. We look at some of the key terms in results sections that can readily be understood without having an advanced degree in statistics and discuss how to determine what you need to really understand and intelligently use nursing research in practice.

To prepare for Chapter 4, summarize some of the data from your in-class study exercise in a way that makes it easier to understand or that makes sense of it. When doing this, think about why your method of organization helps to make it easier to understand. If you did not have an in-class study, your faculty may provide you with some data to use for this out-of-class exercise. Once you have completed this exercise, you are ready to read Chapter 4.

Reference

Hsieh, C., Sprod, L., Hydock, D., Carter, S., Hayward, R., & Schneider, C. (2008). Effects of a supervised exercise intervention on recovery from treatment regimens in breast cancer survivors. *Oncology Nursing Forum, 35–36*, 909–915.

Resources

Locke, L. F., Silverman, S. J., & Spirduso, W. W. (2009). *Reading and understanding research* (3rd ed.). Thousand Oaks, CA: Sage Publications.

Polit, D. F., & Beck, C. T. (2007). *Nursing research: Principles and methods* (8th ed.). Philadelphia, PA: Lippincott Williams & Wilkins.

4

Descriptive Results

Why Did the Authors Reach Their Conclusion—What Did They Actually Find?

LEARNING OBJECTIVE

The student will analyze the relationship between the descriptive results of research reports and the selected conclusion of the reports.

Differentiating Description From Inference

Understanding the Language of Results Sections
   Language Describing Results From Qualitative Studies
   Language Describing Results From Quantitative Studies

Connecting Results That Describe to Conclusions

Common Errors in the Reports of Descriptive Results

Critically Reading Results Sections of Research Reports for Use in Evidence-Based Nursing Practice

Published Report—What Would You Conclude?

KEY TERMS

Bivariate analysis	Mean
Categorization scheme	Measure of central tendency
Coding	Median
Content analysis	Mode
Data reduction	Normal curve
Data saturation	Predictor variables
Demographic	Skew
Dependent variable	Standard deviation
Distribution	Theme
Frequency distribution	Univariate analysis
Independent variable	Variable
Inferential statistics	Variance
Inference	

Clinical Case • N.B. is a 64-year-old man whose wife experienced a major stroke 6 months ago. Though his wife completed rehabilitation and came home from the hospital 2 weeks ago, she still has difficulty communicating, has an indwelling catheter, and requires assistance to dress and eat. An RN has been assigned to provide home health care to N.B.'s wife, as she needs weekly injections and catheter care. N.B. is very caring with his wife and asks many questions, but after just two home visits, the RN can see that N.B. appears fatigued, lacks interest in life, and has lost weight. The RN wonders what can be done to assist and support N.B. in managing his role as caregiver, recognizing that his health is intertwined with the health of his wife. The nurse takes a few minutes at work to search ProQuest using the keywords "stroke," "caregiver," and "health" and finds a citation in a journal that appears to be relevant to N.B.'s situation. The article is entitled "Predictors of Life Satisfaction in Stroke Survivors and Spousal Caregivers After Inpatient Rehabilitation" (Ostwald, Godwin, & Cron, 2009). This article is presented as Appendix A.4. We will be using the information in the results section of this report as examples throughout this chapter and in Chapter 5. Table 4.1 summarizes the RN's question for this clinical case.

■ DIFFERENTIATING DESCRIPTION FROM INFERENCE

At the end of Chapter 3, we decided that to base clinical decisions on the conclusions of a research report, we need to have a better understanding of the study results. The results are the specific findings of a study that can provide an answer to the second question we are using to organize this book: Why did the authors reach their conclusion—what did they actually find? This chapter and Chapter 5 address this question.

The results sections of reports summarize findings with two broad goals: (1) to describe or explain the phenomenon of interest and (2) to predict aspects related to that phenomenon. Because qualitative studies approach knowledge development with an expectation of increasing understanding to inform practice, their results use data analysis methods to provide description and explanation. In contrast, quantitative studies may predict, as well as describe and explain, because the assumption behind them is that there is generalized objectivity. Quantitative data analysis aims not only to describe and explain but also allows us to infer what would happen with other similar groups based on what was found in the present study. Inference is the reasoning that goes into the process of drawing a conclusion based on evidence and is common in research work. It refers to the statistical procedures used in most quantitative studies, which therefore are called inferential statistics.

It is important to differentiate between results that merely describe what the researcher found and results that are intended to allow inference, because it directly affects

Table 4.1

Statement of Clinical Question From the Clinical Case	
WHAT INTERVENTIONS ASSIST AND SUPPORT THE CAREGIVER'S HEALTH AND FUNCTIONING?	
The *Who*	Caregiver
The *What*	Health and functioning
The *When*	While caring for stroke survivor
The *Where*	In home
Key search to find research-based evidence for practice	Stroke Caregiver Health

what we can conclude from a study. The knowledge we gain from description can assist in the understanding of a situation or phenomenon, and that understanding can help us in our clinical practice. Description does not allow us to predict the future or to understand what causes the phenomena that we have described.

To understand cause and effect and to make predictions, we must know not only what is present at a given point in time but also the order of factors or events and the timing of such events or factors. Why can't description allow us to predict? When we describe the presence of two or more factors, we know that they are present concurrently, but we do not know if one came before the other, if one caused the other, or if some other outside event caused both. Take the simple example of driving a car. If one were to describe the factors involved in driving, one would think of a car, a key, a driver, and a license. However, which factor must come first is not necessarily obvious from that description. Do we need a driver first to get a license? Or, do we need a car before we can have a driver? Description does not give us order and timing, so it does not allow us to predict.

CORE CONCEPT 4.1

Results that allow us to predict include information about the order and timing of events or factors.

Only results that allow us to infer provide information that is useful to predict future responses or situations if the same set of circumstances applies. Results that allow us to predict include information about the order of events or factors and the timing of those events or factors. Therefore, results that are intended to allow inference may be used in clinical practice to predict future health-related outcomes under similar circumstances. The article about caregiver experiences found by the RN in the clinical case for this chapter uses inferential statistics in the results section. These results show that couples who had a good marital relationship (higher mutuality scores) and felt prepared for providing spousal care had higher life satisfaction. These results could be used by the RN in the clinical setting to predict that because N.B. and his wife have a good relationship as well as his interest in learning about his new role as caregiver, and that they are both receiving follow-up care, he is likely to experience a higher life satisfaction score.

Not all inferential statistics lead to an understanding of causation, but all are used to infer that what was found in the specific results is also likely to be found in similar cases. Understanding some of the language that is used in the description of results and in inferential statistics is the first step in understanding what results mean for evidence-based nursing practice (EBNP). The article in Appendix B uses quantitative methods, which we will use in this chapter to gain a better understanding of the language in the results sections of research reports that reflect descriptive data analysis. We will look at the language of inferential statistics in Chapter 5 and will continue to use the fictional article and the article found by the RN as examples in both chapters.

CORE CONCEPT 4.2

Research results that only describe or explain cannot be used to predict future outcomes or to directly identify the cause of the findings.

■ UNDERSTANDING THE LANGUAGE OF RESULTS SECTIONS

To discuss the language in the results section of research reports, we must take a closer look at data and data analysis. As mentioned in Chapter 2, data are the information collected in a study. This information may take several forms—it may be numbers, words, or drawings, and it may be written, spoken, or observed. Once the information is collected, it has to be sorted and organized to be meaningful in answering the questions addressed in the research.

Most research reports' results sections begin by providing a summary of information about individual study variables. A variable is something that varies: It is not the same for everyone in every situation. Therefore, a variable is an aspect of the phenomenon of interest or research problem that differs among people or situations. Research aims to understand, explain, or predict those differences or variations. A variable may be some attribute of a person, such as age, health, or beliefs. It may be a test score, such as a score for anxiety level, or a physiologic parameter, such as body temperature. It may be an environmental aspect, such as community resources, family support, or employment rates. In all of these examples of variables, we know that there will be differences among people or situations.

Research attempts to gain new knowledge about variables that have been identified as important. In the research articles for Chapters 1 and 2, the major variables studied included hunger, satiety, sleep hours, self-esteem, stress, coping, social support, eating behaviors, depressive mood, and demographic and environment. Think about these for a moment. We can say that these are variables because we expect different people to have different levels of self-esteem and eating behaviors.

The goal of the depressive mood, self-esteem, coping, and eating study was to understand and describe relationships among self-esteem, stress, social support, and coping and how they affected eating and mood in teenagers. In contrast, the purpose of the sleep and hunger in adolescents study was to investigate relationships among sleep, hunger, food cravings, satiety, and caloric intake. The researchers hoped to find key factors or connections that could guide them in the provision of care. The variables for the study found by the RN in the clinical case for this chapter are identified in Table 4.2.

In Chapter 2, we said that multivariate analysis indicates there are more than two variables being discussed, and, in fact, most studies will probably include more than one variable. However, analysis of data at a given point that focuses on only one variable is called univariate analysis. When you worked with the data from your in-class study, you were doing univariate analysis—that is, you were organizing data about individual variables.

Another word that you will often see in results sections is *bivariate*. Bivariate analysis refers to analysis with only two variables. Notice that the words themselves reveal their meanings: *uni* means "one," and *variate* means "to vary," so univariate is analysis of one variable; bivariate is analysis of two variables; and multivariate is analysis of more than two variables.

Table 4.2

Identification of Specific Variables in the Life Satisfaction in Stroke Survivors and Spousal Caregivers Study

DEPENDENT VARIABLES	INDEPENDENT VARIABLES
Life satisfaction—stroke survivors	Time
Life satisfaction—spousal caregivers	Age
Life satisfaction—changes over time	Level of depression
	Mutuality score
	Stroke impact
	Health status
	Perceived stress
	Preparedness level

Both qualitative and quantitative studies have variables, but information about the variables for studies using these two approaches differs in how data are collected and how they are organized and reported in the results section of a report. The purpose of qualitative studies is to increase our understanding about some aspects of experiences. The results of those studies describe what was found, usually by organizing the data into concepts or themes and then by providing examples of the specific language used by participants to support and clarify the meaning of those concepts. The results describe findings about single variables, usually without using many numbers. Because quantitative studies use numbers to represent variables of interest and then often apply statistical tests to allow inference, we expect to see mostly numbers in the results section of a quantitative report.

CORE CONCEPT 4.3

Both qualitative and quantitative studies have variables, but information about variables for studies using these two approaches differs in how data are collected and how they are organized and reported in the results section of a report.

Language Describing Results From Qualitative Studies

In the Out-of-Class exercise in Chapter 3, you were asked to organize some numerical data so that it would be more informative. If the data had been words instead of numbers, the task of how to create some kind of order would not have been immediately obvious. For example, if you were given written paragraphs from a number of students and were asked to organize this data, you might break down the paragraphs into units that you could organize, such as individual sentences or groups of sentences that address the same idea. You could then organize the sentences according to shared ideas and determine how many different ideas occurred and how much agreement there was about the ideas. The goal of data analysis in a qualitative study is the same as that in a quantitative study: to organize the data and create some kind of an order so that meaning can be found.

Box 4.1 lists excerpts of data that might have been collected in response to "What experiences in your life have led to your anticipated choice for field of nursing practice?" the question identified in the fictional article as the measure used to collect subjective responses to help understand why students chose their fields of practice. Take a moment and read through those responses. Reading data in this form is even less helpful than reading a long list of individuals' ages. For the qualitative researcher, the organizing, ordering, and synthesizing of the data collected represent the heart of the research method. In fact, in most qualitative studies, data are analyzed throughout the process of implementing the study, and the results of this analysis are then used to guide additional data collection. This is in contrast to quantitative studies, in which the researcher usually does not analyze the data until all have been collected because changing the way data are collected, or changing which data are collected, undermines the results of the study.

Another difference between data analysis in qualitative studies and quantitative studies is that no absolute formulas are consistently applied to the data. Qualitative data analysis requires understanding, digesting, synthesizing, conceptualizing, and reconceptualizing descriptions of feelings, behaviors, experiences, and ideas. *Content analysis* is often the term used to describe this process of data analysis. Content analysis is the process of understanding, interpreting, and conceptualizing the meanings in qualitative data. To do this, the researcher starts by breaking down the data into units that are meaningful and then develops a categorization scheme. A categorization scheme is an orderly combination of categories

---

Box 4.1

Examples of Qualitative Data Collected in Response to the Question, "What Experiences in Your Life Have Led to Your Anticipated Choice for Field of Nursing Practice?"

"I have always loved movies where the nurses save the lives of people during a disaster. I guess, well, it seems like the best place to do that, you know, is, well, the emergency room."

"Nursing is all about caring for people. I mean, I don't know how I would have gotten through my son's illness without the nurses."

"The one thing I remember when I had my tonsils out was the nurse giving me ice cream. It made me feel safe."

"I come from a family of nurses who have all worked in hospitals, mostly the surgical or medical ICU."

"It was the nurse holding my hand when the doctor in the emergency room told me about my brother that made it possible for me to keep going."

"My roommate in college was a nursing student, and she always helped any of us who came to her, whether it was if we were sick or just feeling down."

"Every time I have had to go to the hospital with one of the kids, it was the nurses who really listened to me and made a difference."

"My aunt was a nurse. She always was so strong and sure of herself—I wanted to be just like her."

"The shows I've seen about the flying nurses—that is just such an exciting thing to do, I guess I figured I would never get bored."

"My best friend in high school was in a car accident and I was so scared to go see her. But the nurse, he just really helped me relax and not freak out seeing all the machines and things."

"There was no one like my Grandma Jane—she was the most caring person I ever knew; she nursed about everyone in the family until it was her turn to get sick and die."

---

carefully defined so that no overlap occurs. In qualitative analysis, the categorization scheme is developed based on the ideas found in the data; then pieces of data—units that reflect distinct ideas—are put into the categories. This process of breaking down and labeling large amounts of data to identify the category to which they belong is called coding or data reduction. When this coding or data reduction occurs, the researcher is also refining the categorization scheme and using the categories to guide further data collection.

One might say that there is a spiraling nature to the process of data analysis in qualitative studies, as illustrated in Figure 4.1. The process is not circular because it does not simply return to where it began but rather evolves to eventually identify key themes or concepts that reflect the meaning of the data. *Theme* is another term that is often found in the results section of a qualitative report. A theme is an idea or a concept that is implicit in and recurrent throughout the data. Themes are not the concrete, explicit words contained in the data; rather, they are the underlying ideas behind the words. Qualitative data analysis seeks to categorize and understand the data and the relationships among the categories to eventually conceptualize the data into themes. The spiral of qualitative data analysis occurs, in part, because as categories are developed through analysis, they are used to collect additional data, which is then coded and categorized. Eventually, data saturation occurs. Data saturation in qualitative research is the point at which all new information collected is redundant of

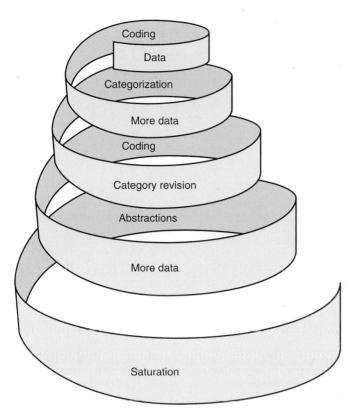

FIGURE 4.1   Spiraling process of qualitative data analysis.

information already collected. Data saturation occurs at a time when all new information fits into the newly established coding system so that the new information is saying the same thing as the data already collected. Therefore, no new information is being generated through continued data collection.

Look again at the data in Box 4.1, which have already been broken down into units, mostly sentences—and in a few cases, more than one sentence—that combine to express one idea. Content analysis to develop a categorization scheme might start by using a category for "Caring Experiences" and another for "Television and Movies." As the researcher examines the data and codes them into these two categories, you see that only two of the units fit under the "Television and Movies" category, whereas all the rest belong to "Caring Experiences." The researcher might then notice that, in some cases, the data under "Caring Experiences" suggest a desire to follow in someone's footsteps. This idea can be refined to a category called "Experiences With Nursing Role Models." Once the data that reflect role models are moved into the new category, further analysis of the data that remain suggests that not only caring experiences but also personal caring experiences are being described. Thus, three themes can be derived from the data.

Figure 4.2 shows this process of content analysis in schematic form. This is a simplified example of how a qualitative researcher might analyze data to identify themes. Notice that the final three themes identified are never explicitly addressed in the actual data. That is, no piece of data says that it was the nurse role model that led to the choice of field of nursing. The themes identified are implicit; that is, the ideas are repeated differently by different people.

The themes or categories derived from qualitative data analysis are usually reported in the results sections of qualitative research reports. The author of this type of report cannot provide averages or other statistics to describe the data. Rather, the themes or categories are described, often using specific examples from actual data to help make the implicit ideas within the themes clearer.

FIGURE 4.2
Schematic.

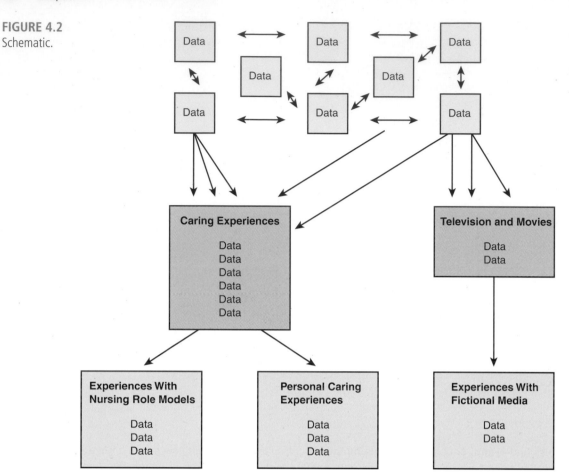

Language Describing Results From Quantitative Studies

We have said that qualitative research examines at least one variable. Quantitative research differs from qualitative research in that there are two types of variables: dependent and independent (or predictor). Because the purpose of quantitative research is to explain or predict a particular variable, we call that variable the dependent variable, which is determined by, or depends on, other variables in the study. It is the outcome variable of interest. In the fictional article about nursing students' preferences for practice, the outcome that the research is trying to explain or predict is choice of field of nursing practice, so it is the dependent variable.

Independent variables are those variables in a study that are used to explain or predict the outcome of interest, that is, the dependent variable. In the fictional article, the independent variables included age, perceived well-being, race, and marital status. These were factors that differed among students and that may explain or predict their choice of field, the dependent variable. Independent variables also are called predictor variables because they are used to predict the dependent variable.

Notice that Table 4.2 classifies the variables from the predictors of life satisfaction study as dependent or independent. This study is quantitative and attempts to explain the caregivers' satisfaction with life while considering characteristics of both the stroke survivor and the caregiver. In some studies, you may notice that the variables may be identified as both a dependent variable and an independent variable. This is an example of a research term being "gray" rather than clearly "black and white." For example, if the authors first looked at how mutuality for the caregivers differed from what has been found to be normal for a general population and examined how characteristics of the stroke survivor and the caregiver impact mutuality. If both these analyses looked at mutuality as a dependent variable with the authors examining what mutuality is dependent on. The authors would then look at how caregivers' mutuality impacted overall life satisfaction. In these analyses, they examined mutuality as a factor that may affect life satisfaction. Thus, life satisfaction was the variable that depended on mutuality, and that would have made mutuality an independent variable in those analyses. We discuss types of variables in quantitative research in more detail in Chapter 5.

In preparation for this chapter, you were asked to organize data from your in-class questionnaire to make it easy to understand. What did you do to make the information more understandable? Probably, your first thought was to create some kind of order in the data. The data that you were given consisted of numbers. A logical way to create order is to list the numbers from smallest to largest (or vice versa). Doing so gives a sense of how alike or different people are in the values of the numbers, such as in age or marital status, by showing how many numbers are repeated or are close together and what the smallest and largest numbers are. The next thing you may have done was to determine the most common responses. This could be done by simply counting how many times each response was given, by calculating the percentage for each response out of the total responses, or by calculating an average of all the numbers.

Another approach to making sense out of a group of numbers includes using graphs, bar charts, or pie charts. This approach provides a visual representation of the data, which allows us to see the difference between the smallest and largest numbers as well as the most common responses. Figure 4.3 is an example of a histogram (a type of bar chart) that could have been included in the fictional article on students' choices for clinical practice.

Hopefully, you found that organizing the data helped you to increase your understanding of what that information meant. Regardless of the approach taken, the product

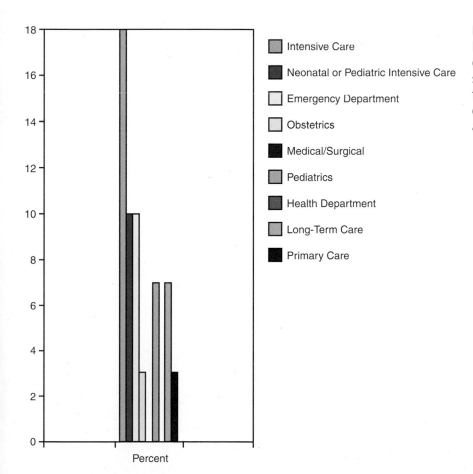

FIGURE 4.3

Histogram for the frequency distribution of students' choices of field of practice based on results in fictional article.

probably helped you to see two things: (1) how much diversity or difference occurred in the data and (2) the most common responses.

Variance, Standard Deviation, and Distribution

In the language of statistics, the diversity in data for a single variable is referred to as the variance, which reflects how the values for a variable are dispersed. The most common or frequent responses in a set of data are statistically described as the measures of central tendency. Each is discussed individually.

Variance is a statistic—a number—that can be used to show how much difference or variety exists in a group of numbers. Table 4.3 lists the ages of nursing students from three different classrooms. With short lists like this, you can look at the numbers and determine that there is more variety in the ages of students in classroom 2 than in classroom 1 or 3. But how do you objectively measure the variety or describe that variety in a way that can be consistently understood and interpreted by anyone? Obviously, just saying that classroom 2 has more variety in age than does classroom 1 or 3 is nonspecific—how much is "more?" You could also say that the ages range from 19 to 21 in classroom 1, compared with ages ranging from 18 to 24 in classroom 2. This is certainly more specific and gives us a better sense of the differences, but the ages of students in classroom 3 also range from 18 to 24 years, yet there is more variety in ages in classroom 2 than in classroom 3. Therefore, there must be some way to represent the values in between the two numbers that give us the age range.

The variety in a group of numbers is explained statistically by computing a number appropriately called the variance, which is the sum of the squared differences between each value in the set of numbers and the mean (average) of those numbers, divided by how many numbers there were in the set minus 1. That can be understood by using the age of students in classroom 1 as an example. The variance is computed by subtracting the average of all 10 students' ages (20) from each student's age and squaring the difference, then adding those squared differences and dividing by 9. We square the differences between the mean to avoid negative and positive differences canceling each other. Therefore, the variance statistic is an average of the squared deviations from the mean. This is a mathematical definition, so you may still be wondering what it is you know when you see a value for a variance.

Table 4.3

Ages of Students in Three Different Classrooms With Variation and Central Tendency

CLASSROOM 1*	CLASSROOM 2*	CLASSROOM 3*
20	20	18
21	24	20
20	19	20
20	21	24
19	18	20
21	23	20
20	18	20
20	19	18
19	18	20
20	20	20
$SD = 0.67$	$SD = 2.11$	$SD = 1.63$
$M = 20$	$M = 20$	$M = 20$
Mode = 20	Mode = 18	Mode = 20
Median = 20	Median = 19.5	Median = 20

*Age in years.
SD, standard deviation; M, mean.

Whether or not you understand the formula for computing the variance, you can understand that variance tells you how much variety there is within a set of numbers. For example, the variance for the ages in classroom 1 is 0.44 ($s^2 = 0.44$), the variance for the ages in classroom 2 is 4.44 ($s^2 = 4.44$), and the variance in classroom 3 is 2.66 ($s^2 = 2.66$). These statistics reveal that there is more variety in age in classroom 3 than in classroom 1, but less variety in classroom 3 than in classroom 2. Although you can see the variety in the ages by looking at the short list of numbers in Table 4.3, if the list contained 100 numbers or 1000 numbers, it would be much more difficult to get the variety without computing the variance. The variance gives us a specific statistic that represents differences or variety when reporting results for a single variable.

Thus far, we have discussed the variance for a single variable; however, more often the results section of a research report will use a statistic called the standard deviation instead of the variance. The standard deviation is simply the square root of the variance, so it also reflects variety among all the numbers. Remember that to compute the variance, we squared differences in values from the mean. This computational process results in the values for the variance being squared units of measurement, such as 4.44 squared years for the variance in classroom 2. The idea of "squared years," however, does not make much sense. If we take the square root of that variance, we get a standard deviation of 2.11 years (not squared years). The standard deviation is, in a sense, the average difference in ages from the overall average age. You can see by looking at the values for the ages in classroom 2 that it makes sense that the variety in ages can be accurately communicated by saying that there is an average of 2 years' difference from the overall average. This makes more sense than 4.44 squared years. In contrast, the standard deviation for the ages of students in classroom 1 is 0.67 years (or less than 1 year), and the standard deviation of the ages of the students in classroom 3 is 1.63 years. Standard deviation is usually abbreviated in research reports as SD, so a research report giving the standard deviation for classroom 3 would write "$SD = 1.63$." Although classrooms 2 and 3 both have a youngest and oldest student of 18 and 24 years, respectively, the average deviation from the overall average age is clearly greater in classroom 2.

Why do we care about variance and standard deviation? To understand the meaning of results for clinical practice, we must understand how much variety there is in the results. For example, if you were reading a research study that examined the effectiveness of an intervention to relieve pain, and the report tells you that the average rating of pain on a 10-point scale after the intervention was 2, that sounds good. Suppose that two different interventions each led to an average rating of 2, but the first had a standard deviation of 3.5, whereas the second had a standard deviation of 0.7. Although the first intervention led to the same average as the second intervention, the standard deviation tells us there was a great deal more variety in pain ratings with the first intervention. This means that some of the people who received the first intervention had higher scores or more pain as well as possibly lower scores or less pain. Although lower scores may be better, our goal in nursing is to consistently improve pain, and higher scores in some of our patients definitely are not desirable. The second intervention led to much less variety in ratings of pain, which means that most of the subjects scored their pain close to a rating of 2 after the intervention. As a clinician who understands standard deviations, you might decide that the second intervention is more consistent in relieving pain because it has a smaller standard deviation and choose to use that intervention rather than the first one.

A pain intervention study is an example in which we may not want variety because our clinical goal is to consistently decrease our patients' pain levels. In other cases, however, we may want variety to make the information useful clinically. For example, in the predictors of life satisfaction article, the authors reported that the mean age of the caregivers in their sample was 63, with a standard deviation of 10.6 ($SD = 10.6$) (Ostwald et al., 2009). This means that the average deviation around the age of 63 was 10.6 years, telling us that the individuals in the sample had a wide range of ages. Although N.B. is within this age range, the RN in the home health agency works with patients who are mostly over the age of 60, so the nurse must decide if the large range of ages of caregivers in this study will affect the usefulness of this study for EBNP.

Distribution is another term that is used in results sections to indicate the variety or differences found. In research, distribution refers to how the findings are dispersed. The variance and standard deviation for a set of numbers give us a clear sense of the spread of those numbers. However, it is not appropriate to compute the statistics of variance and standard deviation for variables that fit into discrete categories, such as type of job preference, rather than variables that are real numbers, such as age. For simplicity, often a researcher will assign numeric values to categories, such as 1 = professional employment, 2 = blue-collar employment. However, the actual numbers "1" and "2" are not a true measure of type of employment, and adding or subtracting the numbers will not tell us the "average" type of employment.

In cases where the variable is a category, we may find distribution described by using a table of percentages, histogram, or pie chart. For example, Table B.1 in Appendix B (the fictional article) shows us the frequency distribution of choices of field of nursing. A frequency distribution is the spread for how frequently each category occurs or is selected. We see from the table that 60% of students choose intensive care as their preferred field after graduation, and another 10% choose neonatal intensive care and emergency department fields. Figure 4.3 shows the same frequency distribution in a histogram format. Figure 4.4 shows what the frequency distribution would look like in histogram format if none of the students had selected the neonatal and emergency room fields and, instead, had selected the health department and long-term care fields. You can see that the distribution of choices would have looked different even with 60% still selecting intensive care. Just as the statistic for standard deviation can tell us about the distribution or variety in a numeric variable, a frequency table or histogram can tell us about distribution and variety in a categorical variable.

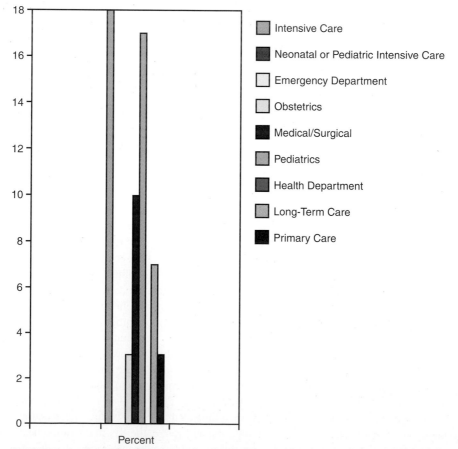

FIGURE 4.4   Example of histogram for distribution of field of study choices if health department and long-term care were endorsed more frequently.

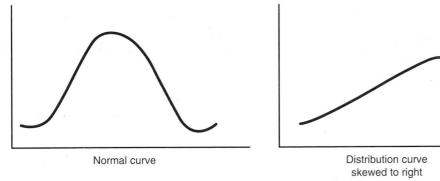

Normal curve   Distribution curve
                                  skewed to right

FIGURE 4.5   Examples of a normal curve and a curve that skews to the right.

An important statistical concept that you may remember from your statistics courses is the normal curve. A normal curve is a type of distribution that is symmetric and bell shaped. Figure 4.5 shows two graphs with distribution curves; the one on the left is the familiar normal curve. Many of the variables in life that we are interested in understanding or using in research are distributed similarly to the normal curve. For example, height can range from small, in the case of a neonate, to tall, in the case of a few extraordinary individuals, but most people fall somewhere in the middle, with a relatively even balance on each side of the average height. The normal curve is a theoretical distribution. That means that if we could measure a variable, such as height, for every human on earth and plot all the heights, the result would be this perfectly symmetric bell-shaped curve. One thing that makes the normal curve unique is its symmetry; the normal curve can be folded in half at the center, which is the average, and the two sides will match. On the right side of Figure 4.5 is an example of a distribution that has a curved shape but is asymmetric. Much of inferential statistics is based on the assumption that the distribution of a variable would be normal or bell shaped if all the possible values for the variable were known. This assumption is based on experience with many variables of interest that are normally distributed. Therefore, when reading results, you will find references to a distribution of a variable being "approximately normal."

In summary, one of the important aspects of data that we expect to see described and summarized in the results section of reports is the diversity or variety in the data. This may be described by a univariate statistic called the *standard deviation* (or possibly the *variance*) or a frequency distribution, histogram, or pie chart. In any case, the variety for each study variable is important for us to understand because it affects the clinical decisions we can make based on the study.

Central Tendency

In addition to wanting to know about the diversity in a set of numbers for a variable, we almost always want to know the most common or average response or value for a variable. In quantitative research, a measure of central tendency shows common or typical numbers. Central tendency measures reflect the center of a distribution or the center of the spread. Three univariate statistics, called the mean, the mode, and the median, are the most commonly used measures of central tendency. Table 4.3 shows that the mean value for the ages of the students in each classroom is 20 years. The mean is simply the average of all the values for a variable—that is, the sum of all the values divided by the number of values summed and may be reported as $\bar{x}$.

The mode is the value that occurs most frequently: In classrooms 1 and 3, the mode is 20 years, but in classroom 2, the mode is 18. Although the mean of the ages in the three classrooms is the same, suggesting that the center of the distributions is the same, the center of the distribution of ages in the three classrooms differs when one looks at the mode.

The median is the value that falls in the middle of the distribution when the numbers are in numeric order. Although 20 years is the median age in classrooms 1 and 3, the median age for classroom 2 is 19.5 years (the average of 19 + 20, the two most central values for age in that classroom). Although the mean, mode, and median are all measures of central tendency, comparing the three for a single variable also tells us something about the distribution. Looking at the mean (20 years), mode (18 years), and median (19.5 years) for students' ages in classroom 2, we see that although the average age was 20, more students were younger than age 20 than were older than age 20. The age distribution "leans" toward the younger ages. This leaning is described as skew when reporting research results. We have said that the mean, mode, and median are measures of "central" tendency, but if there is a skew in the distribution, these measures will have different values. This tells us that the middle of the distribution is not in the exact center of that distribution; it is off to the left or right of center. The second curve of Figure 4.5 has a skew to the right, which means that the middle of the distribution falls more to the higher range of the possible values. A normal curve does not have a skew. In fact, part of what defines a normal curve is that the mean, median, and mode are all equal.

Now, look at Figure 4.6, which shows curves drawn around the distribution of ages for the three classrooms we have been using as an example. Notice that the curve for classroom 1 is perfectly bell shaped and symmetric and that the mean, mode, and median are equal. The curve for classroom 2 is skewed to the left, is not symmetric, and the mean, mode, and median are not equal. The curve for classroom 3 looks similar to that for classroom 1, but it is narrower and not symmetric.

Again, why do we care about measures of central tendency? We care because a long list of numbers for a variable, such as a long list of ages or pain ratings, is difficult to make

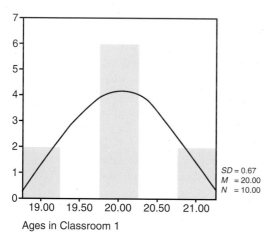

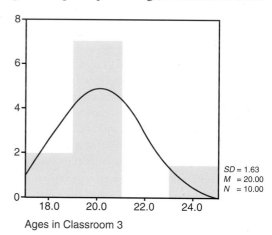

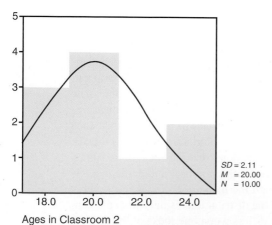

FIGURE 4.6 Frequency distribution histogram and curves for ages of students in three classrooms. *SD*, standard deviation; *M*, mean; *N*, number in sample.

much sense of without some type of organization. A summary of those numbers that tells us the central tendency and distribution also allows us to quickly understand important aspects for the individual variable, such as the most common or frequent value and how much variety there is in the values. This, in turn, allows us to gain more understanding of how the results may or may not apply to real clinical practice.

The data from the in-class study exercise provide an excellent example of how much more we can learn about a variable when the data are summarized to give us the distribution and the central tendency. A second example is shown in Table A4.4 (Ostwald et al., 2009) of Appendix A.4, the predictors of life satisfaction report found by the RN from our clinical case. (Had the authors simply given us a list of the scores of the 131 male and female caregivers, it would have been both tedious and frustrating to try to get a sense of their socioeconomic status [SES].) However, when the author tells us that the range of scores on the Hollingshead scale is from 13 to 66 and that the mean and standard deviation for SES of caregivers is 43.5 and 12.0, respectively, we have information that immediately tells us the SES of caregivers in the study. A common way to report the mean and standard deviation results is to provide the mean with the standard deviation inside parentheses: 13 to 66 (12.0) (Ostwald et al., 2009).

CORE CONCEPT 4.4

Measures of central tendency and distribution are univariate statistics that summarize information about a variable.

The description of the variables in a study is always an important part of the results section of research reports. Description of data aims to summarize it in a way that makes it understandable and meaningful. Description of only one variable is called *univariate analysis*, and in quantitative research, that description almost always includes information that tells us about the distribution and central tendency for the variables. In reports of qualitative research, the entire results section is descriptive, taking units of data (words, pictures, and sentences) and developing categories and themes to describe that data.

■ CONNECTING RESULTS THAT DESCRIBE TO CONCLUSIONS

The RN in our clinical case has read the results and discussion sections of the research report about stroke survivors and caregivers' life satisfaction. Some demographic data—descriptive information about the characteristics of the people studied—were provided in the results section of the report; additional data were presented in the methods section as well. The second paragraph of the results started with a description of the life satisfaction scores in this study at 12 and 24 months. These results provide the RN with an understanding of any differences in life satisfaction for both the stroke survivor and caregiver that appear to be present over a 24-month period following the stroke survivors' discharge from the inpatient rehabilitation setting. So, if the RN read only the results and conclusions sections, the nurse would not know much about the subjects in this study. Both quantitative and qualitative studies almost always include demographic data, although the reports of qualitative studies may not use statistics to describe those characteristics. However, the article found by the RN does include both the mean and the standard deviation for participants' ages, along with percentages for other categorical variables, such as gender and race in Table A4.4 located in Appendix A.4 (Ostwald et al., 2009).

Checking the descriptive results in Table A4.1 of the article (Appendix A.4), we find the variables that have been shown to be associated with life satisfaction in other research studies, while Tables A4.2 and A4.3 (Appendix A.4) list only those variables that were found to have a significant impact on life satisfaction scores for stroke survivors and care-givers, respectively, for this study. Without reading the instrument and analysis sections of the report, we would not know how the variables/results were selected to be included in the tables. Tables A4.2 and A4.3 (Appendix A.4) titles may be confusing to the reader. Each table's title suggests two sets of data: one at 12 months and the other at 24 months. The specific results described are the basis for the new knowledge identified in the results and discussion sections. Without reading the results, we would not know the actual scores of how the stroke survivors and caregivers rated their life satisfaction. The reader is provided with tables and descriptions in which to understand the results of the study. These results then lead to inferences for clinical decision making and are reported in the implications section of the report. The conclusions section of the predictor of life satisfaction study notes differences in results between this study and previous studies leading the nurse to seek more evidence.

■ COMMON ERRORS IN THE REPORTS OF DESCRIPTIVE RESULTS

Two kinds of problems may be found when reading descriptive results in a research report: (1) incomplete information and (2) confusing information. We have emphasized the importance of understanding the distribution and central tendency in variables from quan-titative studies to make clinical decisions. One problem that sometimes arises when read-ing the results is that this descriptive information cannot be found. The authors may fail to provide any univariate statistics about some of the variables in the study, or they may fail to provide all the information needed.

For example, a report may include only a measure of central tendency for an impor-tant variable without giving a range of values or the standard deviation. This absence of information about the variation in the variable makes it difficult to know how to interpret the findings related to that variable and can even lead to incorrect conclusions. The previ-ous example of a study that examined two interventions to help pain whose results are a mean pain score of 2 for both interventions is a good example of this. Given the mean scores alone, one might conclude that the two interventions have exactly the same effect. This con-clusion would be incorrect, however, because the standard deviations for the mean pain scores in this example (0.7 and 3.5) are different.

Another example of a report with incomplete descriptive results is the fictional article. One of the variables that the author later indicates was important relative to the students' choices of field of practice was their health rating, but the only univariate information provided about the variable is that 20% of the subjects rated their health as fair or poor. We learn neither how the percentages broke down for ratings of "excellent health" or "good health" nor whether most of the 20% of subjects who rated their health at the lower end chose "fair" or "poor." This lack of information affects our ability to interpret the results that are reported later.

Aside from incomplete results, a second problem that may be found in the results section is a confusing presentation of the results. Descriptive results are often reported in tables, and sometimes those tables are not labeled or organized clearly. A table may use titles or identify variables that are inconsistent with the wording used in the text of the report. In fact, sometimes the text of a report fails to refer to the table at all. Another problem is that too much informa-tion may be put into the text, rather than used in a table. For example, the information provided in Table B.1 in Appendix B (the fictional article) would have been confusing and difficult to understand if the author had instead written a paragraph reporting those results as follows:

> Students chose several fields immediately after graduation, with 18 (60%) choosing inten-sive care, 3 (10%) choosing neonatal or pediatric intensive care, and 3 (10%) choosing emergency departments. One student (3%) chose obstetrics for field of study immedi-ately after graduation, and no students chose either medical/surgical or health department. Two students (7%) chose pediatrics, two students (7%) chose long-term care or nursing home care, and one student (3%) chose primary care.

Although this information could be sorted out by the reader, it is presented much more clearly in the table. A similar problem may occur in a qualitative report if the author does not give us clear descriptions of the categories or themes developed from the study. Look at the fictional article again and at the three themes identified that represented the meaning of experiences students identified as affecting their choice of practice. If the author had simply listed the themes as "personal life experience," "experiences with nursing role models," and "experiences with fictional media," it would be difficult to know how these types of experiences differ. The definitions and examples given in Table B.2 of Appendix B make it clear what those themes mean.

■ CRITICALLY READING RESULTS SECTIONS OF RESEARCH REPORTS FOR USE IN EVIDENCE-BASED NURSING PRACTICE

It should be clear from the examples just given that critically reading the descriptive results section of a research report is important. Box 4.2 presents a set of six questions that can be used when critically reading results sections. The first question, "Did the report include a clearly identified results section?" may seem simplistic, but some reports do not present results in a specific section. The answer to the second question, "Were the results presented appropriately for the information collected?" refers to whether or not descriptions included information about distribution, central tendency, and variation that were appropriate for the study's variables. For example, was information about categories such as marital status presented as percentages, and were both the mean and the standard deviation included in information about variables such as age or scores on a measure? The third question is, "Were descriptive versus inferential results identifiable if this is a quantitative study?" When we consider the results in the predictors of life satisfaction article, we find that it combines descriptive and inferential results in both the written and tabular presentation of results in a way that could be confusing to readers.

If the study that you are reading used a qualitative method, a question to ask yourself in order to critically read the results section is, "Were themes or structure and meaning identifiable if this is a qualitative study?" Not all reports of qualitative studies will be as clear. This leads us to the next question, "Were the results presented in a clear and logical manner?" For example, the predictors of life satisfaction report organizes the results by using headings that represent the specific objectives established for the study. This is a logical and clear approach to present results. The last question to ask yourself as you read the results section of a report is, "Did the results include enough information about the final sample for the study?" We have already discussed the importance of including demographic information in the report of results of a study, whether it is qualitative or quantitative. We also have identified that the authors of the predictors of life satisfaction study did include demographic information but most of it was covered in the methods section. We will revisit four of the

---

Box 4.2

How to Critically Read the Results Section of a Research Report?

Do the results answer the question, "Why did the authors reach these conclusions—what did they actually find?"

1. Did the report include a clearly identified results section?
2. Were the results presented appropriately for the information collected?
3. Were descriptive versus inferential results identifiable if this is a quantitative study?
4. Were themes or structure and meaning identifiable if this is a qualitative study?
5. Were the results presented in a clear and logical manner?
6. Did the results include enough information about the final sample for the study?

six questions for critically reading results sections of research reports at the end of Chapter 5, after we finish learning a bit about inferential statistics.

■ PUBLISHED REPORT—WHAT WOULD YOU CONCLUDE?

Understanding what to expect in the reports of descriptive results makes it possible for you to know whether the research is something that might apply to your clinical practice. The RN in our clinical case began the search with an interest in gaining a better understanding of what factors influence life satisfaction for both the stroke survivor and caregiver. After reading the results and conclusions sections of the predictors of life satisfaction article, the RN has an increased understanding of how measures of life satisfaction may or may not change over time. We will continue to look at the language of results sections of research reports in the next chapter, which will add to the RN's knowledge when planning care for N.B. and his wife.

OUT-OF-CLASS EXERCISE

Making Inferences About Well-Being and Marriage

Before proceeding to Chapter 5, look at the data collected from your in-class practice study, focusing on two variables: rating of well-being and marital status. Complete a univariate analysis of data for each of these variables to summarize distribution and central tendency. To do so, you will need to decide what is appropriate in terms of measure of central tendency (mean, median, or mode) and how to summarize distribution (range, standard deviation, and percent). Then, determine what the data tell you in terms of answering the question, "Do married students have higher levels of well-being than unmarried students?" Based on the data obtained, answer the question and explain how you arrived at your answer. If you are not using an in-class study, a practice set of data about well-being and marital status is provided in Appendix D, which can be used for this exercise. Remember, this is an exercise to motivate you to think more about how results are presented in a research report and what they mean. You will then be ready to begin the next chapter.

References

Ostwald, S., Godwin, K., & Cron, S. (2009). Predictors of life satisfaction in stroke survivors and spousal caregivers after inpatient rehabilitation. *Rehabilitation Nursing, 34*, 160–174.

Resources

Locke, L. F., Silverman, S. J., & Spirduso, W. W. (2009). *Reading and understanding research* (3rd ed.). Thousand Oaks, CA: Sage Publications.

Polit, D. F., & Beck, C. T. (2007). *Nursing research: Principles and methods* (8th ed.). Philadelphia, PA: Lippincott Williams & Wilkins.

Salkind, N. J. (2007). *Statistics for people who (think they) hate statistics* (3rd ed.). Thousand Oaks, CA: Sage Publications.

5

Inferential Results

Why Did the Authors Reach Their Conclusion—What Did They Actually Find?

LEARNING OBJECTIVE

The student will interpret inferential statistical results in relationship to their meaning for the conclusions of the study.

KEY TERMS

Analysis of variance

Beta (β) value

Confidence intervals

Correlation

Covary

Factor analysis

Nonparametric statistics

Null hypothesis

Parametric statistics

Probability

Regression

Research hypothesis

t test

Clinical Case • The RN works in a home health agency and has recently started working with N.B.'s wife, who suffered a major stroke 6 months ago. The RN has also taken care of a number of other families where one member of the family has a major role as caregiver. The nurse has noticed that N.B. appears to be experiencing fatigue, lack of interest in life, and weight loss, which the nurse suspects is secondary to his responsibilities of caring for his wife. The RN has found an article that seems relevant in supporting spousal caregivers of the stroke survivors and has read it. The article used a quantitative method to examine predictors of life satisfaction for spousal caregivers of stroke survivors and stroke survivors (Ostwald, Godwin, & Cron, 2009). This article used several statistical terms, such as mean, standard deviation, and significance, in the results section, which the RN must interpret to decide what the results mean for N.B. and his wife and consider whether the evidence in the study can be used to guide nursing practice in this situation. Since the article used in this chapter is the same as that used in Chapter 4, the box describing keywords and the clinical question will not be repeated in this chapter.

■ THE PURPOSE OF INFERENTIAL STATISTICS

Chapter 4 discussed the meaning of the language used in research reports when descriptive results—those that describe or explain a variable or variables—are presented. This chapter continues the discussion of how to understand the results sections of research reports but focuses on inferential results—those intended to explain or predict a variable or variables. Note that the word *explain* is included in both of these definitions. This is because there is an overlap between simple description—a description that explains—and explanation that can be used for prediction. We are looking at a continuum of statistics that build from simple knowing, to understanding and explaining, and finally to predicting, as shown in Figure 5.1.

Let us look at a simple example using the results about the ages, gender, and degree status of students in a nursing class shown in Table 5.1. The mean ($M = 27$) and standard deviation ($SD = 6$) for the age of the students is an example of simple description. Remember, the mean can also be represented as $\bar{x}$. Note in Figure 5.1 that the mean is followed by the standard deviation in parentheses. This is often the form used to report the mean and standard deviation in the results of a research report. This example of descriptive univariate statistics tells us that the students are relatively old and that there is a fair amount of variation in

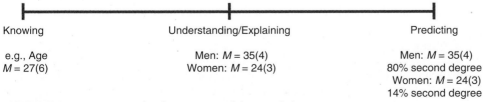

Knowing	Understanding/Explaining	Predicting
e.g., Age $M = 27(6)$	Men: $M = 35(4)$ Women: $M = 24(3)$	Men: $M = 35(4)$ 80% second degree Women: $M = 24(3)$ 14% second degree

FIGURE 5.1   A continuum for the purposes of data analysis.

Table 5.1

Fictional Data for Ages, Gender, and Degree Status of a Nursing Student Class

SUBJECT NUMBER	AGE (IN YEARS)	GENDER	DEGREE STATUS
1	20	F	1st
2	23	F	1st
3	33	M	1st
4	21	F	1st
5	25	F	1st.
6	40	M	2nd
7	32	F	2nd
8	20	F	1st
9	26	F	1st
10	25	F	1st
11	37	M	2nd
12	26	F	1st
13	23	F	1st
14	22	F	1st
15	24	F	2nd
16	30	M	2nd
17	35	M	2nd
18	21	F	1st
19	25	F	1st

the ages, but we have no idea why the variation exists. To have some explanation of the variation, descriptive statistics might be used to give us information about the age of the men versus the age of the women in the class. In the example, the mean age for the male students is 35 (SD = 4), whereas the mean age of the female students is 24 (SD = 3). We now have a partial explanation of the variation in ages: There are both men and women in the class, and the men in the class are older than the women. The variation in age is explained to some extent, but we do not assume that we can use students' gender distribution to predict the age of students. However, if we discover that 80% of the male students are second-degree students, whereas only 14% of the females are second-degree students, this additional information can potentially be used for prediction. We can speculate that men may be more likely to pursue nursing as a second career and that the more second-degree students there are in a class, the older the students will be. To test whether we can use the number of second-degree students to predict the age of students in a classroom, we must use inferential statistics.

Why use inferential statistics instead of just descriptive statistics? Because at this point, we do not know whether the differences and relationships among variables found in this classroom occurred by chance alone. We know that there are differences in this particular classroom, but we cannot know whether, in general, second-degree students are more likely to be men and older. Descriptive statistical results allow us to know and explain variables that we are interested in understanding, but we have to go a step further to use that explanation to predict or infer how those variables may occur in the future. This can be done through the use of inferential statistics, which are based on the concepts of probability and statistical significance. Therefore, to understand results that use inferential statistics, we must understand these terms.

■ PROBABILITY AND SIGNIFICANCE

As the RN in our clinical case starts to read the section of the report titled "Predictors of Life Satisfaction in Stroke Survivors," the nurse encounters the language of inferential statistics in the statement within the second sentence of the section that states "A significant decrease in life satisfaction occurred between 12 and 24 months ($p = .04$)" (Ostwald et al., 2009, p. 163). In Chapter 2, we defined *significance* as a low likelihood that any relationship or difference found in a statistical test occurred by chance alone. Quantitative research often attempts to take what has been found in a specific situation, that is, one study, and infer that similar results would occur in other similar situations. The RN in the clinical case not only is interested in what happened in the study by Ostwald et al. but also wants to predict that the same thing will happen in the practice setting if the information from the study is used to guide nursing practice.

In inferential statistics, we test for relationships, associations, and differences among variables that are statistically significant. We do this by creating distributions of test statistics that reflect variables having no connection between them, are unrelated, or are not different. In Chapter 4, we said that a distribution refers to how the findings are dispersed. A distribution of test statistics shows how the statistics from hundreds of samples would look if plotted on a graft. Then, we compute a test statistic for the results in our particular study and compare what we found in our sample or specific situation to what would be predicted to be found if there were not a relationship or difference in the variables. By convention, researchers say that if the test statistic falls into the range where we would expect 95% of all statistics to fall, given that there is no relationship or connection, then it is a nonsignificant statistic. Stated in the opposite way, if a test statistic falls *out of the range* of values that we would expect to occur 95% of the time, if there were no relationship among the variables, then we say it is a statistically significant value.

To illustrate this idea, we will use the statistic reported in the fictional article from Appendix B about the difference in ages of nursing students who choose acute settings versus nonacute settings. The article states that there was a significant difference in age and gives a test statistic of "$t = 2.1, p < .05$." The "t" value is a test statistic for differences in means between two groups, which we will discuss later in this chapter. In this case, the statistic was computed for the differences in the average ages of students who did and did not select an acute care setting for field of practice. Now look at Figure 5.2, which shows a distribution that is a normal curve, in this case a t distribution. Notice that for the t distribution, zero is at the center, and the possible values for the t test become larger at either end. A t distribution shows how the t tests for hundreds of different samples of two variables *that did not differ from each other in the "real" world* would be distributed. Now, returning to age as a variable of interest, if in the real world the ages of two groups are *not* different, then most of the time we would not get a big difference for the ages in any particular sample, and the t-test statistic would be a small number. However, occasionally, by chance alone, we get a large difference in age between groups in a sample (perhaps because a 12-year-old genius is in a particular sample).

Using the example from the fictional article, if students in the real world who did and did not pick acute settings were approximately the same age, then most of the time, if we took a sample of ages of students, choosing the two types of settings and computed a t test, the value would be plotted on the distribution somewhere toward the middle, in the green

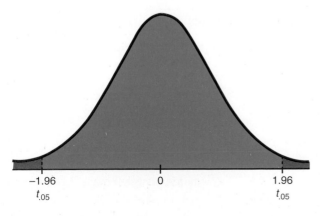

FIGURE 5.2 The t distribution for differences in two means in a sample when there is really no difference in the "real" world; green zone shows where 95% of values will fall, and two red zones show where 2.5% of the values will fall.

zone. In fact, the green zone marks where a t-test value will fall 95% of the time if the two variables tested are not different. The red zones at either end of the normal curve are the areas where the t values will fall by chance alone 2.5% of the time if, in the real world, the two variables tested are not different. When we say that a test statistic is significant, we are saying that we will achieve that statistic only a small percentage of the time if there is no difference or connection between the variables.

When the RN in the clinical case reads that the scores on the "Satisfaction with Life Scale (SWLS)" decreased significantly for stroke survivors from 12 to 24 months poststroke, the nurse knows that what was found in this study probably did not happen by chance. How much "probably" means, or what the probability is that whatever was found happened by chance is reported by a p value. The p value represents the probability and is defined as the percentage of the time the result found would have happened by chance alone. In the predictors of life satisfaction study, the authors indicate that the p value to the significant decrease in life satisfaction scores was .04, which translates to 4%. This means that the statistic computed for the difference in scores from the first to last interview would only happen 4 out of 100 times by chance alone. If the p value were .01, then the statistic would only occur by chance 1 out of 100 times (1%), and if the p value were .001, the statistic would only occur by chance 1 out of 1000 times (1/10 of 1%). Statistical significance, no matter what test has been used, means that the results are unlikely to have happened by chance alone. Therefore, we infer from the finding of statistical significance that the difference, association, or relationship that we tested statistically is one that exists in the real world because we were unlikely to get our statistic by chance alone. Remember that inferential statistics are only used in quantitative methods because only in quantitative studies do we assume that the absolute truth can be found.

Statistical significance is also sometimes described in the results sections of research reports in the form of confidence intervals. Confidence intervals (CIs) state the range of actual values for the statistic we are computing (such as the difference in the mean ages of nursing students who do and do not choose acute care settings), in which 95 out of 100 values would fall. A CI for the differences in ages between nursing students choosing the two types of settings might be 0.8 to 6.2, and a research report might state that the differences in the means of ages for the two groups was 4.2, with a 95% CI (0.8–6.2). This means that given the difference found in the study, 95 out of 100 times, the difference in ages between the two groups of students will fall between 0.8 and 6.2 years. Note that this range does not include zero, so there is a low likelihood that there is zero or no difference. For example, "95% CI" refers to a 95% CI. CIs are almost always stated for the 95% range, whereas the probability of getting the result reported if there really were no difference or relationship is usually reported as one of three possible percents: 5% ($p < .05$), 1% ($p < .01$), and 0.1% ($p < .001$). Table 5.2 summarizes the differences between p values and CIs.

Table 5.2

Comparison of p Values and Confidence Intervals

	p VALUE	CONFIDENCE INTERVAL
Assumption	The relationship or difference tested is zero	The relationship or difference is that found in the data
Meaning	Gives the percentage of the time that we would get the test statistic by chance alone	Gives the range of values (biggest and smallest numbers) that would occur 95% of the time for the relationship or difference found
Interpretation	The smaller the value, the less likely that the test result occurred by chance alone	The smaller the range, without zero in it, the more confident we can be that the test statistic reflects the "real" world

CORE CONCEPT 5.1

Inferential statistics are used to report whether the results found in the specific study are likely to have happened by chance alone. Statistical significance is not an absolute guarantee that the values are really different or related in the real world. Rather, statistical significance means that there is less than 5% chance that the amount of relationship or difference found happened by chance.

CORE CONCEPT 5.2

Whether the report includes *p* values or CIs, the authors are telling you how likely it is that the results from the study were due to chance and, therefore, how likely it is that these results can be used to infer that there would be similar results in similar future situations.

■ PARAMETRIC AND NONPARAMETRIC STATISTICS

Before we begin to discuss some of the specific statistical tests that you are likely to find reported in the results sections, you must understand the difference between *parametric* and *nonparametric statistics*. These terms refer to the two broad classes of inferential statistical procedures that can be applied to numeric results from studies. Parametric statistics can be applied to numbers that meet two key criteria: (1) the numbers must generally be normally distributed—that is, the frequency distribution of the numbers is roughly bell shaped and (2) the numbers must be interval or ratio numbers, such as age or intelligence score—that is, the numbers must have an order, and there must be an equal distance between each value. Nonparametric statistics are used for numbers that do not have a bell-shaped distribution and are categoric or ordinal. Categoric or ordinal numbers represent variables for which there is no established equal distance between each category, such as numbers used to represent gender or rating of preference for car color. In the predictors of life satisfaction study, gender would be a nonparametric statistic, whereas life satisfaction scores would be a parametric statistic.

Understanding that there is a difference between parametric and nonparametric statistics is important for two reasons. First, although it is the researcher's responsibility to decide which type of inferential statistics should be used, as an intelligent reader of research, you should understand that the decision is not always clear-cut. In fact, whole books are written about which types of statistics should or should not be used with selected data. Therefore, the author of a research report may include a sentence or two stating that either parametric or nonparametric statistics were used and the rationale for that decision. Second, types of statistical tests used in research differ depending on the kind of numbers in the results. Thus, more than one type of statistical procedure is needed to look for the same kind of relationship. For example, often research is looking for differences between two groups. If the variable that we expect to be different in the two groups has interval or ratio numeric values (and is distributed roughly normally or bell shaped), such as age, then the researcher can use a *t* test. But if the variable that we expect to be different for the two groups is a category, such as choice between red or green cars, then the researcher cannot use a *t* test and may use something called a Kruskal–Wallis one-way analysis of variance (ANOVA) test. The *t* test is a parametric statistical test, and the Kruskal–Wallis is a nonparametric test, but both help us to look for differences between groups. As we discuss some of the more common statistical tests that may be described in the results section of a research report, we will identify parametric and nonparametric statistics so that you will recognize and understand some of each class of statistical procedures.

CORE CONCEPT 5.3

Researchers use different types of statistics to test for the same kind of relationship, depending on the form of data collected. The research report may tell you why a particular type of statistical test was applied.

■ BIVARIATE AND MULTIVARIATE TESTS

The RN in our clinical case is not interested in becoming a statistician, but does want to know how and perhaps what predicts life satisfaction for caregivers of stroke survivors and stroke survivors. Table 5.3 summarizes some of the most common statistical tests used in nursing research by three general purposes for tests. In general, we use statistical tests to (1) look at differences between groups for one or more variables, (2) look at relationships among two or more variables, or (3) look at relationships of factors within a variable itself. Each of these general purposes addresses a different type of question. When we perform statistical tests to look at differences, we are asking some version of the question "Are groups unlike one another on a given variable or variables?" When we perform tests to look at relationships among variables, we might ask "Is there some natural connection between two or more variables?" For example, in the predictors of life satisfaction study, the authors are looking for connections between mutuality, self-rated health status, depression, stress, preparedness, and stroke impact on life satisfaction. Finally, when we look at relationships within a variable, this question might come to mind, "What are the natural components that make up a variable?" The statistical tests used when we are only looking at two variables or two groups are different from those we use with three or more variables or groups. We will first look at bivariate statistics—that is, statistical tests that are used with just two variables.

Tests Looking for Differences Between Two Groups

In our discussion of significance and probability, we used an example from the fictional article from Appendix B in which the author wanted to explain or predict choice of field of practice. To do so, the author divided the students into two groups: those who chose an acute care setting and those who did not. The author then looked for variables that were significantly different between the groups, hoping that they might help to understand and predict which students would select nonacute practice settings. A *t* test was used to test for significant differences. A *t* test computes a statistic that reflects the differences in the means of a variable for two different groups or at two different times for one group. The two groups being tested might consist of anything of interest to nursing, such as men and women, single-parent families and two-parent families, those who quit smoking and those who did not, or hospitals with level-one trauma centers and hospitals without them. In all of these examples, one variable differentiates the two groups. Alternately, the "groups" might be the same unit at different points in time, such as families before and after a divorce, smokers before and after a smoking cessation program, or hospitals before and after a level-one trauma center is added. The variable tested can be anything that can be measured as a continuous number, such as age, family functioning, self-efficacy, or cost per patient visit.

Table 5.3

Common Statistical Procedures Categorized by Type of Relationship Tested and Number of Variables Included

TYPE OF RELATIONSHIP TESTED	TWO VARIABLES—BIVARIATE	THREE OR MORE VARIABLES—MULTIVARIATE
1. Differences—are groups unlike one another on a given variable or variables?		
Independent groups	• t test (parametric) • Sign test or median test (nonparametric) • Mann–Whitney U (nonparametric) • Wilcoxon rank test (nonparametric) • Fisher exact test (nonparametric)	• ANOVA (parametric) • ANCOVA, MANOVA, one-way ANOVA (parametric) • Kruskal–Wallis one-way ANOVA (nonparametric) • Chi-square for independent samples
Related groups usually overtime	• Paired t test (parametric) • McNemar change test (nonparametric)	• Repeated measures ANOVA (parametric) • Friedman two-way ANOVA (nonparametric)
2. Relationships between variables—is there a natural connection between two or more variables?	• Pearson r (parametric) • Spearman rho (nonparametric) • Kenndall tau (nonparametric) • Contingency coefficient (nonparametric)	• Multiple regression (parametric) • Canonical correlation (parametric) • Path analysis (parametric) • Structural equation modeling (parametric) • Discriminant analysis (parametric) • Logistic regression (nonparametric)
3. Relationships within a variable—is there a structure within a variable?		• Factor analysis (parametric) • Cluster analysis (nonparametric)

ANOVA, analysis of variance; ANCOVA, analysis of covariance; MANOVA, multiple analysis of variance.

The fictional article reports the results of two t tests. The two groups for both of these tests were the same: those who chose an acute setting and those who did not choose an acute setting. However, the tests looked for differences in two different variables. In the first test, the researcher tested to see whether age differed between the groups, and in the second test, the researcher tested to see whether health rating differed. In both cases, there was a statistically significant difference between the groups in the variables. The author also tells the reader that "there was no significant . . . differences in number of years of postsecondary education and field of study." Because the test was not statistically significant, no test statistic is reported here, but the author believes it is important to tell you that the possibility of this difference was tested and was found not to be present. When using research in clinical practice, it is equally important to understand whether or not a difference or relationship is significant. Findings that there are no significant differences or relationships help us rule out factors that will affect our clinical care.

In the results section of the sleep and hunger in adolescents study in Appendix A.1, the authors state "independent t tests showed that mean nocturnal sleep for those who napped was significantly lower than for those who did not nap ($t = 2.03$)" (Landis, Parker, & Dunbar,

2009, p. 119). Other statistical tests that examine differences between two groups are mostly nonparametric and include the Fisher exact test, Mann–Whitney test, Wilcoxon signed rank test, McNemar test, and sign or median test (Table 5.3). It is not necessary to understand exactly how these tests are chosen and applied, but it is important to understand that whenever one of these tests is reported in the results section, it is being used to examine differences between two groups. If the *p* value that is reported with the test is less than .05, then there was a difference between the groups that probably did not occur by chance alone. In the predictors of life satisfaction report section "Instruments," the authors state "only instruments measuring variables shown to be significant predictors of life satisfaction for stroke survivors or their spouses in the final models are discussed" (Ostwald et al., 2009, p. 161).

Tests Looking at Relationships Between Two Variables

In nursing research, we often look for relationships or connections between two variables. When two variables are connected in some way, they are said to covary. Two variables covary when changes in one are connected to consistent changes in the other. For example, height and weight covary in healthy growing children. As the height of a child increases, the weight usually increases as well. Another example of covariance is found between the amount of practice of a procedure, such as urinary catheterization, and the number of errors. In this case, as the variable "amount of practice" increases, the variable "number of errors" consistently decreases. The statistical test used to examine how much two variables covary is called a correlation.

Two things are important to notice about a correlation statistic, also called a *correlation coefficient*. First, it is important to notice whether the number is negative or positive. In the example of the correlation between height and weight in children, the number for the correlation will be positive because the two variables move in the same direction—that is, they both increase. In the second example, the correlation between practice and errors will be negative because the two variables move in opposite directions. Figure 5.3 shows two graphs that can represent the two examples. Note that in the first graph, the points all fall along a line that moves diagonally from the bottom to the top. This shows that there is a positive connection or relationship between these two variables because as one goes up, the other goes up. In contrast, on the second graph, the points fall along a line that moves diagonally from the top and down toward the opposite end. This shows that there is a negative connection or relationship between the two variables because as one goes up, the other goes down.

Second, it is important to note the magnitude of the number for a correlation coefficient. Because of the way a correlation coefficient is calculated, it can only have a range of

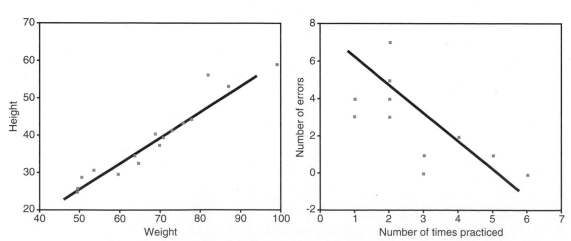

FIGURE 5.3 Scatter plots showing a positive relationship between height and weight in children and a negative relationship between practicing a procedure and number of errors.

values from -1 to $+1$. A relationship between two variables that is "perfect"—as one goes up, the other goes up or down in exactly the same amount—will have a value of either -1 or $+1$. The lines drawn in the middle of the two graphs in Figure 5.3 show what perfect correlations look like. In real life, there is almost never a perfect correlation. Returning to the example of height and weight in children, we can observe that some children will become taller and not gain very much weight, and others will become only a little taller and gain more weight. Therefore, there will not be a consistent increase in weight each time there is an increase in height, as is shown in the scatter plot in Figure 5.3, where each spot represents one child, and the spots do not all fall along a perfectly straight line. However, the bigger the value of the correlation coefficient, the more consistent and stronger the relationship is between the two variables.

To test whether or not two variables covary, a correlation statistic is computed and tested to see whether the computed value is likely to have occurred by chance. The predictors of life satisfaction report does not include any correlation statistics; however, the depressive mood, self-esteem coping, and eating article discussed in Chapters 1 and 2 (and shown in Appendix A.2) provides an example of the use of a correlation coefficient. In the last sentence of the section titled "coping," the authors state "using food to cope was positively correlated with a higher BMI percentile ($r = .26, p = .009$)" (Martyn-Nemeth, Penckofer, Gulanick, Velsor-Friedrich, & Bryant, 2009, p. 103). The r is used to denote a Pearson correlation statistic (to be discussed later in the chapter); so you can see that this statistic shows the covariation between using food to cope and BMI variables. From what we have just learned about correlation statistics, we know this means that using food to cope and BMI were connected to each other and, as one increased, the other did as well. In the "discussion" section of the same article, the authors discuss the relationships among the study variables yet do not report correlation statistics. However, we know that a *correlation* is a statistic looking at covariance or relationships between two variables.

If two variables covary, then they are connected to each other in some way. However, correlation does not tell us how the two variables are connected or whether one of the variables causes the change in the other. For example, if we had no other information besides the correlation statistic for height and weight of children, we would be left wondering whether weight causes growth in height, height causes increased weight, or both tend to increase because of some other factor we have not considered, such as age or nutrition. Therefore, correlations are inferential statistics that explain about relationships but cannot be used to predict because they do not tell us anything about which variable "causes" the other variable to change.

CORE CONCEPT 5.4

A correlation between two variables only tells us that they are connected in some way, not the cause of that connection.

For example, a study shows correlation statistics for each of the possible relationships between different pairs of variables. If we want to know whether there was a relationship between two variables, we would look at the statistical values. Taking the statistical value in the depressive mood, self-esteem, coping, and eating article, $r = .26, p = .009$, this means that in only 9 out of 1000 chances would we get a statistic of 0.26 for the relationship between using food to cope and BMI. Therefore, we decide that there is a relationship between using food to cope and BMI and will expect to find such a relationship in other groups of adolescents who are overweight. We also learn from this number that the connection or relationship between using food to cope and BMI is positive, meaning that as using food to cope goes up, an individual's BMI goes up as well. Finally, we know that the strength of the connection is not all that strong because even though 0.26 falls between 0 and 1 (which indicates no connection at all, and 1, which indicates a perfect connection), the value is not a great deal above 0.

Numerous types of correlation statistics can be computed between two variables, but the one you will probably find most frequently is the Pearson product–moment correlation, which uses the symbol "r" to represent the value of the bivariate relationship. Besides the Pearson product–moment correlation, other types of correlation statistics include the Spearman rho, the Kendall tau, and the phi. In all cases, the statistic gives the strength of the covariance between two variables. Remember a positive correlation occurs when both variables move in the same direction (if one goes up, the other does as well) and a negative correlation occurs when the variables move in opposite directions (one goes up and the other goes down).

For example, let us say you have two variables with the correlation value of $r = .50$, $p < .05$, because the size of the correlation coefficient reflects how strong the connection was between the two variables, we see that there was a moderate relationship between the variables. This would be in contrast to the correlation of variables with these values ($r = -.10$, $p < .01$). Although both of these connections are statistically significant, the strength of the relationships is different. What we understand from these statistics is that although as the first set of variables there is a moderately strong connection between them, in the second set of variables, the connection between the variables is not that strong.

Tests Looking for Differences Among Three or More Groups

Frequently, nursing research addresses questions about more than just two groups. For example, we might be interested in comparing patients who smoke, patients who have never smoked, and patients who have quit smoking for their rates of respiratory complications after cardiac surgery. We can perform three different t tests to examine differences in complication rates between smokers and those who have never smoked, then between smokers and former smokers, and then between those who have never smoked and former smokers. Keeping up with these comparisons makes one's head whirl, and obviously, the number of comparisons required would become more complicated with the more groups we have. In addition, each time we get a result that is statistically significant, a small chance remains that we are wrong in our decision that the result did not happen by chance. These chances of being wrong add up when we do multiple statistical tests to answer just one question, making our chance of an error in our decision much larger when we do three or more tests on the same set of variables. The alternative is to use a different type of statistical test called ANOVA.

Analysis of variance tests for differences in the means for three or more groups. Although it is not necessary that you do the calculations for ANOVA, it may be helpful to know what the test does, which is reflected in its name. The ANOVA compares how much members of a group differ or vary among one another with how much the members of the group differ or vary from the members of other groups. In other words, the test analyzes variance, comparing the variance *within* a group with the variance *between* groups. For example, an ANOVA test of respiratory complications in three groups of patients categorized by smoking status calculates how much variation there is in respiratory complications within the patient group that smokes, the patient group that never smoked, and the patient group that formerly smoked. It then calculates the amount of variation in respiratory rate between the smoking patients, the patients who never smoked, and the former smokers. Finally, the test compares the variation inside the groups with the variation between the groups to see their differences or similarities. The test statistic in ANOVA is usually an "F ratio" value, and like other statistical tests, the final test statistic is then compared with a set of statistics one would get if there were no differences between the groups. The F ratio compares the variation between groups with that within groups, and the larger the F ratio, the more variation between groups. However, the value of F ratios differs depending on the number of groups compared and the number of people studied, so it is not possible to make general statements about the meaning of the F ratio, except within the context of significance testing. If the F ratio value for a particular study falls into the area of statistics that has less than a 5% chance of occurring by chance, then we decide there is a statistically significant difference between the groups. In the example of respiratory complications, if the F ratio were significant, we would be able to decide that smoking and smoking history affect the rate of those complications.

Neither the fictional article nor the predictors of life satisfaction article used ANOVA because neither study needed to compare the means of three or more groups. However, in reading nursing research results, you often find this statistical test, or a variation of it, reported in the results section. Other versions of the ANOVA allow the addition of more variables and various interconnections among variables into the ANOVA. Some of the most common are analysis of covariance (ANCOVA), multiple analysis of variance (MANOVA), and one-way ANOVA. For each of these, the basic purpose of the test is to compare means of an independent variable among three or more groups. Some of the most common nonparametric statistical tests that also test for differences among three or more groups are the Kruskal–Wallis and the chi-square test (Table 5.3).

In addition to comparing three or more groups, we often want to look for differences within groups during three or more points in time. Continuing with the example of patients who smoke and their respiratory complication rates, suppose that instead of comparing them with patients who never smoked, we compared smoking patients' respiratory complication rates before and after pulmonary toilet care over a 3-day period. In this case, we are not comparing different groups, but the same group over time. The statistical test used in this type of situation is a repeated-measures ANOVA. Like other ANOVA tests, it calculates differences in variance within the group at each time point but compares those variances with the variances between the time points. Commonly used nonparametric tests for differences within groups at three or more points in time include Friedman tests and the Cochran Q.

Tests Looking at Relationships Among Three or More Variables

Just as we are often interested in differences among three or more groups, we are also interested in how a group of more than two variables covaries. For example, in the sleep and hunger in adolescents article (Appendix A.1) (Landis et al., 2009), the authors are interested in how a set of variables, such as the adolescent's age, gender, and daytime sleep, all covary in relation to an individual's caloric intake. If each of these variables is connected to caloric intake but is also connected to each other somewhat, how much does each variable independently contribute to the variation occurring in the caloric intake? Our goal is to understand what factors or variables connect to different caloric intake amounts and in what direction and to what extent so that we can use our knowledge of those connections to increase the potential that we can impact caloric intake in adolescents. If individuals' values reflecting their caloric intake were a big pie, each of the factors studied might be a piece of that pie, although those pieces will overlap somewhat. We are interested in seeing not just how much each factor by itself connects, but how the factors overlap so that we know which of the many factors might be the most useful to focus on when planning EBN care. The statistical procedure that we use to look at connections among three or more variables is called *regression.* Regression measures how much two or more independent variables explain the variation in a dependent variable. The regression procedure allows us to predict future values for the dependent variable based on values of the independent variables.

A regression analysis gives the information needed to know how much different factors independently contribute or connect to a dependent variable. Authors can use a table format to report the results of regression analysis in order to examine how much of an effect each of the factors that they had identified contributed to, let us say in this case, life satisfaction. Suppose the table has two columns with results labeled "β" and "R 95% CI." Under the column labeled "β," the statistical value for relative contribution of each of the factors is listed. A beta (β) value tells us the relative contribution or connection of an independent variable to the dependent variable. The R refers to how much of the variation in scores the factor studied explains. The 95% CI refers to what we would expect the β value to be 95% of the time, given the results that we found in the study. In summary, what you should understand is that each variable in a regression analysis is tested to determine whether it is independently connected with the dependent variable. If it is connected, a test of how much or to what extent it is connected is provided. The RN in our clinical case must read the results section of the article to see what factors predicted life satisfaction. From this, the nurse can see that the spousal caregivers and the stroke survivors had different contributing factors for life satisfaction and must take this into consideration when trying to improve the life satisfaction of both N.B. and his wife. In addition to regression analysis, numerous statistical procedures examine relationships among three or more variables. The names of some of the most common types of procedures used in nursing research are listed in Table 5.3 and include canonical correlation, path analysis, structural equation modeling, and discriminate analysis.

Tests Looking at the Structure or Components of a Variable

We have discussed bivariate statistical tests that look for differences between two variables and tests that look at relationships between two variables. We also have discussed multivariate tests that look at differences or relationships among three or more variables, and we have identified several parametric and nonparametric statistical tests for each purpose. The last general purpose for statistical procedures is to look at the structure or components within a variable of interest. These types of statistical tests are used when the variable of interest is complex and not easily measured using a single item or question. The researcher may collect information about the complex variable using several different questions or measures and then want to determine the connections among the questions or measures. For example, a nurse researcher might be interested in studying patient satisfaction associated with care. Several aspects of care may influence satisfaction, such as availability, communication with providers, cost, and whether expectations for care are met. The researcher might develop 60 statements for a survey, each of which affects some aspect of satisfaction. Responses to the survey may be scores on a scale to indicate the respondents' level of agreement with each of the statements. Scores to all 60 statements can be added together to produce a single score for satisfaction, but this does not help us to understand the important components of satisfaction that make up that score. Statistical procedures, called factor analysis, can be used to look for discrete groups of statements that are more closely connected to each other than to the other statements. Factors are the components or discrete groups of measures or statements that covary closely. In our example, the researcher might find that statements about paying bills, insurance, and difficulty getting referrals all covary more closely than statements about communication. These statements might be said to reflect a factor that could be called *barriers to satisfaction.* Factor analysis will identify groups of measures of a single variable that are connected closely enough that the connections are not likely to happen by chance. In clinical practice, a study that uses a factor analysis procedure has the potential to provide knowledge about some of the components or parts that comprise a health-related concept, such as fear, pain, or denial. The nonparametric statistical test that may be used to look at structure within a variable is called *cluster analysis*.

To summarize, several specific statistical procedures are used to test for differences and relationships. The types of tests differ depending on the type of data and whether two, or more than two, variables are to be tested. When any of these tests are applied to specific data, they produce a test statistic that will be symbolized in a unique manner, such as a "*t*" statistic, "*F*" statistic, or "*r*" statistic. The specific statistic from the study is compared with a distribution of statistics that would have occurred in similar data by chance alone if there were really no relationship or difference. If the statistic from the study falls into the range of values that occur less than 5% of the time, it is likely that there was a relationship or difference, and the result is statistically significant. Often, the level of statistical significance is specifically stated in the form of a *p* value or CI.

■ HYPOTHESIS TESTING

In Chapter 2, we defined *hypotheses* as predictions regarding the relationships or effects of selected factors on other factors. Inferential statistics are used to test whether the predictions in hypotheses are "accurate," so hypotheses direct which statistical procedures are used with the data. The results for two types of hypotheses may be described in a research report. The first type, a research hypothesis, is a prediction of the relationships or differences that will be found for selected variables in a study. None of the reports of research that we have read to date have used hypotheses. However, if the predictors of life satisfaction article had used a research hypothesis, it might have stated, "higher health status, mutuality, and caregiver preparedness scale scores and lower stress and depression scale scores will all positively impact life satisfaction for stroke survivors and spousal caregivers." This hypothesis predicts that as health status, mutuality, and caregiver preparedness scale scores go up, and stress and depression scale scores go down, life satisfaction will increase. This is a clear prediction that not only will there be a relationship, but also it will be positive. The authors of the predictors of life satisfaction study did not give us predictions in the form of hypotheses. In some studies in which we are not given predictions in the form of hypotheses, the authors may use research objectives instead, and we will discuss these further in Chapter 10.

The second type of hypothesis that may be tested and reported about in the results section of a research report is a statistical hypothesis that is often called the *null hypothesis*. A null hypothesis always predicts that there will be no relationship or difference in selected variables. Remember that, in general, researchers want to be cautious about jumping to conclusions based on the results of a particular study. This is why researchers agree that statistical test results are acceptable only when they would occur by chance less than 5% of the time. Otherwise, even if we find a difference or relationship in the data, we decide that it was just a chance happening, and we cannot prove that there was a "real" relationship. The null hypothesis reflects this same thinking by stating our prediction about relationships or differences in the negative, predicting no relationship or difference. The researcher must then find enough evidence to reject that prediction, a statistically significant test result being the evidence that is required.

In summary, a research hypothesis is stated in the positive and predicts the nature and strength of a relationship or difference among variables. It is the researcher's hope that the results of a study support the prediction. A statistical hypothesis is stated in the negative, and it is the researcher's desire for statistical tests to be significant so that the null hypothesis can be rejected. Not all quantitative research studies use hypotheses, but if there are one or more hypotheses, they are usually identified in the section of the report that describes the research problem. Chapter 10 discusses hypotheses in more detail.

■ IN-CLASS STUDY DATA

To illustrate the use of inferential statistics, let us look at the data that were collected in your in-class study. If you are not using an in-class study, you can refer to a sample set of data in Appendix D that could have been collected in a nursing class. Suppose that before these data were collected, you had observed that your fellow students who were married were generally healthier than those who were not married. You wonder whether this is true and realize that the data from your in-class study could be used to test this idea because a question about marital status and a question about overall health is included. This means there are two variables of interest: (1) marital status and (2) rating of health. The question of interest concerns differences between two groups and might be stated as "Is there a difference in health rating between married and unmarried nursing students?"

To use the in-class data to answer this question, you must first divide the health ratings into two groups: the health ratings of students who indicated that they were married and those who indicated that they were single, divorced, or widowed. Once this is done, it is easy to get an average health rating for the two groups and to see whether they are different. If they are exactly the same, or close, you probably do not have to look any further for a tentative answer to your question based on this data. If there is a difference, the next question is whether the difference is in the direction you predicted and whether it is big enough that you can believe that it did not happen by chance alone. Looking at the average health ratings will tell you whether single students seemed to have higher or lower health ratings. However, you cannot judge whether the findings prove or disprove your hypothesis because the ratings may have been simply chance findings. This is the place where inferential statistics come in because if this information is entered into a statistical computer program, you can run a t test to calculate differences in the means for rating of health of married and unmarried students.

If you are using an in-class study, predict whether some difference found in your class data will be significant before your professor runs an independent t test to determine the t value for your in-class data. For the fictional data in Appendix D, the computer calculates that the mean health rating for single students is 3.1 and the mean rating of health for married students is 2.3. These ratings look different and are opposite to what was predicted before data were collected. When we do a t test, we get a t value of 2.7 ($p = .011$), so there is a significant difference in health ratings between single and married students. However, from this data, we can conclude that the evidence does not support the hypothesis that married students are healthier; instead, it supports the opposite idea. In this fictional study, single nursing students had significantly higher ratings of their health than did married nursing students. That it was a statistically significant difference tells us that we can be sure that the difference did not happen by chance alone.

■ CONNECTING INFERENTIAL STATISTICAL RESULTS TO CONCLUSIONS

There are several important connections between results and conclusions of reports that have used inferential statistics. If inferential statistics were used, we know that the goal of the researcher is to predict that the findings of the study apply to similar situations or groups in the future. Therefore, we expect to find in the discussion and conclusions statement both how the results can be applied to similar situations or groups in the future and what aspects of the study may limit our ability to draw conclusions about future situations or groups. In the fictional article, for example, the author summarizes the findings and then concludes that "Nursing programs that are particularly concerned about shortages in nonacute settings may be able to expand this workforce by focusing their recruitment efforts on older students and by further developing or expanding RN to BSN and LPN to BSN programs." The author is saying that in the future, age and type of program of study are likely to be connected with choice of field of study, just as they were in the article. Although the author fails to give any statement of the limitations of the conclusion, the size of the sample—one class of 30 nursing students—might be a reason to consider limiting it.

If the results of a report included hypothesis testing, we should also expect a statement in the conclusions of the report about whether the hypotheses were rejected or accepted. Most importantly, the meaningfulness of statistically significant results should be discussed in the discussion and conclusions section. Throughout this chapter, we have talked about statistical significance; however, the presence of statistical significance does not necessarily indicate that the results are meaningful for clinical practice. Conversely, lack of statistical significance does not necessarily mean that there is no clinical significance in the results. The presence of statistical significance depends on several factors, one of which is the number of cases in the study. This is logical, given that we are trying to use probability to help us to infer connections or differences in the real world. If the study only includes a few cases or subjects, then the chances of a "weird" or unusual case affecting the average result is pretty high. The test distribution for a study with only a few cases results in a large "green" zone and a small "red" zone because there is a good chance that a single odd case will change the actual test statistic (Fig. 5.2).

CORE CONCEPT 5.5

The size of the sample, or number of cases, in a study affects the likelihood that a statistical significance will be found.

A study that has a large number of cases has a high likelihood of finding statistically significant findings, simply because whatever is found is not going to be affected easily by the chance that an odd case fell into the sample. However, the difference or connection that is found may not be large enough to have meaning for clinical practice. The author of the fictional article, for example, does not give the average ages of students who selected acute and nonacute settings. It is possible that the difference in age was only 1 or 2 years. A difference of this size may be statistically significant but may also be too small to have any meaning when one is trying to recruit individuals to nursing.

A clinical example of the difference between statistically significant and clinically meaningful findings might be a study of ratings of pain, such as the one discussed in Chapter 4. Suppose that this study has 500 subjects and that after one group receives an intervention, the mean ratings of pain are 2.5 (1.3) for patients getting the intervention and 2 (1.5) for patients not getting the intervention. In Chapter 4, we used an example where the standard deviations were different, although the means were the same. In this example, the means are different, whereas the standard deviations are similar. The researcher might report that there was a statistically significant difference in pain ratings between the group that did and did not get the intervention. This means that the difference in ratings was not likely to happen by chance. However, if you look at the difference, it is not large and may not, in fact, be clinically meaningful. You must decide whether a difference of only one half of a point is large enough to warrant implementation of the intervention, even though you may believe that this difference is unlikely to have occurred by chance. Thus, statistical significance does not necessarily imply clinical significance.

We would expect, therefore, that the conclusions of a research study that used inferential statistics would address whether the statistically significant findings were also meaningful findings. We also would expect that the conclusions would address whether findings that were *not* statistically significant might still warrant further consideration because they appear to be clinically meaningful.

CORE CONCEPT 5.6

Statistical significance does not directly equate with clinical meaningfulness.

■ COMMON ERRORS IN RESULTS SECTIONS

As with the reports of descriptive results, two kinds of problems may be found when reading inferential statistic results in a research report: (1) incomplete information and (2) confusing information. Incomplete information occurs when the results section of reports gives us the statistical test results, including the *p* value or CI, but does not give us the descriptive results needed to interpret the statistically significant result. For example, suppose that the author of the fictional article from Appendix B had told us that there was a significant difference in health rating ($t = 2.1, p < .05$) among students who chose acute versus nonacute fields of practice. The test statistic alone does not tell us which group had the higher health rating, so it is impossible to interpret the meaning of this statistically significant difference.

Another example of incomplete information might be a research report that includes a statement that there was a statistically significant finding but does not provide the test statistic. Because some of the statistics tell us a great deal, the lack of the statistic can limit our understanding of the results. If, for example, the author of the effects of exercise on recovery report in Appendix A.3 had told us only that there was a significant relationship between exercise and recovery, we would have no idea about the direction of that relationship or its strength. It would be conceivable that those who had more exercise had a longer recovery or did not recover as well, which would be a negative relationship with the value for "*r*" being negative. Supposing that the authors do give us the correlation coefficients of *r* (.37) we would know that this tells us that there was a positive relationship and that it was weak to moderate.

A third type of incomplete information is a failure to test for relationships or differences that might be meaningful for understanding the results of the study. The fictional article reports in the results section that age and health rating were both different in students who chose acute versus nonacute fields of practice. One might wonder whether age and rating of health are related. This is a logical question, given what we know about aging and health, and the answer would help us better understand the meaning of the results of this study. However, the author does not test for a relationship between these two variables, so we are left wondering about the possibility of this relationship.

In addition to incomplete information, research reports may present results in a manner that is unclear or unnecessarily confusing. The titles of tables should clearly identify the table's content and should be referenced within the text of the results section. Labels for columns should be consistent with the use of language in the text and with accepted language for reporting statistical results that may be tested and reported about in the results section. Lastly, sometimes a researcher may overinterpret or overgeneralize about results from a study. Similarly, sometimes a researcher actually incorrectly interprets a statistical result. For example, suppose that an author interpreted the correlation between obesity and depression to mean that obesity *causes* depression. A correlation means that there is a connection, but it does not tell us that one of the two connected variables caused the other. These last types of errors are not likely to appear in research reports published in peer-reviewed journals because those types of errors will be found and corrected. However, occasionally, research results in the public sector are overinterpreted or incorrectly interpreted.

> Box 5.1
> **How to Critically Read the Results Sections of Research Reports**
>
> Do the results answer the question "Why did the authors reach these conclusions—what did they actually find?"
>
> 1. Did the report include a clearly identified results section?
> 2. Were the results presented appropriately for the information collected?
> 3. Were descriptive versus inferential results identifiable if this is a quantitative study?
> 4. Were themes or structure and meaning identifiable if this is a qualitative study?
> 5. Were the results presented in a clear and logical manner?
> 6. Did the results include enough information about the final sample for the study?

■ CRITICALLY READING THE RESULTS SECTION OF A REPORT FOR USE IN EVIDENCE-BASED NURSING PRACTICE—REVISITED

In Chapter 4, we looked at six questions that can help you to read critically the results section of a research report. These questions are shown again in Box 5.1. Let us revisit some of these questions now that we have talked about inferential statistics. The second question to consider asks, "Were the results presented appropriately for the information collected?" As we discussed in the previous section, at times, the results presented are either incomplete or confusing. The authors in the predictors of life satisfaction article provided results in table and descriptive format as is appropriate for the purpose of the study. The third question listed for critically reading results also addresses a concern with the predictors of life satisfaction report. That question asks about clear identification of descriptive versus inferential results. This article's tables present descriptive results for each of the measures in the study and discuss inferential results in the results section. The authors probably would have improved our ability to use their research if they had provided descriptive findings, and then had given the results of the t tests.

As we indicated in Chapter 4, this study was quantitative, so we cannot use it as an example for answering the fourth question for critically reading results sections. However, we can decide about the fifth question, which asks how clearly and logically the results were presented. In general, the tables in this report clearly listed descriptive results, and organized the presentation of their results, and clearly indicated this in the readings Therefore, we might decide that the results are presented clearly and logically. Finally, the last question refers to information about the sample. The predictors of life satisfaction report provides a table about the characteristics of the final sample in the study and gives us the details about the sample that we might need, such as age and gender, as well as additional information in the results section. We will have to evaluate this aspect of the results further after learning more about samples and sampling.

■ PUBLISHED REPORT—WHAT WOULD YOU CONCLUDE?

The RN in our clinical case now has an increased understanding of the results and conclusions of the study examining predictors in life satisfaction for spousal caregivers and stroke survivors. The nurse knows that there were several differences in how caregivers and stroke survivors scored on life satisfaction measures. The nurse also knows that selected factors, including depression and mutuality, appear to impact life satisfaction in stroke survivors while caregiver preparedness and mutuality appear to impact life satisfaction in spousal caregivers. The authors also have indicated that they found a statistically significant difference in life satisfaction between 12 and 24 months after hospitalization for stroke. They state two limitations of the study: (1) life satisfaction and mutuality were not measured before the stroke had occurred and (2) life satisfaction was not measured until 12 months after hospitalization; so did the life satisfaction change in the first 12 months? The RN must decide whether the evidence from this study can be used to guide nursing practice with N.B. as well as with other caregivers in the future. However, the nurse does note that the majority of caregivers in the study were female and wonders if some aspect of the approach to sampling led to more female than male caregivers being included. Since the caregiver that the nurse is concerned about is a man, the RN needs to know more about how this sample was selected before a decision can be made on how useful this evidence is for nursing practice. Chapter 6 addresses samples and how they affect the conclusions we can draw from research.

OUT-OF-CLASS EXERCISE

What Do You Want to Know About Samples?

The next two chapters focus on the process of sampling and the meanings of different types of samples. In preparation for reading the next chapter, think about your in-class study sample. Write a list of information that you would like to have about the characteristics of the sample for this study, including a rationale for why you would like that information next to each item. Then, think about what you know about the composition of your class and assume that an interesting result that has implications for nursing education was found in the in-class data. If you were writing the conclusions of a report about this finding, how would you describe the group of individuals to whom the results might be applied in the future? Write a short paragraph describing this group, including to whom the results probably apply and to whom they probably do not apply. If your class did not use an in-class study, you can do this exercise by pretending that a study was conducted using your class group. List what you would want to know about the people in the study and why. Then, given what you do know about those in your course group, write a short paragraph describing to whom the results of a study with this course group probably would apply and to whom they probably would not apply. After you complete one of these exercises, you are ready to begin Chapter 6.

References

Landis, A., Parker, K., & Dunbar, S. (2009). Sleep, hunger, satiety, food cravings, and caloric intake in adolescents. *Journal of Nursing Scholarship, 41*(2), 115–123.

Martyn-Nemeth, P., Penckofer, S., Gulanick, M., Velsor-Friedrich, B., & Bryant, F. (2008). The relationships among self-esteem, stress, coping, eating behavior, and depressive mood in adolescents. *Research in Nursing & Health 2009, 32*, 96–109.

Ostwald, S. K., Godwin, K. M., & Cron, S. G. (2009). Predictors of life satisfaction in stroke survivors and spousal caregivers after inpatient rehabilitation. *Rehabilitation Nursing, 34*(4), 160–174.

Resources

Field, A. (2009). *Discovering statistics using SPSS for Windows* (3rd ed.). London: Sage Publications.

Locke, L. F., Silverman, S. J., & Spirduso, W. W. (2009). *Reading and understanding research* (3rd ed.). Thousand Oaks, CA: Sage Publications.

Pedhazur, E. J., & Schmelkin, L. P. (1991). *Measurement, design, and analysis: An integrated approach*. Hillsdale, NJ: Lawrence Erlbaum Associates.

Polit, D. F., & Beck, C. T. (2007). *Nursing research: Principles and methods* (8th ed.). Philadelphia, PA: Lippincott Williams & Wilkins.

Salkind, N. J. (2007). *Statistics for people who (think they) hate statistics* (3rd ed.). Thousand Oaks, CA: Sage Publications.

Talbot, L. A. (1995). *Principles and practice of nursing research*. St. Louis, MO: Mosby.

6

Samples

To What Types of Patients Do These Research Conclusions Apply—Who Was in the Study?

LEARNING OBJECTIVE

The student will relate the sampling methods and study sample to results, conclusions, and clinical meaningfulness of the study.

KEY TERMS

Bias
Cluster sampling
Convenience sample
Criteria for participation
Generalizability
Matched sample
Nonprobability sampling
Population
Power analysis
Probability sampling
Purposive sampling
Quota sampling

Random assignment
Randomly selected
Response rate
Sample
Sampling frame
Sampling unit
Saturation
Selectivity
Simple random sampling
Snowball sampling
Stratified random sampling
Systematic sampling

Each of the RNs in the clinical cases discussed in previous chapters had an EBN clinical question and sought an answer through evidence in research-related publications. As we reviewed what each could conclude regarding their questions, we had to wonder whether the results and conclusions of the study could be applied to the patient or patients of concern to the RN. Specifically, we wondered:

1. What are the most effective interventions to meet the complex needs of an adolescent who is medically obese and has health and self-image/esteem issues associated with obesity?
2. What nursing interventions should be considered by the nurse when planning care to decrease the fatigue of patients undergoing breast cancer therapies after discharge from a hospital?
3. What interventions assist and support the health and function of caregivers of stroke patients?

   In exploring the topic of research samples, we will use a new clinical case, revisiting the four previous clinical cases as well as the research found by our RNs.

Clinical Case • J.K. is a 35-year-old married army officer who suffered a traumatic brain injury (TBI) while serving in Iraq. He suffered a TBI when his vehicle hit a homemade bomb; he was thrown from the vehicle and hit his head when landing on the ground. He has had substantial recovery of functioning but requires a considerable amount of care to meet daily needs, and he is still wheelchair bound. Although he has recently gone home from a rehabilitation hospital, he has not returned to work and is on disability. The RN works for the hospital and has been assigned to see J.K. and his wife in the home setting. The RN has recognized how difficult all of this has been on J.K. and his wife. Both J.K. and his wife are concerned about his ability to be a "productive member of society" and whether he will ever return to his "normal" life.

   The RN is active in a professional nursing organization, and about a month after starting to care for this family, the nurse attended a local district nursing meeting. While networking at the meeting, the nurse spoke with a colleague who works in intensive care. They discovered that they had a shared interest in the needs of patients recovering from TBI and decided to investigate interventions that address helping patients return to a "normal life" from the moment of hospitalization through the return to the community. They agreed to do a literature search, and the RN from the ICU found an article entitled "The use of narratives to identify characteristics leading to a productive life following acquired brain injury" (Fraas & Calvert, 2009) (Appendix A.5). Table 6.1 identifies the clinical question of the RN and the key search terms used in the literature search.

Table 6.1

Development of a Clinical Question From the Clinical Case Study

What interventions should be included in a plan of care to assist patients who have had a traumatic brain injury to lead a productive life?

The *Who*	Patients with TBI
The *What*	Interventions to help patients lead a productive life
The *When*	After a traumatic brain injury and thereafter
The *Where*	In any setting
Key search terms useful in finding research-based evidence for this practice question	TBI Recovery Productive

Regardless of whether we are using EBN strategies to answer questions related to using research to guide discharge planning or to direct the planning of care, education, or programs, it is important to answer the question "To what types of patients do these research conclusions apply?" We must consider this question because a study may address a clinical problem of interest to you, but it may not have used a sample that reflects your patients. As an RN, you will need to understand the implications of different sample types to your ability to use study results as evidence in EBN to address clinical practice effectively. One of the first things that you will need to understand is the difference between a sample and a population.

■ SAMPLES VERSUS POPULATIONS

As discussed, research is rarely able to include in one study all the cases that might be affected by the research question. A study of cardiovascular risk factors in children with insulin-dependent diabetes mellitus (IDDM), for example, could not possibly study every child with diabetes. A study of male patients with TBI resulting from combat is a smaller group, but it is still impossible to include all of these men in one study. All of the studies discussed so far were interested in understanding something about a larger group of patients than those included in their actual studies. The larger group, called the study population, is all of the individuals that the researchers are interested in studying. The population for any particular study is defined by specific common characteristics. For example, the population of interest in the "Sleep, hunger, satiety, food cravings & calorie intake in adolescents" (Landis, Parker, & Dunbar, 2009) study (Appendix A.1) had four common characteristics: they (1) were adolescents between 14 and 18 years of age, (2) were in high school full time, (3) had the ability to speak and read English, and (4) were able to be reached by telephone (p. 117). The population of interest in the study by Hsieh et al. (2008), "Effects of a supervised exercise intervention on recovery from treatment regimens in breast cancer survivors" (Appendix A.3), shared characteristics of (1) surviving breast cancer, (2) being women, (3) being referred to a specific rehabilitation center, and (4) having had a surgical procedure. In the "Predictors of life satisfaction in stroke survivors and spousal caregivers after inpatient rehabilitation" study (Ostwald, Godwin, & Cron, 2009) (Appendix A.4), the population shared characteristics of (1) both the stroke survivors and caregivers living together and (2) patients completing 12 months of a specific rehabilitation program. Notice that it is possible to clearly identify the common characteristics that comprise each population.

Of course, none of these studies included every member of the population of interest. There are thousands of caregivers for stroke patients. There are thousands of women who have breast surgery every year; so the research will select a smaller, more workable group for conducting their study. This subset of the overall population that is included in a study is called a sample. To understand whether a study applies to your clinical situation, you can start by considering three general questions about the study sample and the related population: (1) Does the population for this study reflect the types of patients or situations that I am interested in understanding? (2) Does the sample in the study reflect or fit with the population of interest? (3) Does the approach taken to choosing the sample limit how much I can use the results of the study?

Most of this chapter addresses the third question, but the first and second questions are also essential to answer in order to understand and use research in clinical practice.

Does the Population for This Study Reflect the Types of Patients or Situations of Interest?

As we have discussed many times, EBN is a process of decision making regarding clinical questions that looks at available evidence to answer a clinical question. If research-based evidence is to be meaningfully considered in your EBN strategy, you will need to decide whether a study addresses a population that is relevant or clinically similar to the patient group you are interested in understanding. To do this, you will need to identify the common characteristics of your patient population. One of the ways to identify clearly the population that fits your clinical question is to use the *Who, What, When, Where* approach to forming an EBN clinical question. As you use this approach, you are, in essence, listing characteristics of the population in which you are interested. This will then give you a comparison of those characteristics of the identified sample within a research report.

Nurses occasionally have a problem using research because they look for studies that exactly fit the specific patients with whom they are working. In the clinical case in Chapter 1, if the RN caring for M.D., the 17-year-old female adolescent who is medically obese, had searched the Cumulative Index to Nursing and Allied Health (CINAHL) for a study that specifically addressed needs of 17-year-old teenager females, who were obese, had specific health issues and self-image/esteem issues, the nurse would have had difficulty finding studies matched to such a narrow population. Or if the nurse had searched for a single study that included all of those characteristics, the nurse would have likely found little or nothing. The combination of gender, age, obesity, health, and self-image/esteem issues associated with obesity as patient characteristics is so specific that no one may have implemented a study focusing on that narrow a population. By broadening the characteristics that define the population to only adolescents with obesity or obesity and self-image/esteem, however, the RN found two studies. When these two studies are taken together, they cover several of the characteristics that could potentially apply to the RN's specific patient care situation. Yet, too broad a definition of the population might have found studies with populations that were too different from M.D., making them useless in planning care for her. For example, a literature search that used only the term *obesity* would yield a large number of studies, many without any attention to adolescents. Although there may be some overlap between the concerns of the population of adolescents with obesity and adolescents with self-image/esteem issues, clearly there are some important differences that affect how useful these studies will be to understanding M.D.'s case.

How do you learn what the population of a study may be? Several places in a research report should identify the population for the study, but in this chapter, we focus on the section of most reports that is labeled "Sample," "Sampling Methods," or something similar. In this section of the report, the author identifies how individuals were selected for the study and lists its criteria for participation. Remember our definition of a sample—that it is a subset of the population; therefore, the criteria for participation in the study should be the common characteristics that define the population of interest. In the study report used in Chapter 1 from Appendix A.2 on self-esteem and eating behavior (Martyn-Nemeth, Penckofer, Gulanick, Velsor-Friedrich, & Bryant, 2009), the authors state that their study included "adolescents…

enrolled in high school, who were able to read and write English" (p. 99) and "... both parents and students agreed to participate" (p. 101). This tells us that the target population was high school adolescents who were willing to participate but does not tell us at what their grade levels were or their grade point averages. In some cases, such as a meta-synthesis study, where the findings of several studies are examined, the actual identification of the sample may be more difficult to find. Also, reports may not have a specific section called *sample*, but the description of the sample may be located under the method or results sections. The statements of sample characteristics above supply us with information that we can compare with the population of interest to the RNs in our clinical cases. In summary, it is important to identify the criteria for study participation in order to understand the targeted research study population and to decide on its applicability to your clinical practice.

Does the Sample in the Study Reflect the Population of Interest?

At first glance, this question may appear to be the same as the first question, but it is not. Once a study defines the population of interest—that is, the larger group we are interested in gaining knowledge about—the researcher must find a way to recruit or get a sample of individuals who are members of that population. This is sometimes more difficult than it might seem. Occasionally, it is not ethical to ask members of the population to submit to the study, and it might be difficult to get members of the population to agree to be in a study. As well, there occasionally may be limits inherent to a setting that make it difficult to get members from the population of interest. We discuss each of these potential problems in getting study samples later in this chapter. For now, it is important to realize that a researcher may define the population of interest for a study one way and end up with a sample that does not fit that planned population.

If you have discovered a lack of fit between the sample and the population of interest in a research article, this should be considered a limitation to the study and may limit your ability to apply the evidence to your clinical concerns. To read intelligently and to use research, it is important to identify (1) the population of interest, (2) the population for a particular research study, and (3) whether the sample reflects that population of interest.

CORE CONCEPT 6.1

A researcher may define the population of interest in one way but end up with a sample that differs from that defined population.

Does the Approach for Choosing the Sample Limit the Usefulness of the Study Results?

Our third broad question considers how the researcher obtained his or her sample and whether that approach limits how you can use the study conclusions in clinical practice. To address this, we must first discuss some of the unique language used in research to describe samples.

The language used differs between qualitative and quantitative studies because the general purposes of the two types of research differ in two broad areas: (1) constraining versus enriching the complexity of samples and (2) rigidity or flexibility in sampling. In general, qualitative research neither tries to predict future occurrences of the phenomena nor attempts to control any aspects of the phenomena as it is studied. Therefore, samples in qualitative research try to derive what is called *rich* samples. These samples contain as many of the complex aspects of the phenomena as possible. Qualitative research samples are also flex-ible. As researchers begin to understand more about what they are studying, the sample may change. These approaches to sampling can be contrasted to quantitative research, where the researcher will often attempt to constrain aspects of the phenomena when studying it and the sample is generally rigid, not changing after it is selected. We will now discuss these significant differences between qualitative and quantitative research in more detail.

■ SAMPLING IN QUALITATIVE RESEARCH

When reading qualitative research, understanding whether the sample fits the population of interest is essential because the subjective experiences of the sample are at the heart of the study. Suppose that a researcher studies homeless patients' satisfaction with health care. The population of interest in such a study would have the characteristics of (1) being home-less, and (2) having had experiences with health care. If the researcher enrolls subjects who have been homeless in the past but are now in some type of housing, even temporary hous-ing, this might alter the fit. The meaning of the experiences for formerly homeless individ-uals is likely to be different from the meanings for those who are currently homeless. Because the goal of this hypothetical research would be to inform our practice by increas-ing our knowledge about the overall satisfaction with the experience of receiving primary health care as a homeless person, a sample of formerly homeless individuals would not have been appropriate and would have entirely changed the population for the study.

In our clinical case, the RN is interested in developing a plan of action to assist TBI patients in perceiving themselves as being productive or returning to normal life. In look-ing for research-based evidence to support EBN practice, the RN finds the "The use of nar-ratives to identify characteristics leading to a productive life following acquired brain injust" report (Fraas & Calvert, 2009) (Appendix A.5). A qualitative study such as this has a goal of broadly increasing our understanding of the population of interest, recognizing that each piece of the picture that we collect gives us a better sense of the whole phenomenon. In order to accomplish this, the sample must then be composed of individuals who have knowl-edge of the phenomena. In our example of the researcher looking at homeless patients' sat-isfaction with primary health care, the phenomenon of interest to the research is satisfaction with care. So, to find a sample of this population, the researcher would need to select indi-viduals who are homeless and who, while homeless, had received primary care services.

As the researcher plans to find such a group of individuals, we will notice one of the first obvious things that differentiate a qualitative sample from a quantitative sample. In qualita-tive research, the individuals who comprise a sample are most often called *participants*, *vol-unteers*, *members*, or *informants* rather than being called *subjects*. Use of these terms reflects the perspective seen in qualitative research that the individuals are an active part of the research process and are sharing their knowledge and experiences with the researcher.

The qualitative researcher is looking for the most content and the most contextually rich sources of data available to understand the meaning of the experiences of interest. Immer-sion in the experience with as much complexity as possible is critical in understanding these realities and experiences. Therefore, the qualitative researcher wants each participant or informant to be different so as to lend additional insight, or richness, about a particular phe-nomenon. The researcher will intentionally seek ways to find individuals who are deeply involved and a part of the phenomenon being studied. In the study of patients with severe acquired brain injury (ABI) (Fraas & Calvert, 2009), the researcher searched for patients who were involved in a specific rehabilitation program. In this sense, they could be assured that they were finding patients who were deeply involved in the phenomenon of interest, patients with TBI. Think about how the sample would have been less rich if they used a small community rehabilitation center for patients needing rehabilitation services for any disease/trauma. Under the "Methods: Participants" heading (p. 316), the authors list the inclusion criteria for obtaining their sample. This criteria identifies the characteristics of the sample, and, therefore, of the population. They identify that (1) participants were survivors of ABI and (2) "members of a community-based, rehabilitation program for adults with ABI" (p. 316). Reading this, we know that the participant sample was composed of patients who were in a rehabilitation program specifically for those recovering from an ABI. There was no attempt to limit the sample. In fact, the authors state, "no members were excluded from participating" (p. 317). Acquiring a sample that reflected diversity was the goal. The type of sample used in this study is called a convenience sample because it includes members of the population who can be readily found and recruited and are "convenient" for the researcher to recruit.

Qualitative research may also use an approach called snowball sampling. A snowball sample is just as the name implies. The researcher will start with one participant or member of the population and will then use that member's contacts to identify other potential participants for the study. The next few participants will share other contacts who may have experiences of interest, thus ever increasing the sample. Snowball sampling is most commonly used when the researcher would have difficulty in finding participants who might otherwise not be identified easily. Snowball sampling often allows the inclusion of several views or experiences.

Another type of sampling used in qualitative research is purposive sampling. A purposive sample consists of participants who are intentionally or purposefully selected because they have certain characteristics related to the purpose of the research. The characteristics sought in the sample will vary, depending on the approach taken by the researcher. Occasionally, a researcher's goal is to obtain as much diversity as possible in the sample, but sometimes the goal is to focus intently on a particular aspect of the phenomenon under study. If researchers are interested in understanding smoking cessation, they may wish to look at a purposive sample of individuals who have quit smoking in the last month. In this approach, they will purposefully not recruit individuals who are still smoking or who have been tobacco free for over a year. But the researchers may also take a different approach and purposefully recruit individuals who have tried three or more times to quit but who are still smoking. From these examples, we can see that different experiences with a phenomenon may be used by researchers to select the sample purposefully.

Strengths and Weaknesses of Qualitative Sampling Approaches

A convenience sample for a qualitative study has the advantages of being relatively easy and inexpensive to acquire but may have the disadvantage of yielding a group of participants that is not as diverse and cannot provide as rich a detail about the phenomenon of interest. For example, a convenience sample of homeless people from just one shelter may yield individuals who have been homeless for only a short time because of the location of the shelter or the type of services offered at that shelter.

Similarly, purposive sampling has its advantages and disadvantages. A purposive sample in a qualitative study actively seeks to enrich the data by including participants who have a particular type of experience, characteristic, or understanding to share. The potential disadvantage to this type of sampling is the possibility of prematurely focusing the data collection on one experience or understanding and missing the broader range of data that may come from a convenience sample.

Sample Size in Qualitative Research

Qualitative sampling strategies are fluid and flexible and are intentionally and thoughtfully revised as the data analysis suggests new avenues to explore or aspects that need additional focus. These strategies are used to seek a detailed and rich understanding of the aspect under study. This process continues until the information shared by participants has become redundant and no new information is being added; at this point, the researcher identifies that sat-uration has occurred. Saturation of data is the point in data collection at which the data become repetitive and no new information or participants is being added.

Sample size is usually dictated by the process of data analysis in qualitative research; data saturation is an example. The size of the sample in a qualitative study is dictated by the method of study and the complexity of the phenomenon of interest. Because the data collection methods in qualitative research yield much data from each participant, the sample sizes in this type of research are usually smaller than in quantitative research. The composition and richness of the setting and participants, rather than the sample size, tell us how useful the results of a qualitative study may be with our own patients. In general, qualitative samples tend to use fewer than 50 participants. Some methods might only require two to five participants. The sampling strategy and the complexity of the phenomenon of interest also dictate sample size in qualitative research.

Summary of Qualitative Sampling

In general, sampling strategies in qualitative research seek to identify participants who have experience with the phenomenon of interest to the researcher and who will bring detail and complexity to the study. Even when a researcher uses a purposive sample to focus on a particular type of experience, the goal remains to have as much depth and detail as possible. As a result, sampling in qualitative research is usually driven by the data being collected and may change as the study progresses. In our above example of smoking cessation research, if the researcher used purposive sampling, he or she might have a sample of participants who have quit smoking in the last 6 months. In collecting data from this sample, the researcher begins to understand that all of the participants had a significant stressor in their lives in the month before they quit. The researcher at this point may begin to seek out new participants who are smokers and who have experienced a significant stress in the last week so that the process of making the decision to quit can be more fully examined. The example highlights how qualitative researchers collect data and analyze it concurrently as well as how they can use insights from the data to guide further participant recruitment.

■ SAMPLING IN QUANTITATIVE RESEARCH

The sampling approaches in quantitative research focus on acquiring subjects who match the population of interest as closely as possible. To accomplish this goal, sampling strategies in quantitative research either attempt to remove extraneous variation from the study subjects or to use strategies that prevent the sample from being limited to any particular group or characteristic. In general, quantitative studies that seek to describe and understand some aspect related to health and health care use sampling strategies that lead to a sample that closely resembles the target population. Studies that seek to predict or to test predictions use sampling strategies focused on eliminating factors that might confuse the results of the study. For example, a quantitative descriptive study of the process of smoking cessation should include subjects who have different economic, educational, racial, and gender backgrounds found in the community of interest. We saw in the qualitative section above that these were not issues of concern to the qualitative researcher. In contrast, a study of the effectiveness of a smoking-cessation program that compares a group using the intervention to a group not using it should ensure that the groups are similar in factors such as race or education. If these factors differ, they might affect quitting success and make it difficult to determine whether the intervention itself made a difference.

In either case, one of the goals in sampling is to avoid bias. Bias occurs when some unintended factor confuses or changes the results in a way that can lead to incorrect conclusions. We say that a bias distorts or confounds the findings, making it difficult or impossible to interpret the results.

The goal of limiting or avoiding the introduction of bias into the study sample is reflected in the consistent use of the term *subjects* to describe the members of the quantitative sample. By using this term, it conveys that the researcher is separate and as removed as possible from those in the sample. The distance and impersonal tone implied by using *subject* are intended to help the researcher to avoid introducing any of the researcher's expectations or interests into the study findings. Just as we saw several different approaches to selecting the qualitative sample, there are many ways to select the quantitative sample. Next, we will look at a few of these approaches.

Nonprobability Sampling

Quantitative studies usually use nonprobability samples. Nonprobability sampling uses approaches that do not necessarily ensure that everyone in the population of interest has an equal chance of being included in the study. These types of sampling strategies are usually used because they are easier or less costly or because it is not possible to identify everyone in the population. Some of the types of nonprobability samples may sound familiar, as they include convenience samples, purposive sampling, quota sampling, and matched samples.

The same processes are used to obtain a convenience sample in quantitative research as in qualitative research. This type of sample consists of subjects who meet the participation criteria and who can be readily identified and recruited into the study. The pool of all potential subjects for a study is also called a sampling frame—that is, the pool of all individuals who meet the criteria for the study and, therefore, can be included in the sample. When the study tells us that the sample was one of convenience, we know that subjects from the sampling frame were included because they could be conveniently accessed, often on a first-come, first-served basis. This means that those who heard about the study first, or were most open to being in a study or happened to be nearby when the researcher came to recruit the subjects, were the ones in the study. If there is not an equal chance for every subject to participate in the study, the sample would be considered a nonprobability sample.

Purposive sampling is used in quantitative research as well, particularly when the population of interest is unusual or difficult to access. Remember that purposive sampling is the careful and intentional selection of subjects for a study based on specified characteristics. Although purposive sampling is used frequently in qualitative research, it is used less often in quantitative research because the potential for introducing unintended bias into the sample can be high. None of the quantitative studies discussed so far has used a purposive sample. This type of sample might be used in quantitative research if the researcher were interested in describing family adaptation when a member survives a lethal health problem. The researcher might intentionally seek out the families of individuals who have survived ovarian and pancreatic cancers because they are two of the most lethal types of cancer. Clearly, other lethal conditions occur in health care, but the categories of ovarian and pancreatic cancer are readily identifiable and consistently have low survival odds. Therefore, the researcher might purposely select families with survivors of these two conditions.

Quota sampling is another type of nonprobability sampling in which every member of the population does not have an equal chance of being included in the study. In a quota sample, one or more characteristics are identified that are important to the study, and they are used to establish limits on or quotas for the number of subjects who will be included. The goal is to make the sample more representative of the population in a situation where all members of the population cannot be identified. For example, the researcher studying nursing students' choices of field of practice might have decided that gender would be an important factor to consider. After discerning that the known percentage of male nursing students in the state was 16%, the researcher might have used quota sampling to ensure that the sample would have a similar gender composition. This may have been done by setting a goal of recruiting 21 female nursing students and 4 male nursing students so that 16% of the sample would be male.

The last type of nonprobability sample often used is a matched sample. In a matched sample, the researcher plans to compare two groups to explain or understand something that differentiates them but knows that some other important characteristics could confuse or bias understanding. To prevent the other important characteristic(s) from making comparison difficult, the researcher intentionally selects subjects whose important characteristics are the same, or matched. An example of this approach might be found in a study of urinary retention care. Suppose the researcher indicates that the original sample for the study comprised 102 long-term care patients who had a permanent indwelling urinary catheter and 102 long-term residents who were intermittently catheterized. The researcher wants to compare indwelling and episodic catheter patients in terms of how often the patients developed infections and did not want the groups to differ on their risk for bedsores, which can also cause infection. Therefore, the specific factors that put a patient at risk for bedsores such as decreased mobilization, poor nutrition, and the presence of skin tears were identified before the study, and subjects were recruited who were similar on those characteristics but differed on whether they had indwelling catheters or were episodically catheterized. This matched the subjects—that is, they had the same risk factors for infections within each group. Again, all acutely ill patients did not have an equal chance of being in the study because they were included only if they had risk factors for urinary infections that were similar to those of other subjects who differed from them in terms of catheter status. Thus, at the beginning of the study, for each subject in the indwelling catheter group, there was a subject who matched him or her in risks for infection in the noncatheterized group.

Probability Sampling

Quantitative studies that intentionally try to predict some aspect of health are more likely to use probability sampling strategies than nonprobability strategies. Probability sampling strategies ensure that every member of a population has an equal opportunity to be in the study. The most common types of probability sampling strategies are simple random sampling and several variations on that sampling: stratified random sampling, cluster sampling, and systematic sampling.

Although simple random sampling is familiar to most people, the principles involved in this type of sampling are important to understand. Here, all the members of a population of interest must be identified and listed, and each member of the population is assigned a number. Therefore, to select a random sample, all members of the population must be part of the sampling frame. After deciding how many members of the population will be in the study, the researcher uses some device, such as a random number table (Fig. 6.1) or a computer program, to select who will be in the study. Box 6.1 discusses the use of a random number table to identify a random sample. Researchers arbitrarily pick a number from a random number table, which consists of rows and columns of numbers, and then continue in any direction in the table to select numbers. Because all possible numbers are represented in the table, it is by chance alone that the number of any particular member of the population is chosen.

In stratified random sampling, the population of interest is first divided into two or more groups based on characteristics that are important to the study, and then members within each group are randomly selected. If a researcher were interested in studying some aspect of nursing students in Wyoming that may be significantly different for undergraduate and graduate students, the population of all nursing students could be stratified—that is, divided according to level of study. Then, the students in each stratum would be listed and assigned a number, and the selection of a random sample would be carried out twice, first with the undergraduate students and then with the graduate students. This strategy is similar to the nonprobability sampling strategy of quota sampling, except that in stratified sampling, members in each stratum have an equal opportunity to be in the sample.

79	75	64	48	5	70	28	68	79	66	64	40	6	59	30	11	42	29	97	9
65	25	22	58	19	27	80	36	63	16	25	20	12	93	47	1	38	42	19	79
58	13	92	29	56	10	51	38	16	0	97	76	65	40	67	34	20	39	86	79
18	97	73	96	28	54	85	80	9	77	43	47	89	13	24	61	6	63	86	99
91	70	17	84	26	21	82	24	42	32	51	94	89	35	93	10	15	28	71	98
81	78	61	93	75	27	17	39	20	18	66	98	12	73	96	88	31	3	57	72
9	7	49	77	38	53	87	86	52	42	12	14	37	5	50	68	80	4	90	15
50	28	27	49	31	67	53	91	15	48	23	83	90	65	25	69	31	14	79	82
72	66	0	83	52	25	93	26	39	23	10	73	44	58	13	85	21	24	22	79
59	27	90	21	52	41	73	40	83	49	93	97	81	40	49	51	7	44	56	39

FIGURE 6.1   Random number table of 200 numbers between 0 and 99.

Cluster sampling is a third type of probability sampling that can make it easier to acquire a random sample. This type of sample occurs in stages, starting with selecting groups of subjects who are part of a larger element that relates to the population and then sampling smaller groups until eventually individual subjects are selected. A cluster sample of nursing students in Wyoming might start by listing every National League for Nursing (NLN)-accredited undergraduate and graduate program in Wyoming. A random sample of 10 of these programs might be selected, and then a random sample of 200 students might be chosen from a list of

---

Box 6.1
Using a Random Number Table to Identify a Random Sample

In order to identify a random sample, the researcher must enumerate the entire population. Then, the researcher arbitrarily picks a number from a random number table, which consists of rows and columns of numbers, and continues in any direction in the table to select numbers. Because all possible numbers are represented in the table, it is by chance alone that the number of any particular member of the population is chosen. Therefore, to obtain a random sample of nursing students in Wyoming, a researcher must identify and list all nursing students in the state. If the researcher wants a sample size of 100 nursing students, he or she will assign numbers to each student; pick a number in the random number table; and continue to read off numbers going down, up, or diagonally through the table, until the numbers of 100 students have been picked. Because the goal of quantitative research is to generalize and to avoid bias, a simple random sample is considered the best type of sample because the only factors that should bias the sample would be present by chance alone, making it highly likely that the sample will be similar to the population of interest.

every nursing student in those 10 programs. Every student in Wyoming had an equal opportunity to be selected for the sample, but the researcher did not have to identify and list every student to select that sample. Instead, the larger element of colleges and universities with accredited nursing programs was sampled, followed by sampling from those colleges and universities.

The last type of probability sample that may be used in nursing research is a systematic sample. This strategy is similar to the random sample because the members of the population are identified and listed. However, rather than using a random digit table to select members of the population, the members are selected at a fixed interval from the list. The selected interval may be every tenth member, every fifth member, or any other interval that will lead to a sample of the size desired. When using a systematic sample, it is important to ensure that the members are not listed in some order that creates bias in the sample. For example, the students from every NLN program of nursing in Wyoming might always be listed starting with undergraduate students followed by graduate students. If the researcher were using systematic sampling, taking every fifth student for a total of five subjects from each program, the students selected might all be undergraduates because only the top part of each list would be included in the sample. If, on the other hand, the students in each program were listed alphabetically, selecting the fifth student for up to five subjects would lead to a sample that was likely to consist of undergraduate and graduate students in the proportion that exists in the population as a whole. Table 6.2 summarizes the types of samples used in qualitative and quantitative research. The same strategy is described using slightly different language, depending on whether it is used in a qualitative or quantitative study.

Table 6.2

Sampling Strategies for Qualitative and Quantitative Research

QUALITATIVE RESEARCH

Convenience sample: Participants who are readily available and represent the phenomenon of interest are included in the sample

Snowball sample: Participants who are known to and recommended by current participants are identified and included, building the sample from a few participants to as many as are needed

Purposive sample: Participants who are intentionally selected because they have certain characteristics that are related to the purpose of the research are included in the sample

QUANTITATIVE RESEARCH

Convenience sample: Members of the population who are easily identified and readily available are included in the sample; a nonprobability sample

Quota sample: One or more criteria are used to ensure that a previously established number of subjects who fit those criteria are included in the sample; a nonprobability sample

Purposive sample: Subjects in the sample are limited to those who have certain characteristics that are related to the purpose of the research; a nonprobability sample

Simple random sample: Subjects are selected by enumerating all members of the population, and a completely random process is used to identify who will be included; a probability sample

Stratified random sample: Members of the population are grouped by one or more characteristics, and subjects are selected from each group using a completely random process; a probability sample

Cluster sample: Groups of the population are enumerated and selected by a completely random process, then individual subjects from within these groups are randomly selected; a probability sample

Systematic sample: The members of a population are enumerated and every kth member at a fixed interval is selected as a subject; a probability sample

Strengths and Weaknesses of Quantitative Sampling Approaches

As with qualitative methods, a convenience sample for a quantitative study also has the advantages of being easy and inexpensive, but it has the disadvantage of not having control over factors that may prejudice the study. A convenience sample consists of those subjects who happen to be at the right place at the right time to be included in the sample. What brings those people to the "right" place and time may have to do with their age, economic status, education, illness, or history—factors that may then prejudice the results of the study. In addition, because a convenience sample takes those who are readily available, often on a first-come basis, participants who willingly and readily volunteer may differ in significant ways from those people who would be more reluctant to participate.

In quantitative research, purposive sampling is used to identify a sample that has certain characteristics relevant to the population of interest. The advantage is that selected factors are clearly defined and identified in the sample, but the disadvantage is that the greater a sample is limited and defined by selected characteristics, the less likely it is to reflect the population at large. In the example of a purposive sampling of families with a member who has survived ovarian or pancreatic cancer, for example, both of these cancers occur in relatively young individuals, leading to their families being relatively young and making the results less applicable to older families. A second bias that may be introduced in this sample is that cancer may make unique demands on families that other highly lethal conditions, such as a severe closed head injury or acute pancreatitis, do not.

In quantitative research, nonprobability sampling strategies are usually more likely to allow bias to enter a sample and make it less likely to be representative of the population of interest. This is because all nonprobability samples have the potential for some outside unidentified factor directing who is and who is not included in the study. By definition, probability samples eliminate the potential of some outside factor systematically entering into the sample because all of the members of the population have an equal chance of being included. However, probability sampling strategies have the disadvantage of being complex, costly, or not feasible, given the population of interest. For example, it would not be possible to enumerate all of the homeless individuals in any particular state as one might enumerate all of the nursing students, making a probability sample more difficult. However, it might be possible to enumerate all homeless shelters in a state, use cluster sampling to randomly select shelters, and then randomly select residents of these shelters. This would yield a probability sample of homeless people who are housed in shelters within the state—but not of all homeless people because many homeless individuals do not use traditional shelters.

One approach that is taken to decrease the potential for a bias in a sample using quantitative methods is to assign subjects randomly to different groups. This is not truly a sampling strategy, but more of a research method that is used to offset a potential problem that can occur from nonprobability sampling. Random assignment ensures that all subjects have an equal chance of being in any particular group within the study. The sample may be one of convenience or purposive, so there may be some bias influencing the results. However, because that bias is evenly distributed among different groups, the bias will not unduly affect the outcomes of the study.

Obviously, random assignment is only an option when a study is going to include more than one group of subjects because the process requires giving each subject in the sample an equal chance to be in any particular group. If a researcher were interested in studying HIV prevention for homeless individuals, he or she might use random assignment of different shelters to try to decrease any bias rather than using a convenience sample of one homeless women's shelter. Often random assignment is desirable but not feasible. In our example, if the researcher wanted to test the usefulness of an HIV prevention program for homeless women, there might be great difficulty in creating two groups and in giving such an intervention to some women in a shelter and not to others. Table 6.3 summarizes the advantages and disadvantages of different sampling strategies.

Table 6.3

Advantages and Disadvantages of Sampling Strategies in Qualitative and Quantitative Research

SAMPLING STRATEGY	QUALITATIVE RESEARCH		QUANTITATIVE RESEARCH	
	Advantages	Disadvantages	Advantages	Disadvantages
Convenience sample	Easier to identify participants; often provides a breadth of information	May "miss" a source of information that is not readily available	Inexpensive; easier to recruit subjects	Most likely to include biases that make it difficult to generalize
Purposive sample	Focuses research on the potentially richest sources of information	Only likely to become a disadvantage if the sampling becomes too narrowed	Locates a sample that is hard to recruit or identify	Likely to include many unique characteristics that limit the ability to generalize
Snowball sample	Allows the researcher to locate sources of information that might otherwise not be identified or available	Could lead to focusing the research and understanding prematurely		
Quota sample			Allows the researcher to control the sample on selected characteristics, so that it more closely resembles the population of interest	Open to systematic variations that can bias the sample
Simple random sample and stratified random sample			Eliminates likelihood of a systematic bias in the sample, so that results are more readily generalized	Time-consuming, costly, may not be feasible to enumerate the population
Cluster sample			Same advantages as a simple random sample, but more efficient	Population of interest may not be readily grouped or the groups identified may narrow the population
Systematic sample			Can be easy to implement	May introduce a bias if there is some systematic factor embedded into the list that occurs at regular intervals

Not all samples consist of individuals. A sampling unit is the element of the population that will be selected and analyzed in the study. The unit depends on the population of interest and can comprise individuals, but it can also be hospitals, families, communities, or outpatient prenatal care programs. Occasionally, samples consist of more than one sampling unit. If we continue with our example of a researcher interested in HIV prevention in homeless women, the researcher might use shelters as the sampling unit and compare two or more types of shelters. Then, the researcher might move to the level of individuals in the shelters. When the sampling unit is shelters, there may be only six or eight in the sample; whereas when the unit becomes the individual residents of the shelters, there may be 75 to 100 in the sample.

Sample Size in Quantitative Research

In addition to understanding how the approach taken to sampling will affect to which patients the results of the study will apply, it is important to understand how the sample size affects the ability to draw conclusions from a study. In quantitative research, the goal of generalizability drives the sample size. Probability samples often can be smaller than nonprobability samples because probability samples control for bias through the random selection process. Nonprobability samples must be larger in general so that any unusual or systematic factors that could bias the study will be canceled out by the number of subjects. For example, if the study "Predictors of life satisfaction in stroke survivors and spousal caregivers after inpatient rehabilitation" (Ostwald et al., 2009) (Appendix A.4) had only included 10 caregiver/stroke survivor pairs instead of the 131 used, there would be a good chance that some of those dyad pairs would have unusual circumstances, such as having had significant personal problems prior to the stroke or having been estranged from each other before the stroke, that might bias the results. Even 1 or 2 of the 10 pairs having unusual circumstances or characteristics could have had a significant impact on the study's results. However, with 262 in the sample (131 pairs), the impact of only 1 or 2 individuals with unusual circumstances will not be as great. Therefore, in general, the larger the sample size in a quantitative study, the more likely the sample will be representative of the population of interest, and the more likely the study will apply to our clinical situations.

In addition to the logic inherent in obtaining larger samples to eliminate the effects of odd or unique cases, sample sizes in quantitative research are determined by the goal of having a reasonable likelihood that the inferential statistics applied to the data will yield statistical significance. Remember that inferential statistics are used to calculate a test statistic that is then compared with a distribution for test statistics occurring by chance alone for that particular sample size. The larger the sample size, the more likely we are to get results that are statistically significant—that is, that did not happen by chance alone. However, it is always costly to recruit and implement a study with many subjects, so it is useful for the researcher to know how large a sample is likely to be needed to be able to apply inferential statistics accurately to the data. Quantitative researchers often use a process called power analysis to determine how large a sample they will need. This allows the researcher to compute the sample size needed to detect a real relationship or difference in the phenomenon under study, if it exists. You may see a written statement of power analysis indicating that a specified sample size was adequate. For example, in "the relationships among self-esteem, stress, coping, eating behavior, and depressive mood in adolescents" (Martyn-Nemeth et al., 2009), the authors provide the results of the power analysis in the "sample" section. However, in the "limitations" section, the authors state, "although an adequate sample size was obtained based on the prospective power analysis, observed effect sizes were actually smaller than expected, which reduced the ability to detect mediating effects of avoidant coping." In this way, the authors are telling you why they used the selected sample size and how it may have impacted the study results.

Summary of Quantitative Sampling

The goal of quantitative sampling strategies is to acquire a sample that is as representative as possible of the population of interest so that the findings from the study can be generalized. To accomplish this, quantitative studies control and limit differences in the sample that may bias or distort the results. Quantitative research does not necessarily want everyone in the study to be exactly alike, only that the sample is similar to the population of interest.

Nonprobability approaches, such as quota sampling and matched sampling, limit variations that may bias a study. For example, it is generally recognized that the people who are most likely to agree to participate in research studies are white and educated. There are several social and historical reasons for this, but as a result, researchers may implement sampling strategies that specifically target under represented groups using a quota or matched sample approach.

The goal of probability sampling is to ensure that every member of a population can be in the study so that no systematic factor defines the sample and makes it different from the population.

Quantitative sampling often limits or controls the variety that qualitative sampling seeks. Researchers in quantitative studies remove themselves from the selection of subjects to eliminate personal bias. Therefore, in quantitative research, a sampling plan is identified and strictly followed, and analysis of data usually is not started until the entire sample is identified and recruited. If the sampling plan includes stratifying or matching, then selected characteristics of the sample are identified and analyzed throughout the selection process, but the findings regarding the variables of interest are not examined until the entire sample is in place. While qualitative studies will thoughtfully change sampling strategies in response to data analysis, a quantitative study will usually follow a clearly identified plan that is determined before sampling has started and that is not modified during the sampling process.

■ DIFFERENCES IN QUALITATIVE AND QUANTITATIVE SAMPLING

Earlier, we stated that qualitative and quantitative sampling differ in overall goal and approach. Because these goals are different, the strengths and weaknesses of the different strategies for each approach differ as well. This is important to understand because it allows you to understand better how a sample and the approach taken to obtain that sample affect the usefulness of the research for your EBN practice. A summary of the differences in sampling approaches between qualitative and quantitative research is provided in Table 6.4.

Table 6.4

Differences in Sampling Approaches Between Quantitative and Qualitative Research

SAMPLING APPROACH	QUALITATIVE RESEARCH	QUANTITATIVE RESEARCH
General goal of sampling	To include as many sources as possible that add to the richness, depth, and variety of the data	To ensure that only the variables of interest influence the results of the study by limiting extraneous variations in the sample
Approach to sampling	Usually driven by the data as it is collected; therefore, flexible and evolving as the study develops	Established before beginning the process of sampling and followed strictly to avoid introducing bias into the sample
Language for those in the sample	Participants, volunteers, and informants	Subjects

CORE CONCEPT 6.2

Sampling strategies in qualitative and quantitative research differ in their goals and approaches, even when they are using a similar strategy.

■ PROBLEMS WITH THE SAMPLING PROCESS

As we discussed sampling, it may have crossed your mind that many patients are intimidated by or distrustful of the research process and may decline to participate. This reluctance is a hard reality of research with human subjects: The goal of finding a representative sample might jeopardize the goal of maintaining the rights of individuals. Chapter 7 will discuss in detail the rights of human subjects, but we will mention here that researchers know that the process of seeking informed consent can bias a sample because of some systematic characteristic that causes certain individuals to decline to be in a study. Studies that examine who generally agrees to participate in research studies show that those who are more educated are more likely to participate than those who are less educated. Thus, in research, the sample may have more highly educated patients than those with less education simply because the consent process is intimidating or because research is not viewed as valuable by those with less education. Clearly, the obligation to ensure that the basic human rights of potential subjects are protected supersedes the concern that consent processes may limit study enrollment, but researchers must consider this factor as they examine the results of their studies.

An associated problem that can occur in sampling is the withdrawal of subjects partway through a study. Individuals who agree to participate may withdraw for a number of reasons, such as personal problems, lack of time, or even physically moving out of an area. A researcher will usually plan for subject withdrawal by attempting to include more subjects in a research study than are actually needed. However, if there is some consistent reason why subjects withdraw, then the ability to generalize results of the study is limited. Withdrawal from a study is an active statement of a decision to no longer participate in that study. Sometimes subjects do not formally withdraw but simply drop out without notification or are lost to follow-up. In this case, the subject simply cannot be found to complete a study or does not return study materials. For example, in studies of smoking cessation, there is always a concern that the subjects who do not succeed in quitting may drop out of the study due to discouragement. This can lead to the final sample including a higher proportion of successful quitters than is really the case, biasing the results by yielding an artificially inflated success rate.

Whether a potential subject declined to be in a study, withdrew, or was lost to follow-up, it is important to know as much as possible about what happened during the sampling process in order to make informed decisions about the use of the results in clinical practice. Therefore, as an intelligent user of research, you should expect that the sampling section of a research report will tell you enough about the process of acquiring the sample so that you can judge how that process affected the results. Often, that information includes a statement about the number of potential subjects who declined to be in a study, withdrew, or dropped out. When subjects withdraw or drop out of a study, some information is usually given about them. Researchers can use this information to compare the subjects who stayed in the study with those who did not, and they may be able to tell us whether there is some important difference between those who did and did not stay in a study.

In addition to concern about who agrees to be in a study and who stays in a study, another problem that can affect the sampling process is the exclusion and inclusion criteria. As discussed earlier, sample criteria define a study's population. A criterion for exclusion is a characteristic that makes the potential subject ineligible for the study, and a criterion for inclusion is a characteristic that makes the subject eligible for the study. Researchers choose to focus on inclusion or exclusion, depending on the nature of the desired sample. In a convenience sample in which numerous subjects are being sought, a researcher will generally discuss exclusion because most individuals will be eligible to participate, and only a few will be excluded. A study that aims for a tightly controlled sample will more likely describe criteria for inclusion because the focus is on who can enter the study.

In either case, these criteria define the study's population and may limit how the results can be used in practice. For example, an RN working in home care in a large, multicultural city would certainly find the predictors of life satisfaction study relevant to practice. However, the study on predictors of life satisfaction excluded subjects who were unable to read or write English, thus excluding a large number of the population of interest in this RN's situation. To use the results of the predictors of life satisfaction article in practice, an RN in a large, multicultural city would need to decide whether results with subjects who do speak and write English are likely to be meaningful for those who do not.

The last problem with the sampling process is having incomplete data. This is a problem of data collection, but it is closely linked to how a sample may be changed or limited, which affects how useful it is for clinical practice. *Incomplete data* refers to partial information about the variables in a study. Although the specific problems that can lead to incomplete data are addressed in Chapter 8, the effect of this is that the researcher may drop data about selected subjects from the analysis of the results. This raises the question of whether those subjects had some characteristic or characteristics that led to their incomplete data. If so, then a systematic bias will be introduced into the final sample.

Suppose, for example, that some of the subjects in a smoking cessation study completed only part of a questionnaire used by the researcher and did not answer questions about how much they were smoking after they completed a smoking-cessation program. If the researcher drops these subjects from the analysis (because the amount of smoking after the program is a major variable in the study, and there are no data available for these subjects), then it is likely that the sample is biased in the direction of subjects who were successful and, therefore, willing to report their smoking status. We do not know why the data were incomplete, but we must be concerned that the reason is connected to the variables under study.

In summary, several aspects of the sampling process can lead to problems with the final study sample. The criteria used to identify who will be included or excluded from a study may narrow the sample to the point that the population represented no longer reflects the characteristics of real patient populations. Subjects may withdraw or fail to follow up for some consistent reason that is related to the purposes of the study itself, thus limiting what we can learn from the study. Incomplete information may be collected because of some factor that relates to the study, causing some data about subjects to be dropped from the data analysis and changing the actual sample. As intelligent readers and users of research, nurses must understand not only the strengths and weaknesses of different sampling strategies discussed in this chapter, but also what can go wrong with the sampling process and how that affects the meaning of the study. Table 6.5 summarizes the problems discussed. Other factors that can lead to problems with samples are discussed in the next section.

■ PROBLEMS WITH SAMPLING OUTCOMES

In addition to problems with the sampling process, some problems can occur with the sampling outcomes—that is, the final sample—that are only indirectly related to the strategy used and problems that can occur in the sampling process. Previously, we discussed the importance of avoiding bias, an unintended factor that confounds the findings of a study, in a sample. Some sampling strategies, such as nonprobability sampling, are more open to a bias, whereas others, such as probability sampling, are less open to it. When a researcher

Table 6.5

Potential Problems With the Process of Sampling

PROBLEM	EXAMPLE
Subject withdrawal from study	After starting in a study, subjects may decide that they do not want to continue to participate. If some aspect related to the study leads to withdrawal, it can bias the sample.
Lost to follow-up	After agreeing to be in a study, subjects become unavailable to be in it. This may include not returning questionnaires, missing appointments, moving, or having a change in telephone number. If the subjects lost to follow-up represent a particular characteristic related to the study (perhaps high income), then the final sample may have a bias.
Exclusion/inclusion criteria applicability of the sample	If a sample is tightly controlled or restricted to make the research successful, it may lead to the population being so specific that clinical meaningfulness is limited.
Incomplete data	Data are not provided, are skipped, or are missed, causing the researcher to drop subjects from the analysis of the results. If there is some systematic reason for the data being incomplete, dropping subjects can bias the results.

uses a nonprobability sampling strategy, the process may be implemented correctly, but the resulting sample may still be biased.

One type of bias that can be introduced in a nonprobability sample occurs when a researcher fails to recognize or consider subjective factors or approaches that could influence participation in the study. For example, a researcher may be more comfortable approaching either men or women when trying to recruit subjects, thus unconsciously biasing a study in the direction of one gender. In addition, a researcher may collect data only at a certain time of the day, such as Monday through Friday, between 8 AM and 5 PM, preventing anyone who works 12-hour shifts or night shifts from being in the study. If type of work and hours worked are related in some way to what is under study, then a bias has been introduced.

Another kind of bias may occur as a result of the unique characteristics or perspectives of the person who is actually recruiting subjects. For example, because an RN's main role is to provide care for patients, he or she may not be particularly motivated to provide a patient with information about the potential to participate in a study or may conclude that a patient does not need to be bothered with a study. An example of this introduction of bias into a sample might be a study that is conducted in a clinic that cares for both physical and mental health problems. If the person recruiting subjects primarily works with the mental health patients and recruits familiar patients, then the subjects in the study are more likely to have mental illness than the overall population of the clinic.

A second problem that can occur with samples is selectivity. Selectivity is the tendency of certain population segments to agree to participate in studies. In this case, the bias is not introduced by the researcher but by those people who are willing and interested in being in a study. We have already discussed one kind of general selectivity that occurs in all research: the tendency of more educated individuals to agree to participate compared with less educated individuals. However, selectivity can occur that is more specific to the purposes of a particular study. A particular study may attract people who are worried about the problem under study or those who are lonely and want someone with whom they can talk. It may be that mostly women are willing to participate in a particular study or, perhaps, only people with family members who have experienced a particular problem will return a mailed questionnaire. The difficulty for the researcher and for the user of research is to determine whether some aspect of the study may have led to selectivity in the sample and how this, in turn, affects the knowledge gained from the study.

Limited response rates can be another problem with samples. Response rate is the proportion of individuals who participate in a study divided by the number who agreed to be in a study but did not participate in it. Response rate is not a significant problem when the study occurs in a controlled setting, such as a hospital, because those who agree to participate are essentially a captive group. However, in almost any research survey in which subjects are recruited and asked to return a questionnaire or provide data by appointment, some individuals do not return the questionnaire or keep the appointment. As with the other problems that affect samples, we need to know who the nonresponders are and why they did not respond. Their lack of a response caused by a factor related in some way to the study could bias the sample. In these types of situations, the research report should tell you the response rate so that you have an idea of whether a large or small number of possible subjects did not participate in the study. Withdrawal and dropping out of a study are two reasons why response rates can be low.

All of the problems in samples that we have discussed occur in recruiting subjects for any type of study, but they will cause more problems in nonprobability samples than in probability samples. Although the potential bias of a low response rate can affect a random sample, the effects of selectivity and researcher bias are mostly offset in a random sample because the entire population is enumerated, and all members of the population have a chance of being included in the study. Therefore, it is common to find more detail describing the sampling process and the final sample when nonprobability sampling is used because the researcher wants to ensure to the reader that steps were taken to prevent the potential biases that may be present in the final sample.

In summary, three factors are related to both sampling strategy and the sampling process that can lead to problems in samples. The first is bias *introduced by the researcher* or the individual recruiting the sample that reflects the beliefs or characteristics of that researcher or recruiter. The second is *self-selection by individuals* within the population that can lead to a bias. The third is a *limited response rate* that makes us wonder about the characteristics of those who did not respond and how they differ from those who did. Table 6.6 summarizes these three types of problems with samples.

Table 6.6

General Potential Problems With Samples	
PROBLEM	EXAMPLE
Bias in subject recruitment	Some aspect of the recruitment process allows an unidentified factor to enter into the identification of subjects requested to participate in the study. Examples include time of day of sampling or recruiter comfort level with selected subjects. *Selectivity*: Certain subjects volunteer to be in the study due to some characteristic that could relate to the problem being studied. Examples include subjects who are older and lonely being more available or subjects who care about a particular problem volunteering. This can lead to over representation of one segment of the population in the sample.
Response rate	Many potential subjects or actual subjects do not participate in the study. If a study has a low response rate, then the ability to generalize the results of the study to the entire population of interest is limited.

■ COMMON ERRORS IN REPORTS OF SAMPLES

The most common error that occurs in study reports of sampling is a lack of adequate detail, leading to the inability to decide whether the types of subjects or participants allow us to apply the results of the study to our clinical situation. In qualitative research, this error will most likely take the form of an inadequate description of the study setting and participants. We have been using the example of a researcher examining a study pertaining to homeless individuals' satisfaction with health care. In order to determine whether the results of such a study are useful to our clinical practice, we must have information about the environment of the participants. If this research had only used participants who were housed in substance-free shelters, the understanding gained from the study would be less complete than the understanding gained from a study of participants from several settings, including a clinic, a soup kitchen, and different shelters.

In quantitative studies, the information that may be missing or inadequate in a research report usually involves the process of acquiring the sample. To judge either the representativeness of a sample or whether the sample reflects the clinical population of interest requires knowing the sampling strategy and the sampling criteria as well as how the strategy was implemented. For example, a convenience sample of nursing students exiting a college of nursing building at lunchtime is more likely to be representative of the nursing students in that college than a convenience sample of students from any one particular classroom. This is because students who exit the building are more likely to reflect a range of levels of study, whereas a single class will mostly consist of students at the same level.

Similarly, a random sample of homeless shelters that then takes a convenience sample of homeless individuals is less likely to yield a representative sample of homeless persons than a random sample of those staying at all shelters on a particular night. To use information about sampling intelligently, we must know the setting where the study occurred and the process of implementing the sampling plan. We also must be given the descriptive statistics that relate the characteristics of the final sample acquired.

■ CONNECTING SAMPLING TO THE STUDY RESULTS AND CONCLUSIONS

We started this chapter by asking whether the results and conclusions from the five different studies used so far could be used to guide practice in the different clinical situations described in previous clinical cases. Sampling strategies connect to the results of a study in several ways. In both qualitative and quantitative studies, the characteristics of the sample affect the meaning of the results. The appropriateness and focus of sampling in a qualitative study both are driven by and drive data collection, and the detail and complexity of the resulting themes or theory will reflect that sampling. In quantitative studies, the sampling strategy dictates how certain we can be that the results found represent what exists in the real population. Along with sample strategy, sample size also affects the believability of study results. In the clearest connection between sampling and the potential results, some studies require a certain sample size to use certain inferential statistical procedures.

Sampling should also be connected to the conclusions of a study. The nature of the sample and the sampling strategies used may be either a limitation of the study or an aspect that needs further evaluation. For example, let us take the study we introduced in this chapter, "The use of narratives to identify characteristics leading to a productive life following acquired brain injury" (Fraas & Calvert, 2009) (Appendix A.5). In this study, the authors obtained participants from a "community based postrehabilitation program for adults with

ABI" (p. 316). In the conclusions section, the authors state, "The participants in this study represented a sample of individuals who have made remarkable progress during their recovery from ABI. Analysis of the interviews conducted with these survivors identified several themes congruent with each that were influential to postinjury successes" (p. 232). This conclusion fits with the sample used. If the authors had stated that their conclusion applied to families of patients with any kind of traumatic injury, we would have had to question the connection made.

▪ CRITICALLY READING THE SAMPLE SECTION OF RESEARCH REPORTS FOR USE IN EVIDENCE-BASED NURSING PRACTICE

Box 6.2 provides us with questions to ask when critically reading the sample section of a research report. The first question is "Did the report include a clearly identified section or paragraphs about sampling?" This is fairly straightforward, yet it is surprising that sometimes we have to hunt to find the information about sampling. In the report "The use of narratives to identify characteristics leading to a productive life following acquired brain injury" (Fraas & Calvert, 2009) (Appendix A.5), we can easily find the sample information on page 316 under the heading "Method: Participants." However, in some articles it is more difficult to find information on the sample. Part of this is reflective of the different types of research methods used, and some may be the style of the authors' writing or the format of the journal in which the report is published.

Our second question is "Did the report give me enough information to understand how and why this sample was chosen?" The report found by the RN in the clinical case for this chapter, "The use of narratives to identify characteristics leading to a productive life following acquired brain injury" (Fraas & Calvert, 2009) (Appendix A.5), is a good example to look at to answer this question. It gives us a sense of who the sample represented—survivors of ABI who participated in a community-based postrehabilitation program—and identifies further population characteristics. The article gives a clear sense of who were included in the sample, but do we know why they were chosen? In order to

---

Box 6.2

How to Critically Read the Sample Section of a Research Report?

Does the report answer the question "To what types of patients do these research conclusions apply—who was in the study?"

1. Did the report include a clearly identified section or paragraphs about sampling?
2. Did the report give me enough information to understand how and why this sample was chosen?
3. Is there enough information about the sample to tell me whether the research is relevant for my clinical population?
4. Was enough information given for me to understand how rights of human subjects were protected?
5. Would my patient population have been placed at risk if they had participated in this study?
6. Can I identify how information was collected about the sample?

understand this, we will need to read the literature review section, which will be discussed in Chapter 10.

Our third question is "Is there enough information about the sample to tell me if the research is relevant for my clinical population?" This is an important topic in evidence-based nursing practice. If you plan to use research-based evidence in order to answer clinical questions, you need to critically examine whether the sample is similar to the population in which you are interested. The first part of answering this is based on how well you have formed your clinical question. As you remember from Chapter 1, your question gives a "Who, What, Where, When" that establishes who and what makes up your clinical population. Once you know whom you are interested in, you then need to see what the report tells you about the sample. The clinical case for this chapter yielded a clinical question of "What interventions should be included in a plan of care to assist patients who have had a traumatic brain injury to lead a productive life?" This clinical question tells the RN in our case that the researchers are looking for evidence about a population that includes (1) TBI patients, (2) recovery successes leading to a productive life, and (3) TBI patient ranges from a newly injured patient to patient recovery. If we then check the report, we see that there is a variation between the RN's clinical population of interest and the sample in that the sample included only participants from a postrehabilitation program. However, the data collection contained information from diagnosed injury through recovery leading to the conclusion that is was a nice match between the RN's clinical population of interest and the sample.

As we continue to critically read the sample section of a research report, we come to our fourth question, "Was enough information given for me to understand how rights of human subjects were protected?" The issue of using human subjects will be discussed in detail in Chapter 7, but we probably have some awareness now that sample subjects can be vulnerable and have rights even if they agree to participate in research. All subjects need to know the risks of any research and to have the right not to be coerced into participation. In the "The use of narratives to identify characteristics leading to a productive life following acquired brain injury" (Fraas & Calvert, 2009) (Appendix A.5), the authors tell us about the rights of human subjects. They state, "All participants provided informed consent to allow their responses to be used for research purposes" (p. 317). We will see in Chapter 7 that this may not be enough information to constitute a thorough statement regarding the protections of subjects' rights. We see similar but perhaps more clear statements in other reports that we have read. The fifth question we can ask is "Would my patient population have been placed at risk if they had participated in this study?" In order to answer this, you need to be clear of who your patient population is. Much like we stated in addressing the third question, a strong clinical question needs to be formed with a clear *Who*, *What*, *Where*, and *When* in order to answer this. In our clinical case, our RN is interested in interventions to incorporate into a plan of care that would help a patient with a newly diagnosed TBI through recovery lead a productive life. As the RN reads the characteristics of leading a productive life study (Fraas & Calvert, 2009) (Appendix A.5), the RN will need to think about what the sample was asked to do while they were participating in the study. In the same study, the subjects were asked to participate in interviews to discuss their life stories before and after the injury. As we think about it, there is usually not much risk to the sample when participating in interviews. But what if the researcher had decided to take blood specimens to measure serum cortisol and track the stress level of family members in that manner? We can now see a little more risk is present. The subject may bleed from the site of the blood draw, or the site might become infected. While unlikely, it is not risk free. Finally, what if the researcher in this study had decided to include brain scans using the injection of a contrast dye prior to the scan in order to measure activity in the stress-related areas of the family members' brains as they experienced having a family member in the ICU? We can now see a considerable increase in the risk to the sample. The injection of a dye prior to the brain scan will give the best results, but the dye can be dangerous, people can be allergic to it, and the injection might be the source of significant complications. Thus, to answer our fifth critical question, we need to look at what our sample was asked to do and then decide whether our population could, and would, be willing to do the same procedure.

Our final question is "Can I identify how information was collected about the sample?" This is very important because it begins to speak to your ability to implement an evidence-based change in patient care based on the study. The RN in our clinical case about patients with TBI is interested in finding interventions to help these patients return to a productive life. The RN will want to see whether the information collected during the study could reasonably be collected in his or her population. The authors of the characteristics of leading a productive life study (Fraas & Calvert, 2009) report that they collected information in the form of interviews. They also state how the interviews were conducted, how long the interviews lasted, and who conducted them. What is not as clear is where the interviews took place.

■ PUBLISHED REPORTS—WOULD YOU CHANGE YOUR PRACTICE?

The importance of being able to critically read something like the sample section of a report is to allow you to become comfortable in deciding which evidence you should use in EBN. As your skill at reading research-based evidence improves, the overarching question becomes "Should I change my practice based on this published report?"

In this chapter, we have concentrated on critically reading the sample section as part of reaching a conclusion about EBN. We have seen thus far that sampling strategies discussed in a report are directly connected to results and conclusions and that understanding the language and meaning of sampling in research adds one more piece to the puzzle of reading and comprehending research for use in EBN practice. Once you have decided whether the population for the study reflects the type of patients or situations that are of interest to you, the subjects' rights were protected, the sample reflects your population, and the approach taken to choosing the sample limits the meaning of the study, you are well on your way to knowing whether the study results can be applied to your clinical question.

As we review the reports that we have examined so far, you may be starting to see that the RNs in our clinical cases have not so much changed their minds about practice as much as they have acquired a better sense of how useful these research studies will be for their practice. They have received insight into other issues to consider, and they have raised other questions. EBN provides information, but it will never directly tell you what to do. As the RN, you will always need to think through the evidence and apply it to your practice in the best way.

In summary, information about the sampling strategy and the actual sample are important in understanding which results of a study may apply to your clinical question. Unique language is associated with the sampling process for both qualitative and quantitative research. Sampling in qualitative research gathers as rich and complete a set of data as possible, and sampling strategies are guided by and may change based on the concurrent data analysis. Sampling in quantitative research eliminates potential bias and gathers information from a subset of the population that closely resembles the actual population. Sampling strategies in this type of research are carefully planned, with important characteristics defined and used to limit or control the subjects. Probability samples are considered to be better than nonprobability samples in quantitative research because these types of samples eliminate systematic bias, but they are also more difficult and costly than nonprobability sampling. Sample size depends on the strategy and methods used, with qualitative samples generally being smaller than samples for quantitative studies.

Understanding the language of sampling and the meaning of the sampling strategies helps to make the relationship clear between the sample and the results and conclusions of the study. This chapter focused entirely on the language and process of sampling in quantitative and qualitative research. What we have not discussed is the important subject of the rights of individuals who participate in research. This topic is discussed in the next chapter.

OUT-OF-CLASS EXERCISE

Free Write

Before you move on to the next chapter, take a moment to think about the in-class questionnaire that you may have completed or about some past occasion when you were asked to participate in some type of research. Write a paragraph describing how the study or questionnaire was explained to you and what you were told with regard to filling it out. Then, write your thoughts about whether your rights, safety, and privacy were protected. Finally, write down types of individuals or situations that you feel should be excluded from participating in research. What makes you believe that these individuals or situations should or should not be included in research? Refer to these paragraphs as you read Chapter 7.

_____

_____

_____

_____

_____

_____

_____

_____

_____

_____

_____

_____

_____

_____

_____

_____

_____

_____

_____

_____

_____

_____

References

Fraas, M., & Calvert, M. (2009). The use of narratives to identify characteristics leading to a productive life following acquired brain injury. *American Journal of Speech-Language Pathology, 18*, 315–328.

Hsieh, C., Sprod, L., Hydock, D., Carter, S., Hayward, R., & Schneider, C. (2008). Effects of a supervised exercise intervention on recovery from treatment regimens in breast cancer survivors. *Oncology Nursing Forum, 35*(6), 909–915.

Landis, A., Parker, K., & Dunbar, S. (2009). Sleep, hunger, satiety, food cravings, and caloric intake in adolescents. *Journal of Nursing Scholarship, 41*(2), 115–123.

Martyn-Nemeth, P., Penckofer, S., Gulanick, M., Velsor-Friedrich, B., & Bryant, F. (2009). The relationships among self-esteem, stress, coping, eating behavior, and depressive mood in adolescents. *Research in Nursing & Health, 32*, 96–109.

Ostwald, S., Godwin, K. M., & Cron, S. G. (2009). Predictors of life satisfaction in stroke survivors and spousal caregivers after inpatient rehabilitation. *Rehabilitation Nursing, 34*, 160–174.

Resources

LoBiondo-Wood, G., Haber, J., & Krainovich Miller, B. (2009). Overview of the research process. In G. LoBiondo-Wood & J. Haber (Eds.), *Nursing research: Methods, critical appraisal, and utilization* (6th ed.). St. Louis, MO: Mosby.

Locke, L. F., Silverman, S. J., & Spirduso, W. W. (2009). *Reading and understanding research* (3rd ed.). Thousand Oaks, CA: Sage Publications.

Pedhazur, E. J., & Schmelkin, L. P. (1991). *Measurement, design, and analysis: An integrated approach*. Hillsdale, NJ: Lawrence Erlbaum & Associates.

Polit, D. F., & Beck, C. T. (2007). *Nursing research: Principles and methods* (8th ed.). Philadelphia, PA: Lippincott Williams & Wilkins.

Ethics: What Can Go Wrong?

LEARNING OBJECTIVE

The student will evaluate legal and ethical principles, and potential problems as they apply to research.

Which Nursing Actions Are Research and Require Special Ethical Consideration?

Informed Consent

When Research Is Exempt

Critically Reading Reports of Sampling and Recognizing Common Errors

Published Reports—What Do They Say About Consent and the Sampling Process?

KEY TERMS

Anonymous
Assent
Coercion
Confidentiality
Exempt
Five human rights in research

Informed consent
Institutional review board (IRB)
Practice
Risk:benefit ratio
Withdrawal

Clinical Case • We have thus far looked at several aspects of the process of research as we have followed our RNs in the four clinical cases discussed in earlier chapters. As you can see, there is much to consider as a nurse draws conclusions about clinical questions that are based on research studies. For example, in Chapter 6, we saw the importance of considering the sampling approaches used in studies. In Chapters 4 and 5, we saw the importance of considering inferential and descriptive statistics, or in Chapter 3, the importance of carefully critiquing the discussion and conclusions sections of studies. However, in addition to knowing about the sampling approach, statistics used, or the conclusions reached, we must also understand the legal and ethical principles that guide the conduct of the researcher in today's world. Ethical and legal considerations are important because they help us understand who can be recruited into research studies, how the research can recruit these people, and how the studies are to be conducted. Understanding the ethical and legal issues surrounding research also helps us to understand why we often do not find studies on the specific populations with which we are working, or those that we are interested in knowing more about.

To better understand the connections between legal and ethical principles and the research process, consider the following modified version of the clinical case from Chapters 1 and 2, "Sleep, Hunger, Satiety, Food Cravings, and Caloric Intake in Adolescents" (Landis, Parker, & Dunbar, 2009) (Appendix A.1). In this study, the Institutional Review Board (IRB) for Protection of Human Subjects at Emory University was consulted, and it approved the study. The school district in which the study was conducted was also in agreement with the parameters of the study. You will learn more in this chapter about how important it is to secure IRB approval prior to conducting formal research. To recruit participants, the researcher gave a short presentation about the study, and forms were given out so students could determine whether they were interested in participating. For students who wished to participate, parents (or legal guardians) were contacted to request a meeting between them, the child, and the researcher. Informed consent was then obtained as well as assent (agreement) from the participants.

■ WHICH NURSING ACTIONS ARE RESEARCH AND REQUIRE SPECIAL ETHICAL CONSIDERATION?

One important notion regarding research ethics is being able to understand when a particular nursing action is research and when it is a care practice. Research actions require full patient consent and institutional review board (IRB) authorization (concepts we will discuss shortly). However, practice actions are held to a different standard. Sometimes nurses may be asked to collect new data or to perform their care actions in a different manner. It is important for the nurse to be able to determine whether the new action is research or whether it is new care practice in order to safeguard the patient.

While both research and practice can often look alike and can actually occur together, they are different primarily in the purpose and expected outcome. The Belmont Commission Report (1979) defined ethical principles for the protection of human subjects of research and in doing so provided guidelines for deciding whether an action is research or whether it is practice. **Practice** is composed of actions that are planned and implemented exclusively for the enhancement of health and the improvement of the well-being of an individual. Research, on the other hand, is composed of systematic actions that are planned and implemented exclusively to test a hypothesis, to examine a phenomenon, to allow for conclusions to be drawn, or to generate new knowledge or confirm past knowledge. Research does not have any outcome that specifically improves the patients' health or well-being.

Two professional documents exist to help an RN make decisions regarding the ethics of research. These documents are from the American Nurses Association (ANA) and from the International Council of Nurses (ICN). The ANA's Code of Ethics for Nurses was approved by the ANA House of Delegates in 2001 and provides details on the ethical standards of RNs (ANA, 2001). In 2005, the ANA released Interpretive Statements to accompany the 2001 Code of Ethics for Nurses, which can be found on their Web site (visit thepoint.lww.com/Rebar3e for the direct link). The ANA states that the Code of Ethics for Nurses with Interpretive Statements provides nurses with a framework to use in ethical analysis and decision making (ANA, 2005). The ICN Code of Ethics for Nurses (ICN, 2000) is an international code of ethics for nurses and was first adopted by the ICN in 1953, revised and reaffirmed at various times since, and most recently revised in 2006. Both of these documents assert that nurses have fundamental responsibilities to promote health, prevent illness, restore health, and alleviate suffering. Inherent in these ethical statements is the belief that nursing is integrally involved with respecting human rights, including the right to life, to dignity, and to be treated with respect. Nursing research, as an action in which nurses are involved, carries the need to safeguard these rights of patients.

The two mentioned documents are predicated on three ethical principles important to research. They focus on autonomy, beneficence, and justice. Autonomy, as it pertains to research, is a fundamental ethical principle that underpins both self-determination and the right of every person to give clear and knowledgeable informed consent. If autonomy is not safeguarded, a nurse has failed to uphold the ethical standards of the profession. Remember that a patient may, appropriately, be asked to participate in research that carries great risk. The research is not inherently unethical as long as the person's autonomy rights have been addressed and the person's decision to be involved in research is a fully informed decision. There is no requirement that researchers only propose studies that involve no risk. Researchers and the nurses involved must, however, fully reveal any potential risk and assist patients to be fully informed so that patients can make unencumbered decisions about whether or not to enter the study.

The second ethical principle, beneficence, is the basis of the ability of nurses to act in the best interest of the research subject and to always function in an advocacy role as patients consider becoming research subjects. The third principle, justice, is fundamental in research and identifies how subjects should be recruited and treated during the research study. Justice assumes that nurses will ensure that research subjects are always selected from a wide array of the population and are not recruited in coercive ways.

■ INFORMED CONSENT

The RN in our clinical case has been oriented to the study to be carried out and realizes that a patient's consent to participate is important; the nurse also knows that, as a professional, he or she is ethically obligated to follow the three ethical principles of autonomy, beneficence, and justice. The nurse decides to review the consent form so that he or she can plan how to respond to any questions that a participant in the study might have. Upon review, the nurse realizes that there are three distinct components to the consent form: (1) a description of the study, including specifically what the subject will be asked to do as a research participant; (2) a description of any potential risks and any potential benefits to participating in the study; and (3) a description of the subject's rights if he or she chooses to participate. Each of these sections of an informed consent relates to at least one of the five human rights in research that have been identified by the ANA guidelines for nurses working with patient information that may require interpretation. They are

1. Right to self-determination
2. Right to privacy and dignity
3. Right to anonymity and confidentiality

Table 7.1

Definitions of the Five Rights of Human Subjects in Research (ANA, 1985)	
RIGHT	DEFINITION/DESCRIPTION
Right to self-determination	Individuals are autonomous and have the right to make a knowledgeable, voluntary decision that is free from coercion as to whether or not to participate in research or to withdraw from a study.
Right to privacy and dignity	Individuals have the right to the respect of choosing what they do and what is done to them and to control when and how information about them is shared with others.
Right to anonymity and confidentiality	Individuals should be afforded the respect of having information they share or that is gathered about them kept in a manner that does not connect them to the individual information and the respect of choosing for themselves who knows that they are participating in a research study.
Right to fair treatment	Individuals have the right to nondiscriminatory selection of participants in a study, to nonjudgmental treatment that honors all agreements established in the consent, and to resources to address any concerns or problems that should arise during participation in the research.
Right to protection from discomfort and harm	Individuals have the right to be protected from exploitation and to be assured that every effort is made to minimize any potential harm from a study, while maximizing the potential benefits of the study.

4. Right to fair treatment
5. Right to protection from discomfort and harm (ANA, 1985)

Table 7.1 defines these rights, and we discuss them as they relate to the process of research.

Informed consent is the legal principle that an individual or his or her authorized representative can make a decision about participation in a research study only after being given all the relevant information pertaining to the study as well as being given a reasonable amount of time to consider the decision to participate. The written consent form is a legal document indicating that the principle of informed consent has been adhered to. This document, along with a relatively detailed description of the study, is generated by a researcher before beginning a study and is reviewed and approved by an entity called an **institutional review board (IRB)**. An IRB is a board created for the explicit purpose of reviewing any proposed research study to be implemented within an institution or by employees of an institution. Most hospitals have an internal IRB, whereas small clinics may share one or use one associated with a local hospital or university. The individuals who sit on the IRB always represent a variety of backgrounds and interests and usually include members who are researchers, one or two lay members from the community, and individuals, such as ministers, who have a special knowledge and interest in ethics. The diversity of the members' backgrounds helps to ensure that a proposed research study is evaluated from numerous perspectives. The IRB does not examine the scientific merit of the proposed study, only the ethics of what is being proposed and what is being asked of the study subject.

The establishment of IRBs occurred in response to incidences of unethical and dishonest research practices in the past. Best-known examples include the Nazi medical experiments brought to light during the Nuremberg War Crimes Trial following World War II and the Tuskegee Syphilis "Study" that withheld treatment for syphilis from men from a poor black community in the South without their knowledge in order to study the progression of the disease. To address the concern of ethics in research, the National Research Act, Public Law 93-348, was signed on July 12, 1974. This law created the National Commission for the Protection of Human Subjects of Biomedical and Behavioral Research. This federal commission was empowered to identify the ethical principles that should be included in the planning and conduct of all research involving human subjects. They further were empowered to develop guidelines to ensure that research is conducted in accordance with those principles. The results of this commission still impact research today and include (1) identifying the differences between research and activities that are routine care practices; (2) establishing the importance of reviewing the risk:benefit ratio to determine the ethical nature of planned research; (3) establishing guidelines for the selection of human subjects for participation in research; and (4) identifying what is required in the informed consent process for various types of research. The findings of this commission were released in the previously mentioned *Belmont Report* (1979).

The Belmont Report's name was derived from the Smithsonian Institution's Belmont Conference Center, where the commission met to finalize the report. It remains the most important modern document that identifies basic ethical principles and guidelines that should be applied to all research involving human subjects. The report was published in the *Federal Register* and is still the guiding document whose principles are used by IRBs as they consider research proposals. Although the majority of researchers are honest and ethical, there have been continued occasions when researchers have falsified data, failed to disclose risks, or failed to report adverse events that have occurred during their research. IRBs exist to guard against these types of unethical and dishonest practices.

The function of an IRB is to ensure that the research project includes procedures to protect the rights of its subjects. It is also charged with deciding whether the research is basically sound to ensure that the time and potential risk to the participant is outweighed by the potential scientific gain that could come from the study. A research study that asks anything of individuals is, at a minimum, using their time. A study that is not well planned or has a major flaw will make the results meaningless and wastes its participants' time and effort. It is the IRB's responsibility to make sure, as best can be determined, that this is unlikely to happen.

Beyond ensuring the soundness of a research study, an IRB also looks at the balance between the risks and benefits of the study. This evaluation of the risk:benefit ratio (read as "risk to benefit" ratio) is integral to protecting a study subject from discomfort and harm. A risk:benefit ratio is a comparison of the level of risk present for subjects compared with the level of benefit. A study that proposes to ask healthy college-age students to take an experimental acne drug that has a high potential of causing kidney failure has a very poor risk:benefit ratio and would not be approved. But a study that asks terminal cancer patients to take an experimental cancer drug that may cause kidney failure has a much better risk:benefit ratio and would likely be approved.

Researchers are obligated to identify any potential risks to participation in their study and describe how they will try to prevent these risks, how they will monitor for their occurrence, and what they will do if they occur. If the researcher's plan is considered inadequate, the proposed research will not be approved. Some studies entail risks to life or health that simply are too great, regardless of their potential benefit and despite efforts made to minimize those risks.

CORE CONCEPT 7.1

It is unethical and illegal to implement a research study that uses animal or human subjects without IRB approval.

One potential risk to research participants is considered so important that it is viewed as a separate right. This is the risk of a breach in anonymity, confidentiality, or both. A participant in research is considered **anonymous** when no one, including the researcher, can link the study data from a particular individual to that individual. **Confidentiality** is related to anonymity because although the researcher knows the identity of the participant, it ensures that neither the identities of participants nor any information that participants provide individually will be revealed to anyone. Because many nursing studies examine sensitive areas such as abusive relationships, HIV status, sexual function, anxiety, and substance use, merely being identified as a participant in a study can reveal personal and private information about an individual. A study that follows subjects over time cannot ensure anonymity until the study is complete because the researcher must know who the participants are to stay in touch with them throughout the study. However, researchers can guarantee that participation in and responses of individuals in the study are kept confidential and that only the researcher(s) has access to the data. Once a study is completed, all links between individuals and specific data can be destroyed; this ensures that future work with the research data will be anonymous. As with any potential risks in a study, a researcher must tell the IRB in writing how the confidentiality and anonymity of subjects in the study will be achieved and how the security of any collected data will be maintained.

The IRB members address the subject's right to fair treatment by reviewing the researcher's plan for recruiting subjects. A subject recruitment plan must give all the members of the population of interest an opportunity to participate and may not target vulnerable groups simply because it is "easier" to get their participation. Vulnerable populations include groups such as (1) prisoners, as they are available and may feel compelled to participate as a show of good behavior; (2) the homeless, who may be unduly influenced to participate because of such incentives as payment rather than from a true desire to participate; or (3) the mentally ill, who may be less able to fully consent to treatment or who may feel coerced to participate. Additionally, researchers cannot avoid inclusion of individuals who are more difficult to recruit or who have more risk considerations. An example of this would be women. Women, especially during reproductive years, always carry an increased need to consider risks, as they may become pregnant and may be unaware of this during their early participation in a study. Because women have been actively avoided in past research, new studies must now include women and children as well as men, if at all appropriate to the research question, and must include individuals with diverse economic and racial characteristics. Additionally, the researcher must make the IRB aware of the location for data collection, the strategies used to recruit subjects, and any criteria for participation.

In Chapter 6, we discussed that the criteria for participation define the population and are used to either purposely seek diversity or to limit and control for factors that may confound the study findings. In the depressive mood, coping, and eating study used in Chapters 1 and 2 (Appendix A.2), participants were adolescents currently enrolled in high school who were able to read and write English. The researchers purposely limited their sample to adolescents because they were interested in exploring how depressive mood, self-esteem, coping, and eating behaviors related to this limited population. Whatever the criteria for inclusion in a study, the IRB will review them carefully to be sure that they are fair.

CORE CONCEPT 7.2

The goal of the research with human subjects is always to minimize the risks and maximize the benefits.

Ensuring the right to self-determination as well as the right to privacy and dignity are also the IRB's responsibility. These rights are reflected in the informed consent document by providing a clear explanation of the study, what will be required of individuals who participate, and the actual or potential risks and benefits of participation. The intent is that a potential research subject can make a knowledgeable decision based on the information provided in the consent form. In addition, respect for the potential subject is indicated through allowing them the freedom to decide what they will or will not do or share. Self-determination is also included as a direct right within any study consent form in a statement that says that the subject has the right of withdrawal from the study at any time, without penalty, until the study is completed. Once a study is complete, all data become anonymous, and it is no longer possible to withdraw information received from any specific individual. All research consent forms are expected to clarify with subjects that if they start in a study and later change their mind about participating, for any reason, that they retain the right to self-determination and are free to withdraw.

Another aspect of self-determination is the right to decline participation in a study without consequences. A researcher must assure the IRB that individuals who either decline to participate in research or later withdraw after initial consent will not be punished. This is particularly relevant if the study is being conducted in a health care setting where it is possible that a patient might feel direct or indirect coercion to participate. Coercion involves some element of controlling or forcing someone to do something. In the case of research, coercion would occur if a patient felt forced to participate in order to receive a particular test, service, or treatment; to "please" a provider of care; or to receive the best quality of care. Even if not forced to agree to participate in a study, a potential subject still experiences coercion if he or she feels that the best possible care will not be given if the choice is made not to participate. Therefore, any consent form for research where withholding or modifying treatment would be possible will include a clear statement that treatment and care will not be influenced by whether the individual participates in the study. Of course, the researcher is responsible for conducting the study in keeping with that statement, ensuring that action is taken so that treatment and care are not influenced by the individual's decision about whether to participate or not.

The right to privacy and dignity is also related to the right to anonymity and confidentiality. A researcher must inform a potential subject whether participation in a study will involve invasive questions or procedures, again ensuring the respect of being in charge of deciding what will or will not be shared or exposed without the subject's approval. This reflects the participant's right to privacy. Clearly, once data become anonymous, there is no longer a risk of breaching privacy, but until that point, it is the responsibility of the researcher to ensure the right to privacy.

The last aspect of informed consent is a statement about the rights of the participant to care whether some untoward effect should occur from participating in the research and the provision of the specific names and telephone numbers of the researcher(s) and an IRB representative. These sections of the form give the potential participant access to both the researcher and an independent resource, usually the IRB representative, if he or she has questions or problems. Individuals who agree to participate must be given a copy of the consent form so that they can contact the researcher or IRB representative as needed throughout the research and after it is completed.

Throughout this section, we have discussed the responsibilities of IRBs, which are in place to guarantee an organization that any research carried out within that organization or by its employees conforms with, protects, and respects the rights of their subjects. Although IRBs have the responsibility for review, it is always the primary responsibility of the researcher to plan for and guarantee the protection of subjects.

Let us return to the RN in our clinical case. Box 7.1 shows an informed consent form that might have been developed had a researcher chosen to perform a replication of a study concerning sleep and hunger in adolescents. As discussed in Chapter 2, a replication study

---

Box 7.1

Fictional Informed Consent Form for Participation in a Study of Sleep and Hunger in Adolescents

Prison Hospital XYZ
INFORMED CONSENT

PRINCIPAL INVESTIGATOR: Jane J. Doe, RN, PhD

TITLE OF PROJECT: Replication study of factors predictive of correlation of sleep and hunger and adolescents.

PURPOSE: The purpose of this study is to examine associations among total sleep time (TST), hunger, satiety, food cravings, and caloric intake in a sample of healthy adolescents.

DURATION: Volunteering for this study will involve being monitored throughout 7-month period. Participation in this study is entirely voluntary, and deciding not to participate will not affect your care now or in the future in any way.

PROCEDURES. Participation in the study means allowing the nursing staff to meet with you (your child) periodically over the 7-month period, excluding school breaks, standardized testing periods, and the week following the transition to daylight savings time. You (your child) will also be asked to keep a 7-day sleep–hunger–satiety diary during the course of the study. These observations and interactions with the nurse will be provided to you (your child) at no cost. In addition, participation in this study means that the researcher will collect some information from your child's chart about your child's diagnoses, medications, general health, and lab test results.

POSSIBLE RISKS/DISCOMFORTS: Depending on your comfort level with discussing your sleep and eating patterns, discussion of these issues may be embarrassing or upsetting to you (your child). There may be some discomfort in discussing these issues. There are no other known risks to participation in this study.

POSSIBLE BENEFITS: The possible benefit to participation in this study is having access to a health professional to whom you (your child) can ask questions and who is interested in how you (your child) are (is) doing. The other possible benefit is the knowledge that you (your child) are (is) contributing to a study that may help people like yourself (himself or herself) in the future.

CONTACT FOR QUESTIONS: If you have any questions or problems, you may call Jane J. Doe at 423-965-0811 or Bob L. Smith at 423-965-0912. You may call the Chairman of the Institutional Review Board at 423-965-7777 for any questions you may have about your child's rights as a research subject.

(Continued)

Box 7.1

Fictional Informed Consent Form for Participation in a Study of Sleep and Hunger in Adolescents (*Continued*)

CONFIDENTIALITY: Every attempt will be made to see that your child's study results are kept confidential. A copy of the records from this study will be stored in the Department of Acute Nursing, Room 100, at ABC University for at least 10 years after the end of this research. Your child's conversations with the nurse may be tape recorded, but all reasonable efforts will be made to protect the confidentially of your child's information. The results of this study may be published and/or presented at meetings without naming you (your child) as a subject. Although your child's rights and privacy will be maintained, the Secretary of the Department of Health and Human Subjects, the ABC University Institutional Review Board, the Food and Drug Administration, and the Department of Acute Nursing have access to the study records. Your child's records will be kept completely confidential according to current legal requirements.

COMPENSATION FOR MEDICAL TREATMENT: ABC University will pay the cost of emergency first aid for any injury that may happen as a result of your child's being in this study. It will not pay for other medical treatment.

VOLUNTARY PARTICIPATION: The nature, risks, and benefits of the project have been explained to me as are known and available. I understand what my child's participation involves. Furthermore, I understand that I am free to ask questions and withdraw my child from the project at any time, without penalty. I have read and fully understood the consent form. I sign it freely and voluntarily. A signed copy has been given to me.

Your study record will be maintained in strictest confidence according to current legal requirements and will not be revealed unless required by law or as noted.

_____

SIGNATURE OF VOLUNTEER OR LEGAL REPRESENTATIVE & DATE

_____

SIGNATURE OF INVESTIGATOR & DATE

essentially repeats an earlier study with a different sample to see whether the same results are found. Having reviewed the informed consent form that will be presented to M.D., the RN recalls that for this study to have been approved by the institution's IRB, the board must have reviewed the basic soundness of the study in addition to its risk:benefit ratio. This provides the nurse with some assurance that M.D.'s participation would not be a waste of time or effort. It also provides some assurance that the risks to M.D. are probably reasonable, given the potential benefits from the study.

When reviewing the first section of the informed consent, the RN sees a description of the purpose of the study, duration of the study, and procedures. The first thing the nurse notes is that the consent clearly states under the purpose that participation in the study is voluntary and will not be connected to M.D.'s care in any way. The nurse knows that this is an important point to convey so that M.D. does not feel coerced to participate in the study. The nurse knows that it is important to read all of the language within the consent form and be prepared to use more common language when talking with M.D., if need be. The RN also knows that the idea of discussing sleep habits and hunger patterns may be uncomfortable to some patients. The nurse must find an approach to explaining the use of procedures that gives a fair and impartial explanation but also allays any unreasonable fears that M.D. may have.

By considering these aspects of explaining the consent form, the RN is honoring the rights to self-determination, dignity, and protection from discomfort. Only by fully and correctly understanding the purpose and procedures of the study can M.D. make a knowledgeable decision with regard to her participation, ensuring self-determination. By being sure that M.D. fully understands the nature of the procedure that may be performed and the reasons for that procedure, her rights to dignity and protection from discomfort will be ensured as well.

CORE CONCEPT 7.3

The five human rights in research are first and foremost the responsibility of the researcher(s) and are linked to the three ethical principles of autonomy, beneficence, and justice.

When the RN reviews the sections describing the possible risks/discomforts and benefits, one finds that these are clearly stated and include an explicit acknowledgment that personal disclosure is difficult. The consent form seems neither to exaggerate nor to minimize the risks and benefits of this study for M.D. The next two sections of the consent form directly address M.D.'s rights by providing her with the names and telephone numbers of the researchers and of an independent source of information, the chairman of the IRB. The consent form also tells M.D. that her records will be kept confidential, the location of those records, and for how long they will be kept.

Finally, the consent form tells M.D. that she has a right to compensation for any emergency care that might be needed because of her participation in the study. This statement may cause alarm in M.D. because nothing in the form has suggested that there could be a need for emergency care. The RN knows that one must explain that this is a legally required statement that may have limited applicability for this particular study. It should be noted that if there are risks involved, M.D. has a right to know about those in detail. The primary researcher should be the one to conduct this discussion with M.D. and her legal guardian, since M.D. is an adolescent.

The last paragraph of the consent form confirms that M.D. has read and understands the study and that she will always have the right to withdraw from the study, if she chooses to do so. The right to withdrawal without any consequences is as important as the right to decline to participate and assures the patient the right to self-determination and fair treatment throughout participation. Table 7.2 summarizes the links between the five human rights in research and the specific sections of the consent form that we have discussed. After a careful and thoughtful review of the consent form, the RN is prepared to approach M.D. professionally for her consent to participate in the study.

One last point must be understood about informed consent. So far, we have been discussing informed consent to participate in a study, meaning agreement based on a full understanding that assumes the ability to understand and make rational decisions. Occasionally, in research, the potential subject is not able to understand fully and make rational decisions regarding participation, as is often the case for children and persons with cognitive disorders or severe mental or physical illness. Under those circumstances, a researcher is obligated to seek consent from a designated legal representative of the potential subject, such as a parent, guardian, or other relative. The researcher must be cautious to ensure that the legal representative is indeed the correct person who is able to provide consent, meaning that they must be the legal guardian of the potential subject. Researchers must also ascertain that the legal representative not only understands the implications of consent, but also that they do not have a personal stake in the interest of their loved one's participation in research.

Table 7.2

Five Basic Rights and Relevant Components of the Informed Consent Form

BASIC RIGHT	COMPONENTS OF INFORMED CONSENT
Right to self-determination	Description of purpose of study Description of procedures in study Description of possible risks/discomforts Description of possible benefits Statement of right to withdraw from study Statement of voluntary nature of participation without consequences if person chooses not to participate Information about contacts for questions
Right to privacy and dignity	Description of possible risk/discomfort Description of confidentiality
Right to anonymity and confidentiality	Description of confidentiality
Right to fair treatment	Description of purpose of study Description of procedures in study Description of any compensation for medical treatment
Right to protection from discomfort and harm	Description of procedures Description of potential risks/discomforts Description of potential benefits

However, the subject may have a level of function that allows the researcher to seek his or her assent. To assent means to agree or concur and, in the case of research, reflects a lower level of understanding about the meaning of participation in a study than consent. Assent is often sought in studies that involve older children or individuals who have a level of impairment that limits their ability but does not preclude their understanding of some aspects of the study. Because M.D. is a minor, her legal guardian is legally designated as her representative, so the RN would explain the study and review the consent form with both M.D. and the legal guardian. The legal guardian's signature would be needed to include M.D. in the study. However, the RN and M.D.'s legal guardian could seek M.D.'s assent to be in the study by asking her briefly if she would mind helping in a study that looks at behaviors and eating. If M.D. agrees, we would consider that she has assented to participate in the study: She has agreed without completely understanding all the aspects of the study, and it will be her legal guardian who will make the knowledgeable decision, assuring M.D.'s full rights.

■ WHEN RESEARCH IS EXEMPT

There are some instances in which research that is submitted to an IRB will be considered exempt, which essentially means that the study falls under a category of research that is free from the some of the constraints that are normally imposed upon research involving human subjects (United States Department of Health & Human Services, 2007). Some examples of research that may be considered exempt include, but are not limited to, research on educational curriculum efficacy, research involving observation of human behavior (without contact with the individuals observed), and research involving collection of publically available data where subjects cannot be identified. It is of critical importance to understand that proposals for any kind of research, even research which is likely to be considered exempt, be forwarded to the appropriate IRB for consideration. The IRB is responsible for determining exempt status, not the researcher. Once approval has been secured from the IRB, then the researcher may continue his or her study.

There are numerous questions that IRB reviewers must consider when determining whether a study is exempt. The Office for Human Research Protections (OHRP) has designed graphic aids to assist IRBs in their processes when determining whether an activity is considered research that must be reviewed by an IRB, whether the review can be performed in an expedited fashion, and whether informed consent may be waived (OHRP, 2004). An example of one of these algorithms is included in Figure 7.1.

■ CRITICALLY READING REPORTS OF SAMPLING AND RECOGNIZING COMMON ERRORS

Informed consent, as well as the problems that can arise in samples described in Chapter 6, can affect the answer to the question "To what types of patients do these research conclusions apply—who was in the study?" The most common error found in a sampling report related to the ethics of a study is the failure to tell us enough to let us judge the occurrence of potential problems. Almost every study report will include some descriptive information about the sample, and most will indicate the source of the subjects or the location of the study subjects. However, this information may not be adequate for evaluating the sampling process for ethical principles.

An example of a study in which additional information about the process of sampling in terms of ethical concerns would have been useful is the "Predictors of Life Satisfaction in Stroke Survivors and Spousal Caregivers After Inpatient Rehabilitation" used in Chapters 4 and 5 (Ostwald, Godwin, & Cron, 2009) (Appendix A.4). The authors tell us that the study was approved by the university IRB and the various hospitals' IRBs, yet they do not provide any detail about the specific observation of ethical principles throughout the duration of the study.

As you critically read reports of research, there are two questions to ask that directly address ethical considerations in sampling. These are the fourth and fifth questions listed in Box 6.2 in Chapter 6. The fourth question asks, "Was enough information given for me to understand how rights of human subjects were protected?" and the fifth question asks, "Would my patient population have been placed at risk if they had participated in this study?"

■ PUBLISHED REPORTS—WHAT DO THEY SAY ABOUT CONSENT AND THE SAMPLING PROCESS?

As we look at the research studies found by the RNs in our six clinical cases, it is important to realize that when considering sampling as a factor in the utilization of research findings, the clinical nurse often is the expert. We have discussed the meaning of several terms used in research to describe sampling strategies and actual samples, and these are important for understanding the conclusions of a research study. What we have not discussed is that often it is the practicing nurse who most readily recognizes the limits to IRB protection and sampling process because those in practice understand their patients' needs, functionality, and characteristics. If the nurse researcher is not directly involved in patient care with the population of interest, he or she may not realize that a certain segment of the population is not represented in the sample or has special ethical needs. Therefore, once the RNs in our clinical cases understand the sampling language and the IRB process, they are likely to be the best judges of whether a study sample reflects real patient populations and is appropriate to a particular research question.

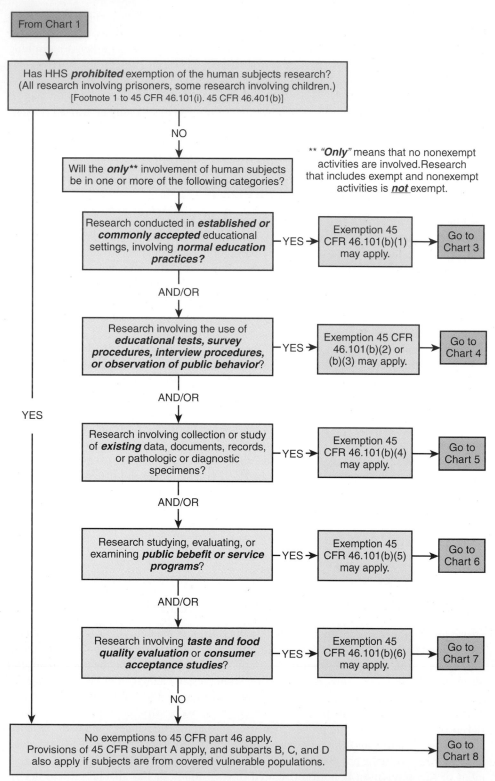

FIGURE 7.1   Chart 2: Is the research involving human subjects eligible for exemption under 45 CFR 46.101(b) (From Office for Human Research Protections (OHRP). (September 24, 2004) *Human subject regulations decision charts*. Retrieved from http://www.hhs.gov/ohrp/humansubjects/guidance/decisioncharts.htm.)

The RNs in the clinical cases now have a much greater understanding with regard to which types of patients these studies can be applied. Legal and ethical principles have been considered and applied appropriately in all of the studies, and all of the samples have strengths as well as some limitations. The next challenge for the RNs is to reach a better understanding of why and how data were collected from the individuals in these samples. Just as the sample affects the meaningfulness of a study for practice, the measures used and approach taken to procuring data can affect the knowledge gained.

OUT-OF-CLASS EXERCISE

What Goes Into a Questionnaire?

Before proceeding to Chapter 8, look at the in-class questionnaire that you completed at the beginning of your course. If you did not have an in-class study, look at the questionnaire included in Appendix C.

As you read the questionnaire, write down your impressions regarding the following questions:

1. As you look at each question, what do you think is the variable of interest?
2. Do some of the questions fit together to measure just one variable? Which variable? Do you think the questions are all logically connected?
3. What makes the questionnaire easy to read and answer?
4. What makes the questionnaire confusing? Are any particular questions more confusing than others? Why?
5. Do any aspects of the organization of the questionnaire or the wording of questions make it difficult for some people to answer the questionnaire?

After you have responded to these questions, to which there are no correct or incorrect answers, you are ready to read Chapter 8.

References

American Nurses Association (ANA). (1985). *Code for nurses with interpretive statement.* Kansas City, MO: Author.

American Nurses Association (ANA). (2001). *Code of ethics for nurses with interpretive statements.* Silver Spring, MD: Author.

American Nurses Association (ANA). (2005). *Code of ethics for nurses with interpretive statements.* Retrieved July 26, 2009, from www.nursingworld.org

Belmont Report. (1979). *Ethical principles and guidelines for the protection of human subjects of research.* The National Commission for the Protection of Human Subjects of Biomedical and Behavioral Research. Washington, DC: Department of Health, Education, and Welfare.

International Council of Nurses (ICN). (2006). *The ICN code of ethics for nurses.* Geneva, Switzerland. Retrieved August 3, 2009, from www.icn.ch/icncode.pdf

Landis, A., Parker, K., & Dunbar, S. (2009). Sleep, hunger, satiety, food cravings, and caloric intake in adolescents. *Journal of Nursing Scholarship, 41*(2), 115–123.

Office of Human Research Protections (OHRP). (2004). *Human subject regulations decision charts.* Retrieved July 26, 2009, from http://www.hhs.gov/ohrp/humansubjects/guidance/decisioncharts.htm#c2

Ostwald, S., Godwin, K., & Crom, S. (2009). Predictors of life satisfaction in stroke survivors and spousal caregivers after inpatient rehabilitation. *Rehabilitation Nursing, 34,* 160–174.

United States Department of Health & Human Services. (2007). Basic HHS Policy for Protection of Human Research Subjects, §46.101(b).

Resources

LoBiondo-Wood, G., Haber, J., & Krainovich-Miller, B. (2009). Overview of the research process. In G. LoBiondo-Wood & J. Haber (Eds.), *Nursing research: Methods, critical appraisal, and utilization* (6th ed.). St. Louis, MO: Mosby.

Locke, L. F., Silverman, S. J., & Spirduso, W. W. (2009). *Reading and understanding research* (3rd ed.). Thousand Oaks, CA: Sage Publications.

Polit, D. F., & Beck, C.T. (2007). *Nursing research: Principles and methods* (8th ed.). Philadelphia, PA: Lippincott Williams & Wilkins.

Data Collection Methods

How Were Those People Studied— Why Was the Study Performed That Way?

LEARNING OBJECTIVE

The student will relate the data collection methods of a study to the meaning of its results and conclusions.

KEY TERMS

Audit trail
Confirmability
Construct validity
Content validity
Credibility
Criterion-related validity
Error
Field notes
Group interviews
Instrument
Internal consistency reliability
Interrater reliability
Items
Likert-type response scale
Member checks
Operational definition

Participant observation
Questionnaire
Reliability
Rigor
Scale
Semistructured questions
Structured questions
Test–retest reliability
Theoretical definition
Transferability
Triangulation
Trustworthiness
Unstructured interviews
Validity
Visual analog

Clinical Case • M.J. is a 74-year-old woman who was discharged from the hospital 1 day after a right mastectomy surgery for stage II cancer. An RN has been assigned to provide home care to M.J., and when the nurse makes the first home visit, M.J. is found crying and expressing feelings of discouragement. While checking M.J.'s incision and her vital signs, the RN listens supportively as M.J. talks about her feelings. The RN has had several cases of postoperative care for women in home care and now wonders how to improve the home care provided to these patients, particularly in the areas of physiologic and psychosocial needs. The RN looks for research evidence that might guide future practice by doing a literature search and finds one report of research that seems particularly relevant titled "Transition to Home Care: Quality of Mental Health, Pharmacy, and Medical History Information" (Brown et al., 2006). This article is presented in Appendix A.6. We will be using the information in the methods section of this report as examples throughout this chapter. Table 8.1 summarizes the RN's clinical question for this clinical case.

■ REVISITING STUDY VARIABLES

The unique language of research associated with data collection is extensive, as a quick glance at the key terms listed at the beginning of this chapter shows. The abstract of the article found by the RN indicates the study tested an approach for care for breast cancer

Table 8.1

Statement of Clinical Question From the Clinical Case

What interventions are effective in supporting home care patients upon discharge from another agency?

The *Who*	Home care patients
The *What*	Physiologic and psychological needs
The *When*	Upon discharge from another agency to the home care environment
The *Where*	In home
Key search terms to find research-based evidence for practice	Home health
	Aging patients home care
	Home care nursing
	Psychosocial well-being

patients that may relate to the needs of M.J. and other patients like her. After reading the article, however, the RN realizes that understanding how complex aspects of health such as "referral documentation," "depression," and "cognitive status" were measured is essential to understanding the results and conclusions of the study. The RN begins to read the methods section to help achieve this understanding.

To examine the measurement approaches taken, the RN first has to identify the variables in the study. We discussed variables in Chapters 4 and 5, defining them as some aspect of interest that differs in a variety of groups or situations. Both qualitative and quantitative studies have variables, but only quantitative studies use the categories of independent and dependent variables. Independent variables are those factors in the study that are used to explain or predict the outcome of interest and are sometimes called *predictor variables* because they are used to predict the dependent variable. In the article, the RN read about the approach for care, based on completeness of referral documentation, and the authors identified completeness of the referral documentation as the primary independent variable. There are other variables that can further implicate the outcome of the study, such as age, comorbidities, and gender, but we will focus on the completeness of referral documentation and the primary independent variable. Dependent variables are the variables that depend on other variables in a study or are the outcome variables of interest. The effect on home care is therefore the dependent variables within this study.

As a review, remember that it is not the variable itself but how it is used that makes it either independent or dependent. For example, in one study, the purpose might be to describe the effects of chemotherapy on patients' levels of stress. In such a study, the outcome or dependent variable is stress. Another study might seek to understand how factors such as education, stress, and perceived benefits lead to nonadherence of diet restrictions. In such a study, we also see the variable "stress," but now it is an independent variable because it is being used to predict the outcome of adherence.

The variables studied in the article about the home care approach are listed in Table 8.2. This article is a quantitative study that uses both the approach itself and demographic characteristics as independent or predictor variables. The outcomes primarily examined medication reconciliation (as it pertains to safety of the patient in the home care environment). In other words, the study examined whether or not the approach and demographic characteristics would predict that variable.

Table 8.2

Types and Definitions of Variables From the Study of Transition to Home Care

VARIABLE	TYPE	THEORETICAL DEFINITION	OPERATIONAL DEFINITION
Information reported by other agencies	Predictor or independent variable	Inadequate communication of patient information between health care providers, when a patient is transferred or admitted to a new health care setting	Clinical information provided by referral sources to visiting nurses for older adult patients admitted to home health care
Type of home care approach employed (e.g., reconciliation of medication, recognition of depressive or cognitive concerns)	Dependent or outcome	None	The type of attention that must be given to home care needs of patients (e.g., medication reconciliation, process by which information is transmitted to ensure accuracy of orders for home care, use of family member to help make decisions, attention to psychological or cognitive deficits and needs)

Before we continue, let us look at how we determine the variables in a study. Although it is logical that variables differ across groups or situations, many research reports will not explicitly identify or list the study variables. For example, the narrative within the study never really lists or clearly states the independent and dependent variables used in the study, but careful reading lets us do this, as shown in Table 8.2. Obviously, variables should reflect the topic of interest, which, in turn, should be described in the purpose, background, and research questions, sections of a research report discussed in depth in Chapter 10. Because a qualitative study usually begins with one or more broad questions and uses open-ended approaches to collecting data, the variables of interest often are clearly identified within the research questions. In contrast, reports of quantitative studies should clearly describe the variables even if they are not explicitly labeled as such because the data collection methods in quantitative research are specifically aimed at measuring study variables as objectively as possible.

The data collection section of a report of a quantitative study should describe how each variable was measured and identify each variable. The RN in our clinical case found the outcome variables identified under a section titled "Measures," and the intervention that was the predictor variable was described under the section titled "Design." Both the measures and the design sections are actually subsections under the general heading of "Methods." By reading carefully the methods section then, the RN should be able to find the description of the measures used and, thus, identify the study's variables.

Variables also can be identified and discussed in terms of their definitions rather than whether they are independent or dependent. Variables can be defined at two levels: the theoretical level and the operational level. A theoretical definition is one that is described and understood conceptually, not concretely. Because it is stated conceptually, this definition is not always clearly measurable. Therefore, a second type of definition called the *operational definition* is needed. An operational definition is one that is defined in specific, concrete terms that allows us to see how we might actually measure the variable. If researchers do not have a clear understanding of the theoretical meaning of a concept, then they may be inconsistent in their measurement of that concept, leading to disagreement about what was actually measured and questions about the overall meaning of the study.

CORE CONCEPT 8.1

The measures in a quantitative study should reflect the specific variables under study.

For example, the variable "stress" can be operationally defined as an individual's perceptions that an event is threatening and that he or she has no way to manage the threat. This definition is conceptual, giving the reader a clearer idea of what is meant by the word *stress*, but it does not tell us how that variable might actually be measured. An operational definition of stress might be an individual's summed score regarding his or her ratings on a four-point scale of the perceived level of threat from 40 life events. Or, still using the same theoretical definition, stress could be operationally defined as the number of beats per minute that the heart rate increases when a person looks at pictures of negative events. These two definitions are concrete and tell the reader exactly how the variable "stress" will be measured.

Although some variables such as temperature or heart rate are concrete and may only be defined operationally, many variables of interest to nursing are relatively abstract and may need both a theoretical and an operational definition if they are going to be used in a quantitative study. Examples of these types of variables include mood and cognitive status. If a researcher believed that we had a theoretical understanding of the mood variable, he or she might break it down into one or more concrete components that would then comprise an operational definition. For example, he or she might operationally define, or operationalize, mood as was done in the article found by the RN in the clinical case. In that study, the researchers operationalized mood as scores on the Structured Clinical Interview for Axis I DSM-IV Disorders (SCID) scale (Brown et al., 2006). Alternatively, a researcher might operationalize QOL as a single item rated on a 10-point scale. Almost any variable can be operationalized, but the correctness and accuracy of that operationalization must be evaluated. You can think of an operational definition, or the operationalization, of a variable as a form of translation: The researcher is translating an abstract theoretical idea into a concrete set of measures.

CORE CONCEPT 8.2

Operationalizing variables is like translating a phrase from one language to another. The researcher is translating an abstract, theoretical variable into a concrete measure or set of measures.

When a variable is not measured with 100% accuracy, we say that there is error in the measurement. In research, error refers to the difference between what is true and the answer we obtained from our data collection. If we operationalized gender as the data collectors' assessment of gender based on observation, that observation might be wrong probably only 1 in 1000 times. Think about that: If we had a data collector sit in a hospital waiting room and record the gender of a person walking in the room, occasionally he or she might misperceive or be confused by odd dress or appearance. In almost all measurement, there could still be some error because an observational assessment would be wrong occasionally. The difference between the gender of 1000 people and the measurement of gender through observation would be the error in the measurement of that variable. In Chapter 2, we compared qualitative research with creating an artist's rendition of a new home as well as compared quantitative research with developing the blueprints for that home. An artist can misunderstand the specifications for a new home and create distortions or illusions in a painting, just as an architect can make errors in measurement that can lead to plans that are inaccurate, incomplete, or wrong. In both cases, error in measurement will occur.

Remember that we said measurement is about translation. If you have experienced having someone translate your words into another language, you know that translation is open to interpretation and even error. Qualitative research does not operationalize variables because it does not presume to know enough about the variables of interest to be able to select appropriate and accurate concrete measures. Yet, qualitative research does translate specific experiences or observations into theoretical concepts or descriptions of variables during the process of data collection and analysis. Therefore, qualitative research is open to errors in interpretation during the data collection process. For example, a researcher may get focused on an idea that one or two participants who are trying to quit smoking discuss, such as "fear of failure," and start looking for that theme in other interviews. The researcher may then hear statements about discouragement as well as about disappointing significant others as variations of the fear of failing when, in fact, discouragement and disappointment are important and different themes that warrant exploration.

Because quantitative research often examines abstract variables that require both a theoretical and an operational definition, the opportunities for error in measurement can be even greater. Error can occur in the translation from theoretical to operational, and it can occur in the operationalized measurement process. Therefore, both qualitative research and quantitative research are open to problems in the translation of variables. We will discuss how those potential problems with translation can affect the meaning of the results of a study for practice later in this chapter.

Before looking at specific approaches used to collect data for studies, let us apply the ideas of theoretical variables and operational definitions to the fictional article in Appendix B about nursing students' choices of field of practice. The author of the article tells us in the first paragraph, under the heading of "Measures," that the questionnaire used in this study had three sections: one that asked about demographic characteristics; one asked about education, well-being, and career choice; and one asked about automobile preferences. Demographic variables are usually fairly concrete and commonly understood, so the author does not offer theoretical definitions of them. However, the author does tell us indirectly that these variables were measured by self-report because they were measured through a questionnaire that was completed by the students. Therefore, the operational definition of age in this study is the actual reported age. The variable age then might be translated to be "the subject's report of his or her age in years." Age also could have been operationally defined by asking for the subject's birth date, which the researcher could then have used to compute age to the day using a computer calculation that subtracts date of birth from the current date. The fictional article does not tell us whether the questionnaire asked for age in years or for birth date, so we do not know exactly how the age variable was operationalized.

The second section of the questionnaire was used to operationalize several variables in the study, including educational background, well-being, and student preference for clinical practice after graduation. Educational background was operationalized by the answers to two questions: (1) if the student was currently licensed to practice as an RN or a licensed practical nurse (LPN) and (2) the total number of years of the student's postsecondary education. Well-being was operationally defined as the student's rating of his or her health on a four-point scale. Anticipated field of choice was operationally defined as choice from a list of career options. In each case, a variable has been translated into a specific measure or measures, and alternate translations could have been used. Equally important, there is room for error both in the translation of a variable to a measure and in the measuring process itself. The remainder of this chapter discusses the measurement process and how error may occur.

Finally, the researcher in the fictional article included in the questionnaire an open-ended question regarding life experiences that led to choice of field of practice. In this last question, the researcher does not concretely translate a variable but asks the subjects to share experiences that may help his or her to develop a definition of the variable "life experiences affecting choice of field." Because this variable is not concrete, the researcher will have to start by developing a theoretical translation or definition before considering an operational definition. The fictional article provides several examples of operationally defined variables but includes no theoretical definitions. As we discuss some specific methods for collecting information about variables, we see examples of theoretical definitions that were in the article found by the RN in the clinical case (see Table 8.2 for the theoretical and operational definitions of those variables).

■ METHODS FOR CONSTRUCTING THE MEANING OF VARIABLES IN QUALITATIVE RESEARCH

A study that is using a qualitative approach should examine variables and increase understanding of something that is abstract and unknown by asking for, or looking for, specific examples, experiences, or perceptions. However, because a qualitative study does not attempt to measure variables concretely, we do not expect to find operational definitions included in a report of the study methods. The primary purpose of many qualitative studies

is to develop a clear theoretical definition of a variable so that it might eventually be operationally defined and concretely measured. For example, the theoretical variable of family
needs is the focus of the qualitative study we are using as an example. Because the purpose
of that study was to increase our understanding of family needs, neither a theoretical nor an
operational definition was offered. A concrete definition would presume that we already
had a relatively clear understanding of family needs and could concretely measure it.
Whereas, in fact, the researchers were trying to construct a theoretical definition of family
needs that then could be translated into an operational definition.

In qualitative research, the study methods used to collect data are intended to allow
the researcher to construct a description of the meaning of the variable(s) under study.
Remember that a qualitative approach assumes that truth is a moving target. The more we
can know, feel, or understand about a variable of interest, the closer we will come to a full
and complete meaning, but that meaning will always be context laden and, therefore, changing and evolving. A qualitative method for data collection, then, does not aim to measure
specifically or make concrete a variable of interest. Rather, these data collection methods aim
to expand our understanding about a variable or variables on as many levels as possible.

Qualitative methods of data collection depend on the participants' open sharing of their
thoughts, feelings, and experiences verbally, visually, in writing, with music, and within
life activities. Although it may not be surprising that participants can share through speaking and writing, other means of expression, such as music or cooking a meal, are probably
less frequently considered but can be meaningful avenues for understanding a participant's
experiences or feelings. Therefore, the data methods include interviews, journaling, participant observation, and art analysis. Interviews are probably the most frequently used methods for collecting data in qualitative research, with two broad categories of interviews used:
those that are unstructured and those that use groups.

Unstructured interviews involve asking questions in an informal and open fashion,
without a previously established set of categories or assumed answers, to gain understanding about a phenomenon or variable of interest. Unstructured interviews in qualitative
research assume that the product of the interview reflects the interactions among the interviewer, participant, and interview environment or setting. Depending on the type of qualitative study, the researcher may identify and purposely set aside or bracket his or her
knowledge, beliefs, or expectations about the variable, or he or she may not bracket and
instead may carefully document and incorporate his or her knowledge, beliefs, and perspectives into the data collection process. In any case, data collection using an unstructured
interview includes not only the actual words of the participant but also notes the participant's tone, expressions, and associated actions, and what is occurring in the setting. These
notes are often called field notes because they are a record of the researcher's observations
about the overall setting and experience of the data collection process while in that setting
or field itself. Field notes are used to enrich and build a data set that is thick and dense.

Not all interviewing techniques are unstructured. However, qualitative research does not
generally use either semistructured or structured interviews because these types of interviews
assume and control options for answers to questions. As such, semistructured and structured
interviews do not fit with the perspective of a qualitative researcher that it is the participant's
own ideas and language that extend our knowledge and understanding of a phenomenon.

Unstructured interviews may take several forms, including in-depth interviews, oral
histories, storytelling, and life reviews. In all forms, the intent is to openly explore the
understanding and experiences of the study participants. Unstructured interviews usually
are tape-recorded or videotaped, then transcribed verbatim into a written form that will
include notes on pauses; vocalizations that are not actual words, such as sighs; and even
voice tone at times.

A related method of data collection is participant observation. In this type of observation, the researcher intentionally imbeds himself or herself into the environment from which

data will be collected and becomes a participant. From the perspective of active participation in the experiences and lives of those studied, the researcher/participant records observations, feelings, conversations, and experiences regarding the phenomenon of interest.

Group interviews also are used to collect data in qualitative research and involve collection of data by interviewing more than one participant at a time. The data collected, then, are not just the participant's responses but are also the responses that occur due to the interaction of the participants as they hear and respond to each other. Group interviews may take the form of focus groups, in which a preset topic is addressed in an open-ended fashion and the researcher keeps the focus of the group on that topic. Another form of group interview is brainstorming, in which no particular focus or direction is established, and group dialogues about a broad topic in an unstructured discussion. Group interviews may occur spontaneously in a setting where a researcher finds or facilitates two or more participants in naturally dialoguing about a phenomenon of interest. For example, a researcher studying the experience of receiving government assistance and observing a group of women waiting for their food stamps might see several women talking about what it is like to shop with the stamps. The researcher might introduce himself or herself, obtain consent, and join the discussion, asking a few questions and listening to what the women have to say. In general, group interviews are rich in data and can be a relatively inexpensive method of data collection. However, use of group interviews may limit hearing and knowing unique individual perspectives or ideas because groups limit some individual expression.

Use of journals is another approach that can be used to collect data in qualitative studies. In journaling, a researcher can ask participants to describe, in writing, their ongoing experiences with a phenomenon of interest. This type of data collection can provide continuous and evolving information from an individual perspective that cannot be collected in face-to-face interviews. However, it clearly depends on the participant's ability and willingness to write on a regular and detailed basis. The researcher also depends on the participant's own description of the setting and interactions related to an experience under study because he or she is not present during the journaling. A more limited form of written data can be collected by directly asking participants to write a response or description about a phenomenon on the occasion of data collection. This approach is often called a *free write*. The fictional article in Appendix B about students' choices of fields of nursing used a limited version of written data collection by asking an open-ended question about students' experiences that had affected their choices of field in nursing. This can be considered to be a form of qualitative data collection because it does not constrain or limit the responses that students can give and lends itself to providing data about the meaning of life experiences for future life choices.

A similar form of data collection involves the use of expressional media or art forms such as art, music, or poetry. Here, data such as drawings or photography are collected, as it is assumed that they reflect the participant's perception and interpretation of certain experiences. When art is used, an interview often is included so that the participant can share or interpret his or her art to the researcher. For example, homeless individuals might be given disposable cameras and asked to take photographs that reflect their experiences of being homeless. The researcher might then analyze the photographs for common subjects or common reflected moods.

Another form of data collected in qualitative research is documents and records. These types of data are used in historical research and may include personal and business letters, logs, contracts, accounts, and other written records. These data are compiled and examined to create a clear picture of some past aspect and are particularly useful when the phenomenon of interest has evolved over time, such as the elimination of wearing nursing caps in the clinical setting.

In all of these methods, the researcher is not collecting discrete, clearly defined, and limited information. Qualitative data are used to develop theoretical meaning by creating a verbal, a visual, or an auditory picture of a variable of interest. Although data collection in qualitative research is not structured and objectified, it is carefully planned and thought through, and it involves clearly identified methods for the overlapping processes of collecting, handling, and analysis.

■ ERRORS IN DATA COLLECTION IN QUALITATIVE RESEARCH

In qualitative research, error can be introduced into a study in two major ways. Problems can occur with the processes of data collection and analysis, or both. When considering the aspects that can create error, qualitative researchers aim to ensure the rigor of both processes. Rigor is a strict process of data collection and analysis as well as a term that reflects the overall quality of that process in qualitative research. It is reflected in the consistency of data analysis and interpretation, the trustworthiness of the data collected, the transferability of the themes, and the credibility of the data. Qualitative researchers use several tools and processes to guarantee that each of these aspects of rigor is ensured.

Trustworthiness

Trustworthiness refers to the honesty of the data collected from or about the participants (Lincoln & Guba, 1985). To collect trustworthy data, the researcher must have a meaningful relationship with the participants, which may require time to develop. Participants also must want to share information so that they can communicate their feelings, insights, and experiences without feeling pressured or wanting to censor what they share (Lincoln & Guba, 1985). People who participate in research studies are not as likely to share their experiences and perceptions honestly and openly unless they believe that the researcher has a real interest in their perceptions and an acceptance of them and their life experiences. Participants do not develop such openness without first getting to know the researcher, at least to some extent. Trust and a respectful relationship must be established early in the study process.

Trustworthiness of data collection may also be supported by using a consistent protocol in data collection. Use of a protocol may seem contradictory to the open-ended nature of most qualitative data collection methods. However, a protocol can provide a broad framework for data collection and ensure a similar setting and interaction, without structuring the data collected.

Confirmability

A second aspect of ensuring rigor in qualitative data collection is confirmability—that is, the consistency and repeatability of the decision making about the process of data collection and data analysis (Lincoln & Guba, 1985). One approach taken to ensure confirmability of data in qualitative research is developing and maintaining an audit trail. An audit trail is an ongoing documentation regarding the researcher's decisions about the data analysis and collection processes. Documentation from the audit trail may include field notes about the process of data collection, theoretical notes about the working hypotheses or developing ideas during the analysis, or methods notes regarding approaches to categorizing or organizing the data. The audit trail can be used to assist the researcher in being consistent as well as to demonstrate the presence of consistency when sharing the data.

Qualitative researchers often use computer software programs, such as ATLAS.ti, QDA.miner, NU.DIST, and N.VIVO, to help them to organize and analyze data. These programs do not perform the thinking and conceptualizing that is at the heart of qualitative data analysis, but they can be used to examine the data efficiently, to organize it around themes and dimensions as they are identified in the data, and to synthesize large volumes of data. As the researcher begins to identify a data theme, different units of language or observations can be categorized under this theme. As new themes arise, the data can be reorganized consistently by the software. In addition, a record of the evolving decisions about themes and the classification of data are maintained, ensuring that the researcher is consistent in the analysis of all the data and assisting the qualitative researcher in maintaining an audit trail.

Taking a simple example, suppose that the researcher for the choice of field study reported in the fictional article (Appendix B) had broken down the students' written answers describing experiences that contributed to their choices of field into units that were the individual sentences and then stored them within a computer program. The researcher might decide that whenever students described some kind of experience with fiction about health care, such as a novel or television series, that this reflected a theme. The researcher now must explore the data to decide what are and are not examples of experiences with fiction about health care. For example, novels, plays, movies, and television series may all clearly fit into the theme of fiction, but are advertisements that depict health care also part of this category? As the researcher decides and tells the program that references to television, radio, literature, film, and theater all reflect exposure to media, the computer will find and place into a category and sentences with those references. When the researcher later adds some additional data from another class of students, it might also be decided that identification with selected actors or actresses is a separate theme from the broader media exposure. The computer can be told to reorganize the data, looking for references to particular actors or actresses, but it will also retain the information about how the original category was formed. This provides the researcher with a powerful ongoing record of decisions, enhances the ability to work with large data sets, and decreases the possibility of the researcher defining or describing a category inconsistently from one time to another.

Transferability

A third aspect of rigor in a qualitative study is the transferability of the concepts, themes, or dimensions identified. Transferability refers to the extent to which the findings of a study are confirmed by or are applicable to a different group or in a different setting from where the data were collected (Lincoln & Guba, 1985). Transferability is different from generalizability because the focus is not on predicting specific outcomes in a general population. Rather, the focus is on confirming that what was meaningful in one specific setting or with one specific group is also meaningful and accurate in a different setting or group. One of the methods used to ensure transferability is to describe themes that have been identified in one sample to a group of similar participants who did not contribute to the initial data collection to determine if the second group agrees with the themes. This procedure is sometimes called *external checks*. Transferability also can be ensured if the researcher actively seeks sources of data that contradict the ideas that are emerging from the data. If disconfirming data are found, they can be used to modify or reinterpret the total body of data to develop more comprehensive and credible findings. Findings that reflect the breadth of experiences or ideas will then be more easily transferred or related to different groups.

Credibility

Credibility, the fourth aspect of rigor of concern to qualitative researchers, overlaps with transferability and trustworthiness. Credibility refers to the confidence that the researcher and user of the research can have in the truth of the findings of the study. Lincoln and Guba (1985) suggest that the credibility of qualitative data can be supported by a researcher performing several actions, including seeking feedback from participants regarding evolving findings and interpretations and seeking participants whose perceptions differ from those already included in the study. The former activity is often referred to as *member checks*. Member checks means just what it sounds like—that the data and findings from data analysis are brought back to the original participants to seek their input concerning the accuracy, completeness, and interpretation of the data.

Table 8.3

Aspects of Rigor

ASPECT	DEFINITION	METHODS
Trustworthiness	The honesty of the data collected from and about participants	Establishment of ongoing or meaningful interactions Use of a protocol
Confirmability	The consistent repeatable nature of the data collection and analysis	Use of computer software to organize and analyze data Audit trails
Transferability	The extent to which findings relate to other settings or groups	External checks Seeking disconfirming cases or outliers
Credibility	The confidence in the truth of the findings	Triangulation Member checks

Credibility also is ensured through processes that guarantee trustworthiness and transferability, such as spending time with the participants and maintaining thorough phenomenon-focused observations. It can be further ensured through the use of triangulation. Triangulation is the process of using more than one approach or source to include different views or to look at the phenomenon from different angles (Lincoln & Guba, 1985). This process focuses on the data, seeking different types of sources of information regarding a phenomenon, or it can focus on the use of more than one investigator, the use of several theories, or the use of numerous methods in the study (Denzin, 2001). When multiple sources of data all lead to the same conclusions, the credibility of those findings is increased.

Table 8.3 summarizes the aspects of rigor that we have discussed. As we read and consider using results from qualitative research in practice, we must consider the rigor of the data collection methods and analysis. The greater the rigor in the study, the more we can be confident that the findings are meaningful truths that we can use to understand our patients. What helps us to be confident includes the use of processes to ensure the trustworthiness of the data, such as the researcher's establishment of meaningful interactions and maintenance of ongoing contact with participants. That the data are confirmable can be indicated by the researcher stating that an audit trail was maintained or that selected software was used to assist in data analysis. Use of approaches such as external checks and searching for participants who differ or have dissenting views can help to ensure us of the transferability of the data. The credibility of the data can be supported by member checks and triangulation.

■ METHODS TO MEASURE VARIABLES IN QUANTITATIVE RESEARCH

In quantitative research, the methods used for data collection aim to measure the variables of interest clearly, specifically, and accurately. Earlier, we said that an operational definition of a variable is a description of how it will be measured and that a researcher doing a quantitative study almost always must decide how to measure the variable of interest, even when it is as concrete as a subject's gender. Remember also that the goal in quantitative research is to measure variables numerically so that they can be statistically described and analyzed. Therefore, the methods used for data collection in quantitative research include physiologic measurements, chemical laboratory tests, systematic observations, and written measures containing carefully defined questions, questionnaires, and/or scales.

In quantitative studies, variables often are discussed and defined at theoretical and operational levels because the goal in a quantitative study is to examine discrete factors as concretely as possible. The home care approach study includes variables called *mood, anhedonia, and suicidal ideation.* Because these variables can have many conceptual meanings, the authors provide a theoretical definition clarifying that "mention of mood (e.g., sad, hopeless, depressed, stable mood, euthymic), anhedonia (e.g., diminished interest in activities, lack of motivation or pleasure), and suicide ideation, (e.g., thoughts of death, thoughts of suicide)" constituted definitions of these conditions (Brown et al., 2006). "If any of these symptoms were documented on the RefD, the reviewers considered depression-related information to be present" (Brown et al., 2006). That definition is included in the "Measures" section of the research report.

Although all variables in a quantitative study should have an operational definition, not all variables in quantitative research will have a theoretical definition. Concrete variables, such as gender, weight, platelet count, or oxygen saturation, do not have or need a theoretical definition. There is a common understanding of the conceptual meaning of "gender," so it does not need a theoretical definition. But even concrete variables need an operational definition when they are being examined in research because several approaches can be taken to measure them. For example, we can operationally define gender in at least three different ways (1) the presence or absence of a Y chromosome, (2) a self-reported characteristic, or (3) an observed characteristic. In most cases, we will get the same result no matter which way we define and measure gender. However, in rare cases, some people perceive themselves to be the opposite gender from that indicated in their chromosomal composition, and some people are androgynous enough that a superficial observation might lead to incorrect categorization. Therefore, even a variable as concrete as gender must be operationally defined so that we can understand exactly what was measured.

CORE CONCEPT 8.3

In a quantitative study, every variable should have an operational definition that specifies how the variable was measured.

Physiologic measurement is probably the most concrete type of data collection in quantitative research and may include anything from a simple measurement of blood pressure to the calculation of pulmonary function values. As was pointed out with the gender variable, physiologic measures still must be defined operationally because most of them can be measured in several different fashions and with different levels of accuracy. A research study that examines a physiologic variable should report specifically how the physiologic parameter was measured so that the accuracy and appropriateness of that measure can be evaluated. Similarly, a study that includes a variable measured by a laboratory test should specify the actual test or procedure used to arrive at the study values. For example, if blood sugar were measured in a study, the report should indicate whether it used a capillary sample or a venous sample and what type of control and calibration measures were used to ensure consistency and accuracy.

A second method of measuring variables in quantitative research involves systematic observation of the variable of interest. Measurement by systematic observation differs from the observation data collection methods used in qualitative research because it is structured and defined to ensure that each measurement is accurate and comparable to earlier or later measures. As a result, systematic observation does not try to collect as much detail and variation as possible but has a narrow focus on specific components of the variable under study.

For example, in a study that was trying to describe factors affecting fecal incontinence, the researchers would need to operationalize the variable fecal incontinence, perhaps by stating that the specific observation required to indicate the presence of fecal incontinence is the presence of uncontrolled release of stool and/or soiled clothing. Thus, the variable is clearly defined, and the data collection focuses on the specific components of the definition.

Therefore, data collectors would not be interested in factors such as urinary incontinence, skin condition, type of bedpan, staffing ratio, or the subject's ability to use the call button. Data collectors will look for and record reports by the staff or the client of involuntary release of stool, and they will count the presence or absence of the defined components to give each subject a value of "yes" or "no" for the variable fecal incontinence.

A third method for measurement in quantitative research is use of an instrument. The word instrument is used in research to refer to a device that specifies and objectifies the data collecting process. Instruments are usually written and may be given directly to the subject to collect data or may provide objective description of the collection of certain types of data. The SCID is an example of a written instrument used in the efficacy of home care approach study to measure depressive symptoms and disorders (Brown et al., 2006) (Appendix A.6). Some instruments provide directions for observations, and the measure depends on observers noting certain specified and defined types of behaviors, counting the presence or absence of those behaviors, and converting them into a final numeric score. For example, the authors might have used an observational measure of depression that required visiting the breast surgery patients in their homes and observing for specific factors, such as facial affect or emotional lability. When a researcher uses this type of observational measurement, the components that define the variable have been specified before data collection begins, and the study does not seek to expand the understanding of the components of that variable, as would a qualitative approach, but seeks to count the extent to which they are present.

We have said that instruments are devices that define and objectify the data collection. Some quantitative studies collect data using semistructured questions (Box 8.1) in order to collect data that specifically target objective factors of interest. For example, telephone surveys often consist of semistructured questions, such as "tell me how you use television to relax in the evening." Phenomenologic research continues this questioning process by asking further flexible questions, called probes and inquiries; the answers given help the researcher to broaden the scope of information received from the participants, in an effort to understand a complete picture of their lived experience. For example, in Box 8.1, the researcher is studying the lived experience of nursing students who have obtained their initial nursing degree from studying in a face-to-face environment and are now studying to obtain their bachelor of science in nursing (BSN) degree in an online program. The initial semistructured questions allow the researcher to gain an initial impression of the participants' perspective about this new way of attending school, while the probes and inquiries provide an avenue to understand, in a broader fashion, how students truly have experienced this transition from initial nursing school to a BSN completion program. However, a quantitative study might use a structured question that establishes what data is wanted ahead of the collection and does not allow the respondent any flexibility in how to answer. For example, the question "how many members of the household eat breakfast daily?" is a structured question. In contrast, unstructured questions are like unstructured interviews and seek to determine what data, experiences, or ideas are relevant and meaningful without previous narrowing of the definition or specification.

Many instruments used in nursing research collect data in a written form, provided directly by the subjects in the study. These instruments are also called *questionnaires* or *scales*, and the terms are sometimes used interchangeably. *Instrument* is the broadest term and, as we have said, can include interview questions, directed observations, or written collection of data. A questionnaire is an instrument used to collect specific written data, and a scale is a set of written questions or statements that, in combination, are intended to measure a specified variable. The questions or statements included on a scale are often called items. The language of research when discussing measurement of variables can become confusing, but grasping the basic meanings of some of these terms will allow you to better understand the meaning of a study for your clinical practice. Box 8.2 summarizes and gives an example of frequently used terms in quantitative measurement.

Box 8.1
Examples of Semistructured Questions, Probes, and Inquiries

Questions

1. How do you feel about your experience with your classmates in the online environment, in terms of how much you sensed an atmosphere of camaraderie?
2. How do you feel about your experience with your facilitator in the online environment in terms of how much he or she promoted an atmosphere of camaraderie?
3. How would you describe the social immediacy you experienced in the online environment?
4. To what extent did you fear psychological distance in the online environment?
5. How would you describe the atmosphere of "caring" that you feel that your facilitator in the course had for you?
6. To what degree do you feel that the facilitator created a sense of community for you and your classmates?
7. To what degree do you feel that your classmates interacted with you and respected your feelings?
8. To what degree do you feel that your facilitator interacted with you and respected your feelings?

Probes

1. To what degree do you feel that the sense of community and relationships you experienced with your classmates in this course contributes to your success in this course?
2. To what degree do you feel that the sense of community and relationships you experienced with your facilitator in this course contributes to your success in this course?
3. To what degree do you feel that the sense of community and relationships you experience with classmates will ultimately contribute to your success in the BSN completion program?
4. To what degree do you feel that the sense of community and relationships you experience with facilitators will ultimately contribute to your success in the BSN completion program?
5. How important is the sense of community to you in an online environment?

Inquiries

1. What was your incentive for moving into an online baccalaureate program as opposed to a brick-and-mortar program?
2. What factors do you feel would improve connections (psychological distance and social immediacy) in the online environment?

Many of the abstract concepts that we want to measure in nursing research are operationalized by using written scales of one type or another. Because the concepts are abstract, it is not logical or reasonable that we could measure them with a single question. For example, suppose we want to measure the concept of "stress." One could simply ask subjects "Are you stressed—yes or no?" However, answers to this question alone will not capture levels of stress, negative versus positive stress, sense of managing or not managing stress, or the nature of the stresses. To collect a fuller and more complex measure of stress, one needs more than one simple question, hence the use of scales that consist of several statements or items related to the concept being measured.

The first step in developing a scale to measure an abstract concept is to identify items or questions that are relevant to the concept. Identification of items may be based on previous

---

Box 8.2

Definitions and Relationships among an Instrument, Questionnaire, Scale, and Item

Instrument—a device that specifies (describes) and objectifies (clarifies) the process of data collection

Example: Written instructions for a focused observation of behaviors indicating pain

↓

Questionnaire—an instrument that is completed by the study subjects

Example: Three-page written form that asks subjects about their personal characteristics, medications, past medical history, and pain

↓

Scale—a set of written questions or statements that measures a specified variable

Example: Three questions that ask the subjects to rate how often they experience pain in different situations (e.g., "How often do you experience pain when walking?", "How often do you experience pain when sitting still?", and "How often do you experience pain when playing sports?").

↓

Item—the individual question or statement that comprises a scale

Example: How often do you wake up in the night because of your pain?

0	1	2	3
Never	Rarely	Occasionally	Frequently

---

research about the concept, theory related to the concept, experts' knowledge regarding the concept, or individuals' experiences with the concept. Often, items for a scale are created based on several of the sources described. For example, a list of items to measure stress might first be developed based on a theory of stress and coping, then reviewed by experts in the field of stress and coping for suggestions, and finally, reviewed or tested with small groups of individuals who are experiencing stress to see what they think about the items. The result might be five items such as those listed in Box 8.3. (*Note:* This is not an existing and established stress scale; it is simply intended to be an example.)

In addition to developing items that all are intended to address the same abstract concept or variable, scale development requires deciding how subjects will be asked to respond to the items. One type of response asks subjects to respond whether an item is true or false. A second approach to responding is called a Likert-type response scale. This type of response asks for a rating of the item on a continuum that is anchored at either end by opposite responses.

Box 8.3

Sample Stress Measurement Items

1. How often do you feel anxious?
2. How often do you have difficulty sleeping at night?
3. How often do you feel overwhelmed?
4. How often do you feel tired, even after a good night's sleep?
5. How often do you feel angry for no identifiable reason?

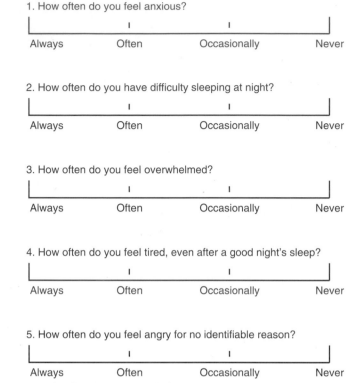

FIGURE 8.1   Example of a Likert-type scale for stress.

For example, a Likert-type response scale that asks subjects to rate the frequency with which they experience what is described in each item that reflects stress from Box 8.3 might range from "always" at one end to "never" on the other end, as illustrated in Figure 8.1. Another example that could be used with the same items intended to measure stress could ask about frequency of experiencing what is described in the item with four options: 0 = never, 1 = once a week, 2 = two to three times a week, and 3 = daily. Likert-type scales may include from three to as many as eight or more choices, although the usual number of responses ranges from four to six. Notice that the answers to these questions are structured so that the subject cannot answer anything that he or she wishes such as "once every other week" or "sometimes." Use of this scale to measure stress would result in a number between 0 and 15, which is a sum of the number for each item. The score on the scale could be considered to reflect the stress of the individual subject with subjects who answered "never" for all items, getting a score of 0, and subjects who answered "daily" for all items, getting a score of 15.

Visual analog is another response format that can be used in scales that differs from true/false, yes/no, and Likert-type scale responses. A visual analog consists of a straight line of a specific length that has extremes of responses at either end but does not have any other responses noted at points along the line. Subjects are asked to mark the line to indicate where they fall between the two extreme points. Often, the line is 100 mm because a line of that length fits easily on a standard piece of paper, and the subject's response is scored from 1 to 100, depending on the placement of his or her mark. For example, a subject might be asked to rate the level of stress that different situations cause for him or her, ranging from no stress to extreme stress, as illustrated in Figure 8.2.

Researchers can use a number of instruments to operationalize the variables in a study, such as the SCID, Mini–Mental Status Exam (MMSE), and the Charlson Comorbidity Index Scale. In the sleep and hunger in adolescents study (Landis, Parker, & Dunbar, 2009) (Appendix A.1), participants rated specific food cravings during the past month on a scale of 1, meaning

Rate your level of stress in each of the following situations by placing an "X" on the line below each situation. The left side of the line represents NO STRESS, and the far right side of the line represents EXTREME STRESS.

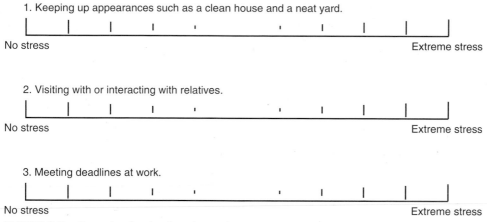

FIGURE 8.2 Example of a visual analog scale.

they never craved a particular food, to 5, meaning they always craved a particular food. The name of each instrument may allude to its use, and a small amount of research through common search engines (e.g., Google, Yahoo) yields a quick definition of what each scale entails.

It is important to recognize that information can be collected in many different capacities, as outlined above. Another format for collecting information in today's highly advanced technological society is via online surveys. There are numerous companies that support the utilization of online surveys, such as SurveyMonkey and Zoomerang. These types of companies provide the user with different survey formats and include survey wizards that will walk the user, step by step, through the creation of a tool. In addition to the creation of a survey instrument for data collection, they also provide services for analysis. Information can be gathered quickly, with data presented in real time. Some of these companies also provide methodologies for linking survey data to other sources, such as integration into kiosks, mergers with professional programs, or incorporation into social networking sites like Facebook.

We have now discussed methods to collect data and specific measurement approaches. We also have mentioned that at times error can occur in the methods or in the process of measurement and in the earlier section talked about potential errors in qualitative measurement. The potential for error occurs in both qualitative and quantitative methods of data collection. Understanding how this error can occur is important so that you can consider what that potential error means for understanding and using research in clinical practice.

■ ERRORS IN DATA COLLECTION IN QUANTITATIVE RESEARCH

In quantitative research, the data analysis process usually is separated from the data collection process. There are two general areas in which error can occur in quantitative data collection (1) in the quality of the measures used to collect data and (2) in the implementation of those measures or the data collection process itself. These two areas are not entirely discrete and do overlap. We start by talking about the quality of the measures used to collect quantitative data.

The Quality of Measures—Reliability and Validity

Accuracy and consistency in measurement are at the heart of successful quantitative research. As an intelligent reader and user of research, you must ask yourself two questions about any measure used in a quantitative study: (1) How consistently does the instrument, questionnaire, or procedure measure what it measures? and (2) Does the instrument, questionnaire, or procedure measure what it is supposed to measure? The first question addresses the reliability of a measure and the second question addresses its validity.

CORE CONCEPT 8.4

Consistent measurement is reliable measurement. Accurate or correct measurement is valid measurement.

Reliability means that a measure can be relied on consistently to give the same result if the aspect being measured has not changed. Consider, for example, measuring the gender of a sample: If three independent observers each record the gender of 1000 adults as they individually walk into a room, there will be a quite high level of consistency in the final count of the numbers of men and women in the sample. However, if even five or six of the sample are androgynous in their appearance, there may be some small differences in the final counts provided by the three observers. We have already said that this leads to some small error in the measure. If we changed our sample to 1000 diapered infants all dressed in white, we would expect much more inconsistency in the final totals because gender identification of infants by observation is much more difficult to do consistently. If, instead, three laboratories conducted genetic testings of each of the 1000 infants, there should be no differences in the final totals for boy and girls (assuming no laboratory error). Thus, the data collection on gender (particularly for infants) using the method of observation is less reliable than the data collection on gender using the method of genetic testing.

The reliability of a measure becomes more difficult to ensure as the measurement process becomes more complicated because complexity allows for more opportunities for error through inconsistency. Several approaches are taken to ensure or examine the reliability of measurement in quantitative research, depending on the type of measurement being used. When data are being collected by observation, a researcher often trains the observers and then tests them with different cases until all the observers agree on their observations the majority of the time. Earlier, we used a hypothetical example of observations to create a score for anxiety. If there were such a measure, the observers might be asked to practice making the observations needed with different "practice patients" to obtain a score on the anxiety scale until they each reached the same score at least 95% of the time.

In addition, when data are being collected by observation, researchers often report an interrater reliability score. Interrater reliability is present when two or more independent data collectors agree in the results of their data collection process. So, perhaps, in our hypothetical case of a rating of anxiety, a researcher might report that actual interrater reliability was 97%. This means that in 97% of the occasions, two independent raters got the same score. By providing this information, a researcher would help the RN in our clinical case to know that this complicated procedure to get a measurement of anxiety was used consistently across the different subjects. That consistency in use decreases the chances that any differences between subjects were due to inconsistent measurement rather than real differences. Assurances of reliability of a measure allow us to be comfortable that little error occurred in the measurement because of inconsistent use of the scale or instrument.

When a measure of a variable in a study is a written questionnaire or scale, two other types of approaches can be taken to ensure that the measure is reliable. The first is to test the measure before it is used in the study by having individuals complete the questionnaire or scale at two or more time points that are close enough together that we would not expect the "real" answers to have changed. This kind of reliability is called test–retest reliability; what we hope for is consistency in the answers in the different time points. If a scale or questionnaire is confusing or does not have a lot of meaning for a subject, his or her responses from one time to another are likely to differ. This means that the scores from the measure will not be consistent, and differences found may occur because of a lack of reliability of the measure rather than because of actual differences.

Similarly, one would expect that nursing students' choices of field of practice would not change much during a week. If the author of the fictional article (Appendix B) had administered his or her questionnaire to the students twice, a week apart, and found big differences in choice, we would believe that the questionnaire was not measuring this variable consistently. That inconsistency would then shed significant doubt on the findings of the study because we could not be sure that the study truly measured choice of field.

A second way that reliability is often measured for quantitative measures is by calculating a statistic called an *alpha coefficient*. This statistic reflects a computation of how closely the answers to different questions or items within a scale are related and is, therefore, often called the *internal consistency reliability coefficient*. Internal consistency reliability is the extent to which responses to a scale are similar and related. Remember that we said that many abstract concepts in nursing and other fields are measured using scales consisting of several items or questions that all relate to the same aspect being studied. If, in fact, all the items or questions address the same aspect or variable, we would expect a consistent pattern in how subjects respond to or answer the items.

Let us go back to the five items that we are pretending were developed to measure stress (Box 8.3). We would expect that a highly stressed person would indicate that most of the experiences listed were happening regularly. If, instead, we found that subjects indicated that one or two of the items were occurring regularly but that others were not occurring at all, there would be a low internal consistency among the items. Alpha coefficients, often called the *Cronbach alpha* after the statistician who developed the test, can range from 0 to 1.0, with a value of 0 indicating that there are absolutely no relationships among the responses to the different items in a scale and a value of 1.0 meaning that the answers to the items were all completely connected or related to each other. In general, researchers hope for an alpha coefficient of greater than 0.7, indicating a relatively strong relationship or connection among the responses to the different items on any particular scale.

To summarize, the reliability of a measure reflects how definite we can be that the measure will yield the same data consistently if the actual or "real" variable stays the same. When quantitative data are collected using observation, the rate of agreement, or interrater agreement, tells us the consistency of the observational measure. Test–retest reliability can tell us if a measure stays consistent over time when the aspect measured has not changed. Internal consistency reliability or a Cronbach alpha coefficient is a statistic that tells us how consistently subjects responded to a set of items or questions. In all three cases, the goal in quantitative research is to use measures that will most consistently measure the variables of interest.

Validity is the second aspect of measurement that must be considered when deciding on use of research in clinical practice. Validity reflects how accurately the measure yields information about the true or real variable being studied. A measure is valid if it measures correctly and accurately what it is intended to measure. Validity becomes more of an issue the more abstract the variable to be measured is; with a concrete variable such as gender, validity is not a great concern. We are generally confident that gender self-report will yield a true measure of gender. However, let us look at another demographic variable that may seem as concrete: the variable of race. To measure this variable, researchers might ask subjects to indicate their race by checking one category from a list that looks like the one in Box 8.4. On initial inspection, we might assume that this list is clear and should yield valid results. However, although the use of the term *Native American* to represent those individuals who represent the indigenous peoples of the Americas is considered politically correct, it also can be interpreted to mean "born in America." If many subjects interpret an item asking about race in this way, then the measure will yield inaccurate information about race.

Box 8.4

Please Check the Item Below That Best Describes You

_____ Black   _____ Latino/Latina
_____ White–non-Hispanic   _____ Asian–not Pacific Islander
_____ Native American   _____ Pacific Islander

A second example of an invalid measure might come from Box 8.3, where we listed five fictional items that a researcher might use to measure stress. Looking at those items more closely, one might wonder if they are really measuring stress or if they more accurately measure depression. Certainly, feelings of anxiety and anger, trouble sleeping, and feeling overwhelmed are classic symptoms of depression. Thus, this measure may be an inaccurate measure of stress because it may actually be measuring depression, which is an entirely different concept. The issue of validity of a measure becomes much more complex in scales used to measure variables such as depression, stress, efficacy, motivation, or coping. Scales or written instruments that are developed to measure abstract concepts such as these must find a way to describe or ask about factors that are specific to the concept and are clear enough to avoid confusion with other concepts. Three types of validity are sometimes described within reports of research: content validity, criterion-related validity, and construct validity.

The simplest of the three, and the one that is most easy for a reader of research to assess, is content validity. Content validity asks whether the items or questions on a scale are comprehensive and appropriately reflect the concept that they are supposed to measure. Put simply, the question becomes "Is the *content* of the scale complete and appropriate?" Researchers who have to develop their own measure of a concept will try to establish the content validity of the measure by asking a group of experts to review the items on the scale for completeness and appropriateness. If researchers are using a measure that has only been used a few times in other research, they may describe what type of assessment was made of the measure when it was developed to ensure content validity. As a user of research, you can assess what is called the *face validity of a measure*, which is simply one person's (perhaps not an expert's) interpretation of content validity. Face validity is a judgment of how clearly the items on a scale reflect the concept they are intended to measure.

As we have said, if we consider the face validity of the items listed in Box 8.3 that were proposed to measure stress, we might begin to question them. In fact, the items listed in that box generally reflect the symptoms that we expect to see when someone is experiencing depression rather than stress. Although depression and stress may be related, we do not necessarily expect everyone who is experiencing significant negative stress to also be depressed. Therefore, the face validity of these items must be questioned. In all likelihood, if a panel of stress experts reviewed these items, they would decide that the items were not valid items for a stress scale.

The RN in our clinical case can make some independent judgments about the face validity of most of the scales used in the efficacy of a home care approach study because the authors give the reader information about the content of the items on several of the scales. In the example of the State-Trait Anxiety Inventory, the authors make this comment: "Research assistants administered the Structures Clinical Interview for Axis I DSM-IV Disorders (SCID) in patients' homes to assess depressive symptoms and disorders. According to SCID criteria, a symptom was rated present if the patient reported that the symptom occurred most of the day nearly every day for any 2-week period in the past month" (Brown et al., 2006).

The RN can think about previous professional experience with depressed patients and decide whether these areas of feelings are inclusive of the major signs and symptoms of depression. In thinking about this, the RN is utilizing clinical judgment about the face validity of the scale; if the nurse decides that it is not valid, it may be decided that the results of the study connected with this variable are questionable for use in practice.

The second type of validity that may be described in a research report is criterion-related validity. Criterion-related validity is the extent to which the results of one measure match those of another measure that is also supposed to reflect the variable under study. The question asked with this type of validity is "Do the results from the scale relate to a known criterion relevant to the variable?" If a researcher were trying to test the criterion-related validity of the five-item "stress" scale in Box 8.3, subjects might be asked to answer those five items and then to rate their stress level on a scale from 1 to 100. If scores from responses on the five items closely matched ratings of stress on the 100-point scale, they might be considered to provide some evidence for the criterion-related validity of the five-item scale. The criterion used in this example is a direct self-rating of stress level, and the example is one of a test for concurrent criterion-related validity. That is, the test looked for a relationship between two measures concurrently, or at the same time.

A second type of criterion-related validity looks for a relationship between the scale being tested and some measure that should be closely related that occurs in the future. This type of validity is called *predictive validity*. An example of predictive validity for the SCID might be found in the fact that the authors recognized that late-life depression is often going unrecognized in the home care environment (Brown et al., 2006) since they picked up on it during their study.

The last type of validity that is sometimes discussed in a report of research is construct validity. Construct validity is the broadest type of validity and can encompass both content and criterion-related validity because it is the extent to which a scale or an instrument measures what it is supposed to measure. The construct validity of a scale or an instrument is supported with time if results using the measure support theory about how the construct (variable) being measured is supposed to behave. This may include predictive validity and concurrent validity but also will include other less direct predictions that arise from theory. Several approaches can be taken to measure the construct validity of a scale or an instrument, including use of statistical procedures such as factor analysis or structural equation modeling, comparison of results from the measure to closely related and vastly differing constructs, and the development of hypotheses that are then tested to provide support for the scale. In all cases, the goal is to build evidence that the construct, or abstract variable, is being measured by the scale.

There is a relationship between the validity and reliability of measures: A scale can be reliable but not valid. However, a scale cannot be valid and also not be reliable. A scale may consistently measure something (reliability) but not the something it is supposed to measure (validity). However, if a scale measures what it is supposed to measure (validity), then it will inherently also be consistent (reliable). So a scale must have reliability in order to have the possibility of being valid. For example, we have suggested that the five items in Box 8.3 have questionable validity as a measure of stress, but it is possible that subjects might answer those five questions consistently, giving us reliable data about something—just not about stress.

One last note about reliability and validity is related to data collection from sources such as medical records. In nursing research, using medical records to collect certain types of data is quite common. However, some unique issues surrounding this data must be considered. As all nurses know, we can be confident that whatever is documented on a record has a high likelihood of having occurred. Therefore, if we are collecting data about pain level and we find notations regarding the patient's pain complaints, we can be sure they are accurate. However, we cannot be as confident that the absence of a notation about pain means that the patient did not have pain. If a great deal happened during a particular shift and a patient's pain was not exceptional in some way, it is possible that the pain was not charted. Thus, the reliability of certain types of data from medical records—that is, the consistency with which the kinds of data are documented—must be considered when choosing to use medical records to measure study variables. This is not to say that records are unreliable, only that there is inconsistency in the documentation of certain care aspects in records.

Table 8.4

Aspects of Reliability and Validity

ASPECT	DEFINITION	METHODS
Reliability—how consistent is the measure?		
Interrater reliability	Agreement between two or more independent data collectors about the results of their data collection process	Carefully structured instruments Practice until a high level of agreement is reached
Test–retest reliability	Consistency in answers on tests when we would not expect the real answers to have changed	Repeated administration of measures or tests to calculate consistency in responses
Internal consistency reliability	The extent to which responses to a scale are similar and related	Calculation of a Cronbach alpha coefficient
Validity—how accurate is the measure?		
Content validity	The comprehensiveness and appropriateness of the measure to the concept it is intended to measure	Expert panel review Face validity
Criterion-related validity	The extent to which results of one measure match those of another measure that examines the same concept	Concurrent validity Predictive validity
Construct validity	The extent to which a scale or instrument measures what it is supposed to measure	Content and criterion-related validity Hypothesis testing Statistica procedures such as factor analysis

In summary, the different types of reliability and validity that must be considered when understanding quantitative studies are detailed in Table 8.4. Although reliability focuses on the consistency of a measure, validity focuses on the accuracy or correctness of a measure. Researchers consider three types of validity. Content validity refers to the extent to which the scale or instrument is comprehensive and addresses the concept or variable of interest. Criterion-related validity can be either concurrent or predictive and refers to how closely the results on the measure in question relate to results on other measures of the same concept in the present or future. Construct validity refers to the overall ability of the scale to measure what it is supposed to measure and is established only after the repeated use of a measure yields results that reflect the theoretical expectations for the concept being measured. An instrument of measurement can be reliable but not valid. However, if a measure has been shown to be valid, then it will be reliable; this is reflective of the ideal of evidence-based nursing practice.

Errors in Implementation of Quantitative Data Collection

We said that error can be introduced into the measurement of variables in quantitative research because of problems with either the quality of the measure or the process of implementing the measure. Although reliability and validity speak to the quality of a measure, even a reliable and valid measure can be implemented incorrectly and lead to error. Implementation of data collection requires careful and detailed planning to ensure that the process is consistent and does not invalidate the measures. For example, a researcher could be using a reliable and valid measure of blood sugars, but subjects may fail to understand the dietary restrictions of fasting before samples are collected, thus introducing errors into the data. A procedure that confirms true fasting status would ensure that the measure yielded meaningful data. Another example of an implementation error occurs when a written scale that may have been shown previously to be reliable and valid is administered with incorrect directions, or the subjects are prompted in a way that sways their responses to a measure. Pointing out that the financial support for an agency depends on positive reviews before asking subjects to complete a satisfaction survey is an obvious example.

The order in which subjects are asked to complete questionnaires also can affect their responses. For example, if subjects are asked to complete a scale that asks several questions about symptoms of depression and then are asked to rate their level of overall depression, the scale likely will have increased their awareness of how depressed they really are, thus affecting their total depression ratings. In addition, different timing and environments affect data collection. For example, asking nursing students about their choices of field when they have just completed an exciting clinical rotation in the emergency room could lead to more of them selecting the emergency room than would have selected it if they had been asked at some time after that rotation.

Other types of error that can occur in the measurement process include sloppy handling of data, resulting in a loss of some of it. Failure to keep careful records can lead to missed opportunities for repeat measures because subjects' addresses or telephone numbers are misplaced or not accurately recorded. This is a problem, particularly in longitudinal studies in which subjects are asked to complete measures at two different time points.

Finally, the implementation of data collection can introduce error by arbitrarily changing a measure through translating it to another language or administering it in a format other than that which was intended. Measures that are reliable and valid have been successfully translated into other languages, but this requires a careful translation process and then translating the measure back into the original language by independent translators to ensure that the meanings of items on a scale remain intact when the language changes. An issue similar to translation to another language exists when a measure that was developed to be read by a subject is instead read to a subject. The subject is then hearing the words rather then seeing them, and this can definitely affect his or her understanding and potential response to the items.

In summary, measurement in quantitative research must be carefully planned and controlled. The variables to be measured must be clearly defined. If the variables are abstract, we should expect to see both a theoretical definition and an operational definition so that we can judge both the meaning of the variable and how well that meaning was translated into data through measurement. Errors in measurement can be present because of problems with the measure itself or incorrect implementation of the measure.

The measurement language in both qualitative and quantitative research can be complex and confusing. Overall, the important points are that data collection must be trustworthy, confirmable, and consistent as well as transferable, credible, and accurate. Both the process and actual measures in data collection must be considered as we decide how to use the results of research in practice. To decide how measurement in a study has affected results and conclusions, we must receive complete and clear information about the measures. This leads us to consider what might be some common problems with written reports of data collection.

■ COMMON ERRORS IN WRITTEN REPORTS OF DATA COLLECTION METHODS

Probably, the most common error that occurs in written reports of research studies is provision of incomplete information. This was somewhat of a problem with the article read by the RN in our clinical case (Appendix A.6) because the report does not provide as much detail about the different instruments used in the study as we might like. For example, we know neither how many items were in the SCID or the Charlson Comorbidity Index nor what the possible range of scores would be. We also do not know from the article much about the MMSE, although this is commonly used in practice; we only know generalities that are addressed.

Similarly, the fictional article (Appendix B) leaves several gaps in the information provided about the collection of the data. For example, the author does not give us a clear theoretical or operational definition of the dependent variable in this study—choice of field. Theoretically, "choice" could be defined as what students would really like to do if all options were open to them, or it could be defined as what students expect to do given current openings and other aspects of their personal situations. The results section of this report does give us some idea about how "field of choice" was operationally defined because those categories that were elected by the students are listed. We know that the students were not permitted to write in their choice but were given a list of nursing career options from which to select. However, the author does not tell us what was included in the original list of options, so we do not know if the final categories reported in Table B.1 from the fictional article included all the possible options or if there were options that were not selected or were collapsed into one of the reported categories. In other words, we are not clear about the operational definition for the dependent variable either. This lack of clear information jeopardizes the usefulness of the research for practice because it becomes difficult to be comfortable with conclusions based on measurement that we do not understand or believe was consistent or accurate.

A second common error with written reports of data collection is a failure to organize clearly the information in a manner that makes it understandable. Although numerous studies do not include a written report of the data collection, the table in the home care study entitled "Sociodemographic and Clinical Characteristics of Sample" helps us visualize the variables and measures used in the study.

A third error that occasionally occurs is a failure to reference the source of measures used in a study. Although the practicing nurse may not choose to do so often, the option of reading other studies that previously used a measure that was used in the new study should be available. Referencing reports of previous studies that indicated the reliability and validity of a measure is particularly important because it gives the reader the option to learn more about that specific measure and increases one's confidence in the quality of the measure.

■ CRITICALLY READING METHODS SECTIONS OF RESEARCH REPORTS

There are seven questions you can ask yourself as you read the methods section of a research report, and these are listed in Box 8.5. The first and probably simplest question to ask yourself is "Did the report include a clearly identified section describing methods used in this study?" The efficacy of the home care approach study included a methods section with several pertinent subsections. The next question to ask is "Do the methods make this a quantitative or a qualitative study?" In this chapter, more than any up until now, we have been able to clearly separate qualitative and quantitative methods because these two approaches to collecting data differ so markedly. Thus, if you read that a researcher is planning a qualitative study using a written questionnaire with 25 items that will measure well-being, you will have to immediately wonder about the match between stated approach and actual methods used. You also will be surprised to find a quantitative study report that does not provide information to operationally define the variables in the study. The article may not call the description of measurement *operational definitions*, but if no explanation of measurement is present or the measurement is openended and unstructured, you may question the fit between approach and methods.

In critically reading the methods section of a research report, you should ask a third question, "Do I understand what my patient population would be doing if they were in this study or a study using a similar method?" If you are not sure what they would be asked to do, or how often they would be asked to do something, then the methods section is probably not as detailed

Box 8.5

How to Critically Read the Methods Section of a Research Report

Does the report answer the question "How were those people studied—why was the study performed that way?"

1. Did the report include a clearly identified section describing methods used in the study?
2. Do the methods make this a quantitative or a qualitative study?
3. Do I understand what my patient population would be doing if they were in this study or a study using similar methods?
4. Do the measures and procedures in this study address my clinical problem?
5. Do I think that the measures used in this study would provide helpful and useful information when used with my patient population?
6. Do I think what the researcher collected and how it was collected was the best way to address the clinical question?
7. Do I think that the researcher(s) should have planned the study differently in order to answer my clinical question?

as needed. Without enough detail about study measurement and procedures, it is impossible to evaluate the usefulness of study results. In particular, if one does not know how a variable was measured, it is not possible to decide whether the measurement was appropriate. A related question is "Do the measures and procedures in this study address my clinical problem?" Again, without enough detail, one cannot answer that question; however, if adequate detail is provided, you will want to ask critically if you think that the methods used address your clinical concern. For example, the RN in our clinical case is interested in home care approaches for physiologic and psychosocial needs. Thus, the methods in this study do seem to reflect the RN's clinical question.

The next two questions to consider address "Do I think that the measures used in this study would provide helpful and useful information when used with my patient population?" and "Do I think what the researcher collected and how it was collected was the best way to address the clinical question?" In a qualitative study, one needs to consider trustworthiness, confirmability, credibility, and transferability of the data based on what is told about the data collection process and the measure used. Similarly, in a quantitative study, reliability and validity of measures used in the study and whether potential error was introduced through the data collection process need to be considered. If the report does not provide enough information for you to answer these questions, then you may not be able to use the findings in your clinical practice.

It is also important to consider "Do I think that the researcher(s) should have planned the study differently in order to answer my clinical question?" Again, the RN in our clinical case might agree with the time intervals and measurement points in the home care study, which reaffirms the nurse's ability to use the information from this study in clinical practice. Similarly, you might decide that a quantitative study that had trouble operationalizing an abstract variable perhaps should have started with a qualitative approach in order to collect data about that concept.

Finally, you should ask, "How can I use this information as part of my evidence-based nursing practice?" Today's nursing practice should be grounded in evidence, and the best way to incorporate this into your own nursing care is by reading, understanding, and utilizing the evidence, from credible sources, that is available to you. This last question directly leads you to consider the overall study design, and that will be the topic of Chapter 9.

■ CONNECTING DATA COLLECTION METHODS TO SAMPLING, RESULTS, AND DISCUSSION/CONCLUSION

At the beginning of this chapter, we said that the RN needed to understand how the study variables were measured to comprehend the meaning of the results of the studies about the home care approach. One thing that may have become clear as the nurse learned more about research methods is that sampling and data collection methods are linked in both quantitative and qualitative research. Particularly in qualitative studies, data collection and analysis drive the sampling because additional participants often are sought purposely to focus on aspects of the phenomenon that are emerging from the data. We also discussed trustworthiness and the use of both member and group checks. These aspects of rigor in data collection require sampling strategies that ensure a trusting and open relationship with the data collector. Further, a researcher may ask the right questions about a phenomenon but may fail to gain access to the right groups to answer those questions; so, as we read about data collection, we must consider the sampling process as well.

In quantitative research, sampling is most connected to data collection in follow-up for repeated measures over time. However, the data collection process also can be affected by the nature of the sample or vice versa. For example, a study of homeless patients that uses measures written in English that have no established Spanish version may exclude a group of Spanish-speaking subjects. Another problem in data collection that is closely related to sampling is the educational level assumed in the measures. A complex written scale that uses language aimed at a high school reading level may become unreliable when used with subjects who have a lower education level. Thus, sampling and data collection can be closely linked in quantitative research as well as in qualitative research.

Throughout this chapter, we have stressed that if variables are not clearly defined or are not consistently and accurately measured, the results of the study must be questioned. Similarly, if rigor is not maintained through both data collection and analysis, the results of qualitative research are jeopardized; the results of a study are only as good as the data that went into those results. Therefore, understanding how data were collected and recognizing how potential sources of error in the data collection were addressed is closely linked to our ability to accept the results of a study. This, in turn, clearly affects our willingness to accept and adopt the conclusions of a study.

A last link between data collection and the rest of the research process is the link between data collection and the section of a research report that speaks to limitations of a study. Despite the best plans and efforts, problems do arise with data collection. These may be mentioned in the write-up of the data collection itself, but the implications of those problems for the conclusions of a study are often addressed when the author discusses limitations. For example, in the discussion of the home care approach study report, the authors identify data collection from a single home care agency, liberal criteria for evaluation of referral information, a small number of subjects with depressive or cognitively challenged symptoms, and age of the data as limitations that may have affected the results of their study (Brown et al., 2006). Thus, the conclusions of a study are directly linked back to the measurement process.

■ PUBLISHED REPORTS—WOULD YOU USE THESE STUDIES IN CLINICAL PRACTICE?

Our RN was concerned about how to help M.J. and other home care patients with their needs after coming home from the hospital. After considering the data collection methods in the efficacy of an in-home intervention article, the RN is comfortable that a home care approach for physical and psychosocial needs intervention has some potential to empower patients in their recovery process. The researchers in the study followed a clearly described procedure and mainly used measures that have reports of validity and reliability. The RN believes that the outcomes examined—the type of home care approach, specifically as it pertains to medication reconciliation (based on information received from referral agencies) and psychological and cognitive states of mind—are clinically relevant in the nurse's experience with patients. Based on this information, the RN decides that this piece of literature will indeed assist her in transitioning M.J. to home care; the information in the study has helped raise the nurse's awareness about the need for thorough attention to medication reconciliation and to assessing M.J.'s psychological and cognitive states of mind. Utilizing these more detailed approaches to create an effective plan of care for M.J., the nurse feels confident that the care M.J. receives will be based on evidence that is credible and useful in practice.

OUT-OF-CLASS EXERCISE

Free Write

The next chapter continues to address the question of why a study included the people it did and it was done the way it was by talking about research designs. Before reading that chapter, consider the question of whether being in nursing school affects the students' well-being. If you were going to conduct a study to address this question, how would you go about it? What do you think would be the best way to conduct a study to answer this question, and what do you think would be the most realistic approach? Are they the same or different, and why? Think about this, then write in as much detail as possible your ideas about how to conduct a study to determine if and how being a nursing student affects well-being. Wherever you can, write your rationale for conducting the study in the manner on which you have decided. After you have completed this assignment, you will be ready to move on to read about research designs in Chapter 9.

References

Brown, E., Raue, P., Mlodzianowski, A., Barnett, S., Meyers, B., Greenberg, R., et al. (2006). Transition to home care: Quality of mental health, pharmacy, and medical history information. *International Journal of Psychiatry in Medicine, 36*(3), 339–349.

Denzin, N. K. (2001). *Interpretive interactionism* (2nd ed.). Newbury Park, CA: Sage Publications.

Landis, A., Parker, K., & Dunbar, S. B. (2009). Sleep, hunger, satiety, food cravings, and caloric intake in adolescents. *Journal of Nursing Scholarship, 41*(2), 115–123.

Lincoln, Y. S., & Guba, E. G. (1985). *Naturalistic inquiry.* Beverly Hills, CA: Sage Publications.

Resources

Campbell, D. T., & Russo, M. J. (2001). *Social measurement.* Thousand Oaks, CA: Sage Publications.

Denzin, N. K., & Lincoln, Y. S. (Eds.). (2007). *Collecting and interpreting qualitative materials* (3rd ed.). Thousand Oaks, CA: Sage Publications.

LoBiondo-Wood, G., Haber, J., & Krainovich-Miller, B. (2009). Overview of the research process. In G. LoBiondo-Wood & J. Haber (Eds.), *Nursing research: Methods, critical appraisal, and utilization* (6th ed.). St. Louis, MO: Mosby.

Locke, L. F., Silverman, S. J., & Spirduso, W. W. (2009). *Reading and understanding research* (3rd ed.). Thousand Oaks, CA: Sage Publications.

Polit, D. F., & Beck, C. T. (2007). *Nursing research: Principles and methods* (7th ed.). Philadelphia: Lippincott Williams & Wilkins.

Research Designs: Planning the Study

How Were Those People Studied— Why Was the Study Performed That Way?

KEY TERMS

Clinical trials
Comparison group
Control group
Correlational studies
Cross-sectional
Descriptive design
Ethnography
Experimental designs
Experimenter effects
External validity
Grounded theory
Hawthorne effect
Historical research method
History
Instrumentation
Internal validity
Longitudinal

Maturation
Measurement effects
Mixed methods
Model
Mortality
Multifactorial
Novelty effects
Phenomenology
Pretest–posttest
Prospective designs
Quasi-experimental designs
Reactivity effects
Repeated measures
Research design
Retrospective designs
Selection bias
Testing

Clinical Case • A nurse is working in the ICU unit of a small rural hospital. The nurse is on duty the night that D.M., a truck driver, is admitted to the unit following an accident, where he fell asleep and ran off the road and into a ditch. D.M. overturned his truck, sustaining a crushing injury to his chest. He was in the ditch for 30 minutes before help arrived, and it took another 30 minutes to extricate him from the vehicle. D.M. specializes in long-distance hauling, and he lives almost 3000 miles from the site of the accident. He is married, has two small children, and enjoys coaching his children's soccer teams. D.M. is still in critical condition and will be in the ICU for some time, as he is currently too unstable to transfer.

The RN assigned to care for D.M. is a recent graduate who has just completed an orientation period to the ICU. The RN wonders how D.M.'s recovery will be impacted by the traumatic circumstances that brought the patient to the ICU and now separates him from his family. The RN is concerned about what nursing interventions will assist with D.M.'s adjustment and how that can be matched to his lack of close psychosocial support. The charge nurse tells the RN there is a nursing article about supporting the psychosocial needs of ICU patients and wonders if the new graduate RN would find it helpful. According to the charge nurse, the study findings indicate that anxiety and depression are most closely associated with critically ill ICU patients. The RN decides to find and read this article, entitled "Psychological Consequences Associated with Intensive Care Treatment" (Carr, 2007) and to search for additional information about the psychosocial needs of ICU patients. This article is available in Appendix A.7. Read it before you continue with this chapter so that the examples discussed will be more meaningful. Table 9.1 identifies the clinical question of the RN and the key search terms that could be used in a search.

We will also return to many of the articles used in the earlier chapters as further examples, so it would be a great idea to review them as well. Remember, all the articles used as examples are available in full text throughout Appendix A.

■ RESEARCH DESIGNS: WHY ARE THEY IMPORTANT?

As we have considered how to interpret and use research findings in nursing practice, we have been moving from the end of research reports toward their beginning. We have learned that the conclusions of a report usually do not provide enough information to allow us to fully understand or apply the findings. The usefulness of the study results depends on the

Table 9.1

Statement of Clinical Question From the Clinical Case

What interventions will assist ICU patients in terms of psychosocial support?

The *Who*	ICU patients
The *What*	Psychosocial support
The *When*	When hospitalized in the ICU
The *Where*	In the ICU
Key search terms to find research-based evidence for practice	ICU, support, adjustment, family, psychosocial, emotional, psychological, intensive care, needs

ICU, intensive care unit.

sample and the methods used to collect data. We have also learned that various approaches to sampling and data collection have differing strengths and weaknesses. Thus, we need to better understand the overall purpose and nature of research designs because they direct the sampling and data collection processes. This chapter discusses research designs to help explain why a study is planned and implemented using a particular design and how different designs affect approaches to sampling and data collection, which, in turn, influence the study results and conclusions.

The RN in the clinical case reads in the psychological consequences article that both qualitative and quantitative research designs have been used in the study of this topic, but the nurse is not sure why one methodology would be selected over the other when choosing a study approach. The RN knows that much of nursing research is qualitative in nature, because nursing deals with the human experience; yet, the nurse also understands that some of nursing research is not qualitative and wonders how a qualitative design will produce information that is useful for his practice. Remembering from nursing school that quantitative research designs, such as randomized or experimental studies, are considered "strong," and whether that might be a better type of design to use when planning care for D.M., the nurse then thinks of the human dynamic associated with anxiety and depression. Based on this knowledge, the nurse decides that qualitative would be the "best" type of design to use in this situation, because care for a psychological concern needs to take the human experience and perception into account.

A research design is the overall plan for acquiring new knowledge or confirming existing knowledge. In Chapter 1, we said that research is characterized by a systematic approach to gathering information to answer questions, which is in contrast to those approaches that use intuition, seek expert advice, or follow tradition. The research design is the plan for that systematic approach, conducted in a way that ensures the answer(s) found will be as meaningful and accurate as possible. The design identifies how subjects will be recruited and incorporated into a study; what will happen during the study, including timing of any treatments and measures; and when the study will end. A research design is selected with two broad purposes: (1) to plan an approach that will best answer the research question and (2) to ensure the rigor and validity of the results. We will discuss each of these purposes in general terms, and then we will look at specific approaches to research design.

Answering the Research Question

The first purpose in selecting a research design is to plan a systematic collection of information that will answer the question of interest. Two considerations are important: (1) the fit of the design to the research question and (2) the functionality of the design for the purpose of the study. Fit refers to how well the design matches the question of interest. It is in considering fit that we begin to address the question the RN in our clinical case has asked

Box 9.1

General Types of Research Questions

- Questions that describe
- Questions that connect or link factors or concepts
- Questions that predict or examine effects of manipulation

about meeting the psychosocial needs of a long-distance trucker. In the simplest terms, not all research questions can be answered through experiments because experimental designs answer questions requiring that we already know a great deal about the topic in order to set up a meaningful experiment. For example, simply setting up an experiment would not answer a research question regarding the characteristics of student nurses who select nonacute settings for their first practice after graduation. Why? Because an experiment assumes that we know some factors that we want to manipulate in order to see if and how they affect an outcome. If we do not know what factors are influencing the outcome of interest—in this example, the choice of practice after graduation—we have nothing to manipulate!

Research questions can be broadly categorized as questions that seek to describe or understand, questions that seek to connect or relate, and questions that seek to predict or study the effects of manipulation (Box 9.1). Generally, if we do not have adequate knowledge about a phenomenon of interest to nursing, we have to start by describing and understanding it, and the researcher will select a design that best allows for meeting that need. Once such studies are done and we have some idea of the meaning of the selected aspects of the phenomenon, we can ask questions about connections or relationships among those aspects. To answer those questions, the researcher will need a different form of design. Only after we know something about the connections and relationships can we begin to ask questions that seek to predict or manipulate aspects of the phenomenon, and there are designs specifically matched to this as well.

Now we are more aware that a research design must fit the type of question asked in order to provide appropriate and effective answers. A research design intended to answer questions about prediction will not be useful or appropriate for questions that seek to describe a phenomenon. Similarly, a design meant to allow meaningful description will not answer questions that seek to predict. The fit of a design to a research question depends on the function of the design and on how much is known about the topic of the study. In other words, different research designs serve different functions and, therefore, are particularly well suited to one type of research question, but not to another.

The functions of specific research designs can be broadly categorized, just as types of questions can be categorized. The functions include

1. Designs for describing or understanding
2. Designs for connecting or relating
3. Designs for manipulation and prediction

CORE CONCEPT 9.1

The type of research question being asked affects the type of research design that will and can be used.

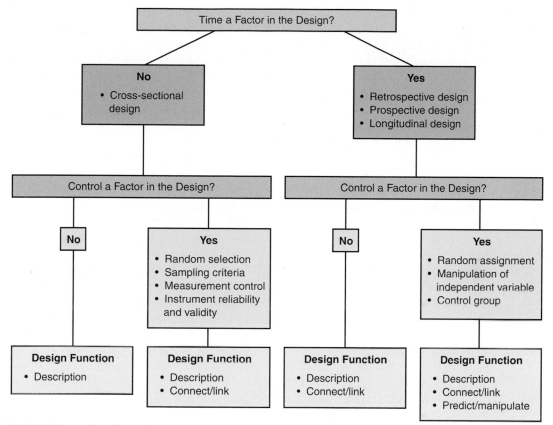

FIGURE 9.1 Three broad factors that affect research design and associated terms.

Two other important considerations are designs that include timing or time as a factor in the study and designs that seek to control or not to control. Although several other factors differentiate types of research designs, the framework we will use for understanding how research designs influence the meaningfulness of research for practice focuses on three factors: (1) the overall function of the design, (2) how time or timing is incorporated into the design, and (3) whether the design seeks to control or not control study factors. Figure 9.1 depicts these broad factors and how they relate. We will discuss specific designs that fit into each category later in the chapter.

In summary, when deciding on a design, a researcher must consider several factors, including the functions of a design and the fit of those functions to the purpose of the research. Research designs differ in terms of the type of questions they can answer, whether they include time as a factor, and whether they focus on control within the study. The fit and functionality of a research design significantly influence whether the study can answer the research question of interest.

Ensuring Rigor and Validity

In addition to examining function and fit to answer the research question, the research design has a purpose to ensure the rigor and validity of a study. In Chapter 8, we discussed these concepts in the context of specific strategies for data collection and measurement. The terms *rigor* and *validity* also are used in a broader sense to refer to the overall study. In Chapter 8, we said that rigor is a strict process of data collection and analysis as well as a term that reflects the overall quality of that process in qualitative research. It is in the broader sense of this quality that we consider rigor when discussing study design. Designs in qualitative research usually are more flexible and often are described as "emerging" to indicate that the design may be altered as the study progresses. Nevertheless, the design must still have a function that fits the research question and provides the foundation ensuring the accuracy of the study.

Like the term *rigor*, *validity* is used in research to refer both to specific ways that measures can correctly and accurately reflect their intended variable and to the accuracy of the overall results. Although use of the word *validity* in reference to measurement and design may be confusing, remember that the validity always has the same general meaning: accuracy or correctness. Content validity, criterion-related validity, and construct validity all refer to aspects of the accuracy of a measure. Validity of a study refers to its accuracy.

Study designs in quantitative research provide the foundation that ensures the overall validity. Two types of validity are mentioned frequently when discussing research design. The first type, called internal validity, is the extent to which we can be sure of the accuracy or correctness of the findings of the study. Thus, it refers to how accurate the results are within the study itself, or internally. The second type, called external validity, is the extent to which the results of a study can be applied to other groups or situations. In other words, external validity refers to how accurately the study provides knowledge that can be applied outside of, or external to, the study. Figure 9.2 summarizes and illustrates the relationships among measurement validity, internal validity, and external validity.

Research designs can affect both internal and external validity, and these two types are related in many research designs. Generalizability, discussed in Chapter 6, is a big aspect of external validity because it refers to the ability to infer that findings for a particular sample can be applied to the entire population. External validity also includes the extent to which the findings from a study in one setting can be applied to other similar settings. Logically, if a study lacks internal validity, it automatically lacks external validity: If the results are not accurate within the study, they clearly will not be accurate in other samples or settings. Similarly, if a study lacks measurement validity, it will lack internal validity. However, a study can have measurement validity and not have internal validity, or it can have correct findings and thus be internally valid but not externally valid. That is, the findings of a study may be real and correct to the specific sample and setting of the study but not applicable to the general population or to other settings. This

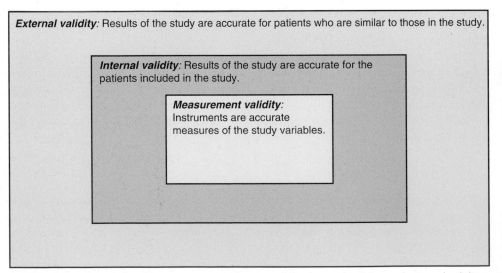

FIGURE 9.2   The relationships among measurement validity, internal validity, and external validity.

Table 9.2

Threats to Rigor and Internal and External Validity

RIGOR—ACCURACY OF FINDINGS OF A QUALITATIVE STUDY	INTERNAL VALIDITY—ACCURACY OF FINDINGS WITHIN A QUANTITATIVE STUDY	EXTERNAL VALIDITY—ACCURACY OF FINDINGS OF A QUANTITATIVE STUDY TO THE SETTINGS AND SAMPLES OUTSIDE OF THE STUDY
Trustworthiness	History	Reactivity effects
Confirmability	Maturation	(Hawthorne effect)
Credibility	Testing	Measurement effects
Consistency	Instrumentation	Novelty effects
	Mortality	Experimenter effects
	Selection bias	

relationship is illustrated in Figure 9.2 by the nesting of the three boxes representing the three types of validity.

Several aspects of study design can potentially lead to problems with rigor and internal and external validity. These problems are referred to as *threats to validity* because they threaten the accuracy of internal findings or the ability to apply the findings to other samples or settings. The threats to rigor and internal and external validity often discussed in research literature are listed in Table 9.2.

Threats to the Rigor of a Qualitative Study

As was indicated in Chapter 8, the rigor of a qualitative study is reflected in the consistency, trustworthiness, transferability, and credibility of the study. Qualitative designs or methods are based on distinct philosophical perspectives and have clearly defined systematic methods associated with each design. When we talked about these concepts in Chapter 8, we focused on the process of data collection, but in this chapter, we will focus on the process of implementing the entire study. For example, when considering these concepts in reference to the overall rigor of a study, we must consider *consistency* in the application of the study design throughout the study or consider *credibility* given the researchers' accurate use of the study method. Thus, the language used to speak about overall study rigor in qualitative research is essentially the same as that used to discuss the data collection process, but the focus is broadened to the implementation of the study as a whole, and method and standards will differ a little.

Threats to Internal Validity

Threats to internal validity are potential problems that can affect the accuracy or correctness of findings within a study. They include problems of history, maturation, testing, instrumentation, mortality, and selection bias. These threats are summarized in Box 9.2.

Box 9.2

Summary of Threats to Internal Validity

Internal validity is threatened because some *outside factor* (**history**) or *time* (**maturation**) affects the dependent variable, because the *measurement process* itself (**testing**) or *changes in a manner* (**instrumentation**) affect results for the dependent variable, or because the sampling process is biased *by loss of subjects* (**mortality**) or *selection of subjects* (**selection bias**).

The threat referred to as history is some factor outside those examined in a study affecting the outcome or dependent variable. The term *history* is used because some past event has influenced the dependent variable.

Maturation refers to a change in the dependent variable simply because of the passage of time. Thus, the natural aging process, a type of maturation with time, might lead to decreased daily functioning, regardless of whether the subjects were providing care to a family member. Those studies with a design that did not include a control group would be vulnerable to maturation. We talk more about the role of control groups shortly.

The threat called testing refers to changes in a dependent variable that result because it is being measured or because of the measure itself. For example, the mere presence of a nurse asking patients about the amount and quality of their psychosocial supports might increase a patient's anxiety, changing his or her self-report. Another possible example is a study in which a pretest of depression might make a subject more aware of how bad he or she feels, thus increasing the depression. A related threat to internal validity, called instrumentation, refers to changing the measures used in a study from one time to another. For example, suppose that the number of injections of pain medication for a postoperative cardiac patient's pain was being examined in a research study. Suppose that the timing of when the researcher collected data on the injections and the way in which the researcher documented the injections changed midway through the study. The change in the measurement might lead to different results; thus, values using the first method would not be directly comparable to values from the revised method.

The last types of threats to internal validity frequently considered when selecting a research design are *mortality* and *selection bias*. We examined both of these threats in Table 6.5, although we did not use that terminology during the discussion of potential problems with sampling. Mortality refers to the loss of subjects from a study because of a consistent factor related to the dependent variable. Occasionally, the loss of subjects is from death. At other times, mortality refers to subjects withdrawing from a study. The author of the psychological support article found by the RN in the clinical case for this chapter does not indicate whether any subjects of the studies commented upon in the article were excluded or lost. Given that the subjects were ICU patients, this loss might be expected. Nevertheless, if even two or three of the critical subjects for this study had died or been dropped from the study, we would have to wonder whether some factor directly related to psychosocial needs may have been associated with their death or being dropped and how that factor then affected the accuracy of the findings.

Selection bias refers to subjects having unique characteristics that in some manner relate to the dependent variable, raising a question whether the findings from the study resulted from the independent variable or the characteristics of the sample. Remember, we examined random assignment in Chapter 6 and learned that the times when we randomly assign subjects, any possible systematic bias in a sample has an equal chance of being present in the subjects of either group. This negates the potential threat of selection bias when comparing two groups.

Suppose that in a study concerning surgical recovery, some patients required additional types of medication. As a result, the researchers might have inadvertently introduced bias into their study by selecting patients who needed additional medication. The bias would occur because additional medications might affect the surgical recovery, thus confounding any differences that might occur solely because of the other variables.

Threats to External Validity

Threats to external validity are potential problems in a study that affect the accuracy of the results for samples and settings other than those of the study itself. As we said earlier, threats to internal and external validity are related, and in fact, overlap exists in the language used to describe the different threats. Because we are discussing the ability to apply the results of a study to other samples and settings, research literature often refers to threats to external validity as the effects of a threat to validity. Several effects are considered when selecting a research study design to ensure external validity. They include the effects of reactivity, measurement, experimenter, and/or novelty.

CORE CONCEPT 9.2

Studies with problems in internal validity automatically will have problems in external validity. Having internal validity, however, does not guarantee that the study will have external validity.

Reactivity effects refer to the responses of subjects to being studied. Threats to internal validity, such as testing, may cause reactivity. However, reactivity also can occur in a broader sense simply because subjects know that they are being studied. Subjects may be aware that their answers could be scrutinized closely, and although they may not know what specific aspects of their answers the researchers expect, the mere fact of their thinking about how their answers could be perceived might change how the subjects respond.

In another example, let us say that the data being collected were based on observations of doctor–nurse interactions. Just because the subjects knew that they were being observed, they may have altered somewhat how they usually would interact. If being observed, in fact, greatly affected the behavior, the results of that study would differ in settings where behavior was not being observed. This then would be considered a threat to external validity. Another term sometimes used to describe reactivity is the **Hawthorne effect**. This name was derived from a study at the Hawthorne Electric Plant in which productivity of workers improved simply because they were being studied, no matter what intervention was applied. Reactivity and the Hawthorne effect are the same concept.

Measurement effects are changes in the results of a study resulting from various data collection procedures. This effect sounds similar to instrumentation and testing (threats to internal validity). Remember that any threat to internal validity automatically affects external validity negatively, and overlaps between internal and external validity can become confusing. Just as there are other forms of reactivity effects besides those inherent in threats to internal validity, there are other forms of measurement effects that are not threats.

For example, suppose that being asked about one's depression when returning to the home care environment (as was done in the "Transition to Home Care: Quality of Mental Health, Pharmacy, and Medical History Information" study) (Brown et al., 2006) (Appendix A.6) led to increased awareness and expectations about how caring for oneself would affect quality of life (QOL) and state of mind. The lack of an effect from an intervention may be valid for patients who have been questioned about depression—that is, those who received intervention measures when returning to the home care environment—but would not be valid for patients who did not receive the evaluation. The measurement of QOL in the study did not jeopardize the validity of the findings since all subjects received the same measure. However, the intervention might have had more effect if the measures had not been used; thus, there might have been a measurement effect on the external validity of the study.

The last two effects for us to consider are novelty effects and experimenter effects. Both involve uncontrolled or unmeasured effects from being in a study. **Novelty effects** occur when the knowledge that what is being done is new and under study somehow affects the outcome, either favorably or unfavorably. Once the independent variable is used outside the context of a study, the enthusiasm or doubts that affected the results are no longer present, so the results are no longer accurate in a setting that is not known to be a study. For example, using a self-help intervention for smoking cessation might be associated with success in quitting smoking, leading the researchers to conclude that the self-help intervention was effective. However, in fact, it was the novelty of the intervention and the subjects' knowledge that it was a new approach that actually led to their success in quitting, and when the intervention was later used in a clinical setting without a study being implemented, the success rate decreased.

Experimenter effects occur when some characteristic of the researcher or data collector influences the study results. For example, subjects may answer the questions the way they believe a researcher wants them to answer so that results change when subjects are not responding to cues from the researcher.

No matter which threat affects external validity, it reflects some problem with the environment or the research process that may make the study results less valid or accurate for other samples or settings. The names of the different effects and threats are intended to reflect the threat or effect, but they can be confusing. What is most important for the RN in our clinical case is not only to know that research designs are selected for their function and fit to the research question, but also to do the best possible job of ensuring the rigor and validity of the study. To review, rigor refers to the overall quality of a qualitative study; internal validity refers to the accuracy of the overall results within a quantitative study; and external validity refers to the accuracy of the overall results of a quantitative study in relation to settings and samples that are different or external to that study. Different research designs have varying strengths and weaknesses in relation to rigor and validity. The next two sections of this chapter describe some of these specific designs considering their functions, timing, and efforts at control.

■ QUALITATIVE **RESEARCH DESIGNS**

Figure 9.3 places qualitative designs within the framework of the broad factors of function, time, and control. As has been said throughout this book, the goal of qualitative research is to gain knowledge that informs our practice broadly and holistically, understanding that all knowing is evolving and contextual. That means that a design or method for a qualitative study will never focus on controlling factors to isolate specific aspects of a phenomenon. Rather, the methods focus on acquiring the richest possible data—that is, data with the greatest complexity and variety. Therefore, the designs intentionally seek to avoid external control over setting and factors.

Earlier, we said that there are three broad types of research questions: those that seek to describe and understand, those that seek to connect or relate, and those that seek to predict or manipulate. Qualitative research questions seek to describe, understand, and connect or relate, but they do not seek to predict or manipulate. Qualitative studies are most often done when we know the least about the topic of interest. As we gain understanding, the researcher will shift to methods other than qualitative.

There are three broad functions of qualitative research designs, including increasing understanding, promoting participation or immersion, and linking ideas and concepts. Designs that function to facilitate understanding answer descriptive design questions. Designs that seek to promote participation or immersion answer questions of both description and connection. Designs that seek to link ideas and concepts answer questions of connection or relationship. We will discuss four general types of designs or methods for qualitative research. Within each method are variations that are often associated with the names of the methodologists who developed them. Some reports of qualitative studies use these specific names rather than the more general method name. It is beyond the scope of this book to describe these variations, but Table 9.3 lists some of the names frequently associated with each of the four methods.

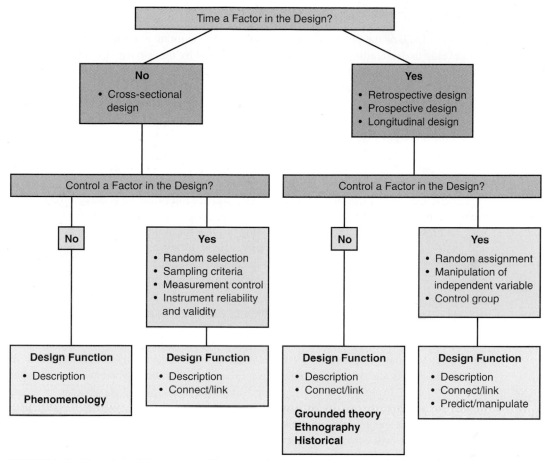

FIGURE 9.3 Three broad factors that affect research design, with associated terms and associated qualitative designs.

Table 9.3

Methodologists Commonly Associated With the Major Qualitative Methods	
MAJOR METHOD	SPECIFIC METHODOLOGISTS
Phenomenology	Parse van Kaam Colaizzi Giorgi Paterson and Zderad Munhall and Boyd van Manen
Grounded theory	Glasser and Strauss Strauss and Corbin Stern
Ethnography	Goodenough (ethnoscience) Geertz (ethnographic algorithms) Sanday (ethnobehavior) Leininger (ethnonursing)
History	Bullough Hamilton

Phenomenology

Phenomenology, or the phenomenologic method, is a qualitative method used to discover and develop understanding of experiences as perceived by those living the experience. As with all qualitative studies, the method seeks to avoid external control by going as directly as possible to those who have lived or are living the experience being studied. The method assumes that lived experiences can be interpreted or understood by distilling their essence.

There are several variations in the phenomenologic method (Colaizzi, 1973; Giorgi, 1971; Spiegelberg, 1976; van Kaam, 1966), but in general, the method includes identifying the people who are living or have lived the experience of interest and seeking, usually through unstructured interviewing, their perceptions. As data are collected, the researcher uses the processes of intuiting, analyzing, and describing to discover essential themes in the experience of the phenomenon (Parse, 2001). Skilled interviewing is needed to promote the most open and rich sharing of experiences as participants lived and perceived them.

As presented in Chapter 4, phenomenology uses a spiraling process of data collection and analysis, and detailed field notes of observations during data collection augment the richness and fullness of data. Time is not necessarily a major factor in phenomenologic methods, except as the participants in the study experience it. In fact, the method supports seeking participants who are both currently experiencing the phenomenon of interest and have already experienced it to get a breadth of perceptions of experiences.

In phenomenologic methods, neither the length of time for collecting data nor the number of participants is defined before the study starts. Rather, data are collected until all information is redundant of previously collected data—until saturation occurs. Sampling in phenomenology is always a convenience sample because only those who have had the experience of interest are sought, and neither limits nor criteria are placed on who can be a participant, other than the ability to communicate about and having lived the experience. Depending on the specific phenomenologic method used, the researcher often starts by identifying his or her own perceptions or expectations about the phenomenon to be studied and then attempts to consciously bracket them—hold them separate—so that they will not color either the data collection or the analysis process (Spiegelberg, 1976).

Ethnography

The second method commonly used in qualitative research is the ethnographic method, or ethnography (Spradley, 1979). A closely related method that was developed by Leininger (1991) within nursing is called *ethnonursing*. This method originated in the discipline of anthropology, and its purpose is for the researcher to participate or to immerse himself or herself in a culture to describe a phenomenon or phenomena within the context of that culture. Ethnography and ethnonursing assume that culture exists, even though it is not visible, and that the only way to know a culture is to get both an insider's view and an outsider's perspective. The insider's view is sometimes called an *emic perspective*.

Let us say in our clinical case that the RN discovers that the trucker was actually drunk at the time of the crash. The RN further finds out that the trucker's family is coming for a visit, and the wife has stated that she plans to bring their 15-year-old son, who is struggling with his emotions regarding his father's drinking while driving. The RN wonders what suggestions could be provided to the mother that would help the adolescent cope. The nurse finds another article reporting a study called "Assessing Adolescents' Understanding of and Reactions to Stress in Different Cultures: Results of a Mixed-Methods Approach" (Nastasi et al., 2007). This article is available in Appendix A.8. The study, in part, used an ethnographic method to understand the feelings, resources, and vulnerability associated with adolescents who have an addicted parent. Reviewing that study report will give you a better understanding of this method.

Again, controlling the environment or aspects of the study is not part of this qualitative method. The researcher tries to become part of the culture studied to acquire an insider's understanding so that he or she can then translate it into a common language understood by those outside the culture (Spradley, 1979). Because cultures are by nature complex, ethnographic methods take time, and the concept of time may be studied within the culture, but there is no set use of time within the method itself. This means that there is no structured plan concerning when data are collected or when the study ends. In general, data are collected as they happen and as opportunities present themselves, although the researcher may seek specific opportunities to interact within the culture. The researcher collects and analyzes data simultaneously so that he or she immediately uses knowledge gained to guide additional data collection. Therefore, there is no structured format for the collection of data.

In the qualitative evaluation of adolescents' stress in different cultures study, we learn that US researchers made several trips to the country and formed partnerships with educational and mental health professions in the area before conducting their study (Nastasi et al., 2007). This information is given to indicate the immersion within the culture that the researchers were studying. The general purpose of this research was to examine what stress means to adolescents with differing stressors, and how they react to that stress. The authors realize that these adolescents are a unique cultural community. Ethnography is prevalent within this mixed methods study, as the cultural implications of these subjects is a driving factor within the study. In addition to studies with recognized cultural groups, ethnographic methods are frequently used in nursing to describe unique subcultures, such as adolescent drug users, people living in homeless shelters, and people residing in halfway houses.

Grounded Theory

Grounded theory is the third qualitative method commonly used in nursing research (Glaser & Strauss, 1967). The function of **grounded theory** is to study interactions to understand and recognize links between ideas and concepts or, in other words, to develop theory. The term *grounded* refers to the idea that the theory developed is based on or grounded in participants' reality rather than on theoretical speculation. Grounded theory is best used to study social processes and structures, hence the focus on links and interactions among ideas or categories.

Grounded theory methods often incorporate time into the study because the focus usually is on processes or change. The method itself, however, does not specify any particular timing to the data collection and analysis process. Sampling in grounded theory usually will be purposive—that is, purposely seeking participants experiencing the process or changes under study (Strauss & Corbin, 1994). Data collection in grounded theory can include interviews and careful observation of interactions and processes. As with all qualitative methods, grounded theory has a goal of avoiding placing limits or external controls on the processes being studied because the function of the method is to ground theory in natural reality.

Historical

The last general qualitative method sometimes used in nursing research is called the **historical research method**. Its function is to answer questions about links in the past to understand the present or to plan the future. Historical research methods require the researcher to define a phenomenon in a manner that can be clearly delineated so that data sources can be identified. For example, a phenomenon that might lend itself to historical research is to understand the process of nurse practitioners' legitimization as health care providers. Nurse practitioner legitimization, however, is too undefined to be approached using the historical method because it is not clear what time period or data sources would be relevant. The phenomenon of credentialing of nurse practitioners as a vehicle to legitimization of the role, on the other hand, defines a focus for data sources as well as a time period because the development of credentialing occurred throughout a definable number of years. Data sources in this example would target the development and implementation of the process of credentialing nurse practitioners and how that process related to perceptions of the legitimacy of the role of nurse practitioners.

Data sources in historical research may include records, videotapes, photographs, and interviews with people involved in the phenomenon or review of published reports. As with the other qualitative methods discussed, the researcher tries to acquire as broad a sample of data sources as possible. Unlike the other methods, in the historical method, a focus of data collection includes evaluation of data sources for their reliability. For example, an editorial in the *Journal of the American Medical Association* regarding the process of nurse practitioner credentialing might reflect a bias that makes the description of the process questionable. That same editorial, however, might be a reliable data source about the professional climate in which credentialing developed. A researcher using the historical method would evaluate the data source and consider this potential bias when deciding how to use it.

We have not had a research study that has used the historical method as an example in this text. However, an article that does use this method, "Pacifiers: An Update on Use and Misuse" (Marter & Agruss, 2007), can be found in Appendix E.

We have now discussed four different methods used in qualitative research, the functions of which vary. Phenomenologic methods provide in-depth data about a particular life experience and, therefore, are particularly useful in answering descriptive questions, especially when very little is known about the topic of interest. Ethnographic methods provide immersion and active participation in a particular culture or subculture and assist in answering descriptive and linkage and connection questions. Grounded theory methods provide data about social interactions, which can be built into a theory based on reality. These methods are particularly useful in answering questions about interactions or links among social processes. Historical methods provide data about past processes to gain insight about the present and future. They answer questions about links and connections.

All the qualitative methods we have examined specifically attempt to avoid introducing external control into the study design because all are interested in gathering data that are as complex and rich as the real world. Nevertheless, all four methods entail a systematic process for sampling, data acquisition, and data analysis. Strict criteria for timing are not part of any of the methods, but time is an inherent component of the historical method, is often a part of the culture studied using ethnography, and is usually an aspect of interactional processes reported in grounded theory studies.

Throughout this section discussing qualitative design, the word *methods* has been used more frequently than the word *design*. This is because design suggests a more formalized and standardized plan than is often present within qualitative methods. Qualitative research designs are consciously and intently unstructured and flexible to reflect the unpredictable and complex nature of phenomena as they occur in life. As we will see in the next section that discusses quantitative designs, the word *design* is more appropriate in quantitative research because quantitative methods seek to standardize as well as formalize the process of sampling, data collection, and data analysis.

■ QUANTITATIVE **RESEARCH DESIGNS**

We will once again use the three broad factors of function, time, and control to categorize quantitative designs (Fig. 9.4). The language used to describe quantitative designs can be confusing initially because terms are used in different combinations to define different methods. Rather than starting with the functions of differing designs, we start by discussing the language used to address time and control when referring to quantitative research design.

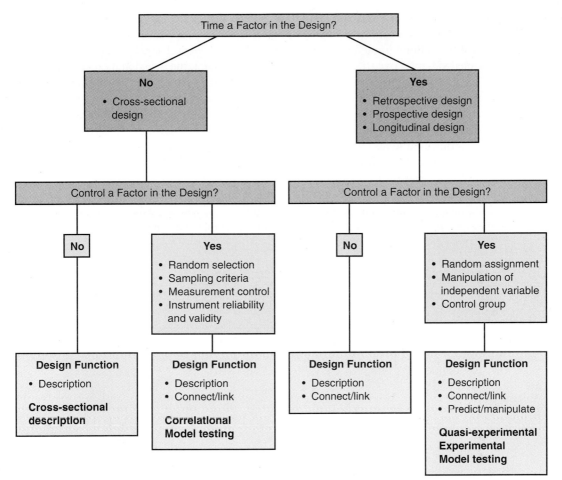

FIGURE 9.4   Three broad factors that affect research design, with associated terms and quantitative designs.

Time

Although time is a factor to study or incorporate into the fabric of a method in qualitative research, time is a specific factor that defines different research designs in quantitative research. Quantitative designs are described as either retrospective or prospective. Retrospective designs are those in which data are collected about past events or factors. Prospective designs are those in which data are collected about events or variables as they occur, moving forward in time. In addition to considering whether data are collected moving backward or forward in time, designs are described in terms of point of time of measurement. Research designs are cross-sectional if they collect all data at one point in time. Research designs are called longitudinal if they collect data at different time points. Therefore, a prospective study automatically is longitudinal as well. A cross-sectional study, however, does not have to be retrospective.

Consider, for example, a study of patient satisfaction with care. A retrospective and cross-sectional study would collect data from patients at some point after they visit a clinic, perhaps 1 or 2 weeks later, and ask them to recall their level of satisfaction during their visit. Data are collected at one time point looking at past experience. A study of patient satisfaction that surveys patients as they leave a clinic also would be cross-sectional because data are collected at only one time point for each subject. However, it would not be retrospective because it is not going back in time; data are being collected about variables in the present. A prospective longitudinal patient satisfaction study might collect data before a visit to a clinic, immediately after the visit, and 1 week later, looking for changes in selected variables over time. At each measurement point, the question might be "How satisfied are you right now with the clinic care?" Thus, data are not being collected about past experiences or perceptions, even when they are collected 1 week after the visit. From this example, it should be clear that it is a combination of factors that define research designs in quantitative research. This idea is important to grasp.

Terms used to describe the use of time in quantitative research designs include those we have discussed and another important term: *repeated measures*. Repeated measures mean just what the words say—a design using repeated measures repeats the same measurements at several points in time. When you see this term, it suggests that a variable or variables were measured more than just two or three times, and you can expect that the analysis of the study examines the pattern of change in the variable over time.

CORE CONCEPT 9.3

The labels for quantitative research designs usually are combinations of words or terms that define the design's function, use of time, and use of approaches to provide control.

Control

In addition to differences in how they consider the factor of time, quantitative research designs differ in the amount of control of extraneous factors that they attempt to impose on a study. Remember that quantitative research seeks to clearly define and measure specific variables. To do so, research designs seek to ensure that outside factors not specifically defined and measured in the study are not allowed to affect what is included in the study. Outside or extraneous factors not considered and measured within a quantitative study are sources of error. In Chapter 8, we discussed error in measurement in relation to measurement reliability and validity. We are now considering error in a broader manner, just as we examined validity of an entire study previously in the chapter. Designs in quantitative research seek to ensure the internal and external validity of the study by minimizing error. They do so by imposing different controls on the sampling, data collection, and analysis.

The areas within which research designs seek to create or to impose control include the sampling and measurement processes. Control in the sampling process can be imposed by establishing criteria for inclusion or exclusion that attempt to prevent some outside difference among subjects from confusing the findings of a study. Another method of control is the use of random sampling, by which the entire population is enumerated, and everyone has an equal chance of being asked to be in the study. A third method is random assignment because all subjects have an equal chance of being included in any particular group in the study. Thus, any differences in the subjects will likely be distributed equally within different groups that will be compared. We reviewed each of these approaches to control in Chapter 6. Quantitative research designs partly reflect and define the sampling approach that a study will take.

Control within the data collection process can be imposed by ensuring the validity and reliability of the measures or by ensuring that the measurement process itself is consistent, avoiding instrumentation threats. Control in measurement also can be imposed by creating comparison group(s) so that either exposure to the factors studied is manipulated in a controlled fashion or the timing of the measurement process is manipulated around a factor of interest. Study designs that include a comparison group create control by comparing subjects in two groups who differ in an independent variable of interest. Inclusion of a comparison group eliminates such threats to internal validity as history and maturation because both groups experience the same history or process of maturation. A design using a comparison group attempts to ensure that two groups are as similar as possible on most factors that could affect the dependent variable of interest and assume that they differ clearly in an independent variable. Therefore, such designs hope to isolate the influence of that independent variable on the dependent variable of interest. Study designs that include a control group create a greater level of control by manipulating the independent variable of interest so that the control group is not exposed to it, whereas the experimental group is. Again, a dependent variable is examined for differences to see whether the factor manipulated affects that dependent variable.

Functions of Quantitative Research Designs

Having considered the factors of time and control, we will now discuss specific quantitative designs considering these two factors as well as overall function. Quantitative research designs vary in the level of control that they impose from limited in descriptive and correlational studies to more control in quasi-experimental studies to the most control in true experimental designs.

Descriptive Designs and Correlational Studies

Descriptive designs function to portray some phenomenon of interest as accurately as possible. Correlational studies use a descriptive design to describe interrelationships among variables as accurately as possible. Researchers generally consider studies that look at correlations to be a subtype of descriptive designs and refer to them as *studies* rather than the broader term *design*. Clearly, descriptive designs are used to answer research questions that seek to describe. Correlational studies are used to answer research questions that seek to link or connect. Both types focus on exerting control through the quality of the measurement— that is, by using reliable and valid measures as discussed in Chapter 8 and through sampling criteria or procedures. Descriptive and correlational studies may impose control by establishing certain criteria for inclusion or exclusion from the study. Remember, this also can be called *purposive sampling* or *use of a convenience sample*. Both types of design can impose even greater control over extraneous factors by using randomly selected samples.

Descriptive and correlational designs can be longitudinal or cross-sectional, and they can be retrospective or prospective. Decisions about how time is a factor are based on the nature of the question, the potential sample, and the measures. Some phenomena, such as growth or productivity, clearly entail a time element that would make it logical for a researcher to use a longitudinal design. However, as we discussed in Chapter 6, finding, following, and maintaining subjects over time can be difficult and costly, so some studies may use a single cross-sectional design to avoid problems of following subjects over time. Certainly, some measures can be repeated easily, whereas others cannot, because they measure stable concepts unlikely to change or because the measurement process is too intrusive to repeat often. For example, the concept of an individual's sense of coherence is a stable sense of the world and oneself within the world and, although a researcher may be interested in measuring this as a variable in a study, it would not be helpful to measure it more than once because it will remain stable. An example of an intrusive measure might be a bone marrow analysis. It could be that data from weekly bone marrow tests would be ideal in evaluating a new cancer drug. However, this test is too intrusive and painful to repeat at that kind of interval.

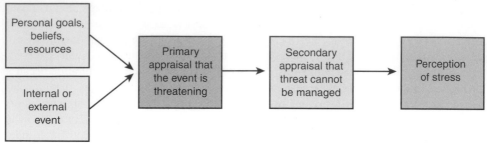

FIGURE 9.5   Schematic model of Lazarus's theory of stress.

A special type of correlational study is a design for model. A model is the symbolic framework for a theory or part of a theory. In Chapter 2, we discussed Lazarus's theory of stress, also shown as a model in Figure 9.5. A design testing such a model identifies measures for each concept and examines how the concepts relate. A study testing Lazarus's theory would identify ways to measure the variables of personal beliefs and resources, the event, primary appraisal, secondary appraisal, and stress. Then, the study would statistically analyze relationships among the results on these measurements of the variables to see whether the relationships found were of the type and direction predicted by the model.

Often, designs for model testing are longitudinal, so some parts of the model are measured at one time point and other aspects are measured at a later time point. This allows researchers to propose causal relationships between concepts in the model. Therefore, model testing designs often attempt to answer questions that predict as well as relate.

In summary, descriptive designs function to portray a phenomenon of interest and may be retrospective, prospective, cross-sectional, or longitudinal. They also may impose varying levels of control through sampling strategies, such as purposive samples or random sampling. Correlational designs function to describe or identify inter relationships among factors of interest; they also may be retrospective, prospective, cross-sectional, or longitudinal. Because correlational designs describe relationships, you will occasionally see them called *descriptive correlational designs*. Correlational designs may use the same range of sampling strategies used in descriptive designs. Model testing designs are a special type of correlational design that usually incorporate time in some manner, either through longitudinal data collection or through use of measures that combine retrospective and concurrent data collection.

Quasi-Experimental and Experimental Research Designs

Quasi-experimental and experimental research designs function to answer questions involving prediction and the effects of manipulation. Quasi-experimental research design differs from experimental research design primarily in the amount of control imposed. Both types include control of an independent variable, but a true experimental design always includes a control group and random assignment to groups. Remember, a control group is a group of subjects who do not receive an intervention so that the control group can be compared with those who do receive the intervention (Box 9.3).

Box 9.3

Components of Experimental Designs

- Manipulation of the independent variable
- Random assignment of subjects to groups
- A control group

R   **O_1**   **X**   **O_2**   **FIGURE 9.6**   Schematic of pretest–posttest experimental design.

R   **O_1**   **O_2**

When researchers discuss quasi-experimental and experimental designs, they often use a set of symbols to diagram the particular form of design used. When they do this, they use the symbol "O" to indicate occasion of observation or measurement, with a subscript number designating the time point of the observation. They use the letter "X" to denote the intervention, meaning the independent variable, and they use "R" to denote that subjects were randomly assigned to groups. Figure 9.6 is an example of this type of diagram. It translates to mean that two groups were formed using random assignment (R). Each group had measurements taken (O_1), one group received the intervention (X), and both groups had a second measurement taken (O_2). This design includes manipulation of the independent variable, random assignment, and a control group; therefore, it is experimental. Because it includes an observation both before and after the intervention, the type of design in Figure 9.6 is called a pretest–posttest experimental design.

Although most quasi-experimental and experimental designs are longitudinal, it is possible for an experiment to be implemented at only one time point. Figure 9.7 shows how a single time point experimental design would look. Because experimental designs always involve manipulation of an independent variable, they are never retrospective. Finally, multifactorial is a term sometimes associated with experimental design that refers to several independent variables being manipulated in a study. The examples we have considered have all had a single independent variable; however, some studies control and manipulate two or more independent variables.

A quasi-experimental design lacks either a control group or random assignment. It may not include two groups at all. Instead, it may involve a series of observations, followed by an intervention and then another series of observations (Fig. 9.8). In this case, there is manipulation of the independent variable but no control group. The threats to internal validity in this type of design include instrumentation and testing as well as selection bias and mortality. There also are quasi-experimental designs that have two groups of subjects, but the groups are nonequivalent because subjects are not randomly assigned to each group. Such a design is referred to as a *nonequivalent control group pretest–posttest quasi-experimental design*, and it entails observations of two groups, followed by one group receiving the intervention and then a second set of observations. Because both groups receive the same measurement, this quasi-experimental design is less threatened by instrumentation and testing but still is threatened by selection bias and mortality. Thus, a rather long name for a design tells us a great deal about how the research study was implemented. What if we were interested, for example, in studying the effect of positioning changes on the pain levels of hospitalized patients? If we were to find a study that randomly assigned patients to two groups and then manipulated a variable for one group but not the other, we would say that the study was most likely experimental in design. A design must include manipulation of an independent variable, a control group, and random assignment in order to be classified as experimental.

Another phrase applied to methods that we need to discuss further is repeated measures. We have already said that this phrase means that multiple measures of the same variable were taken over time. In our hypothetical study of the effect of positioning, let us

R   **X**   **O_1**   **FIGURE 9.7**   Schematic of an experimental design with only one point of measurement.

R   **O_1**

$$O_1 \qquad O_2 \qquad O_3 \qquad O_4 \qquad X \qquad O_5 \qquad O_6 \qquad O_7 \qquad O_8$$

FIGURE 9.8   Schematic of repeated-measures quasi-experimental design.

assume that the researcher chose to measure a variable such as heart rate before turning the person, immediately after turning, and 5 minutes after turning, then 10, 15, and 25 minutes after turning, for a total of six measures. This is a good example of the frequency of measures you would expect if a design is said to use repeated measures. If a study lacked true random assignment to the intervention groups, and/or lacked a control group, the study would be labeled as quasi-experimental.

In summary, the language used to describe quantitative research designs reflects their function, such as descriptive, correlational, or experimental. Other language used to describe designs reflects how time is a component, such as retrospective, cross-sectional, or longitudinal. Finally, the language of designs reflects the level of control imposed in the study, with experimental designs imposing the greatest control over extraneous variables. We have reviewed several of the studies used throughout this book as examples of various designs. To provide familiar examples of several research designs, Table 9.4 categorizes each of the eight studies in this text thus far according to type of research design used.

■ HOW CAN ONE GET THE WRONG DESIGN FOR THE RIGHT QUESTION?

Let us return to the question that our RN in the clinical case was considering about why all studies are not experimental. We have already addressed one part of the answer to that question: The research question must ask about prediction or the effects of manipulation before an experimental design will fit. For a question seeking to examine the effects of manipulation or to predict, we must have certain baseline knowledge already in place. The other reason that experimental designs are not the right design for every question involves the strengths and weaknesses of the design itself. Experimental designs are strong on control; therefore, they have the fewest threats to internal validity. That same control, however, makes experiments dissimilar from the "real" world of patient care, where variety and complexity are the rule. Therefore, the results of a study using an experimental design are generally accurate, and we can trust highly that the findings are correct. However, the findings may not be easily applied or generalized to clinical practice, where many of the factors controlled in the experiment will not be controlled.

For example, if subjects in a study on the effects of a new multiposition bed had to receive a two-dimensional CAT scan or an echocardiograph to confirm physiologic changes when the bed moved, the availability of technology would automatically reflect a certain level of hospital and, in most cases, a certain level of insurance coverage. Thus, uninsured patients and those from rural settings without access to tertiary care centers would more than likely be underrepresented or not represented in such a study. Yet, being uninsured or living in a rural setting are factors that may affect physiologic functioning and resilience. The very controls that ensured that the patients did have physiologic changes related to the multiposition bed also may limit the generalizability of the study. In reality, the controls exerted in this example probably do not greatly influence the utility of the results for more general practice; however, this example gives you an idea of why the aspects that provide control in a design also may limit the clinical usefulness of the results.

Quasi-experimental studies lose some of the internal validity of an experimental design but often gain some applicability to real life. Often, a quasi-experimental design is selected to answer a research question when the implementation of a true experimental design is not feasible. For example, researchers who want to study HIV-prevention

Table 9.4

Categorization of Research Designs of the Eight Articles Used in This Text

CHAPTER AND REFERENCE	RESEARCH DESIGN
Chapters 1 and 2	
Landis, A., Parker, K., & Dunbar, S. (2009). Sleep, hunger, satiety, food cravings, and caloric intake in adolescents. *Journal of Nursing Scholarship, 41*(2), 115–123.	Quantitative with regression analysis
Marytn-Nemeth, P., Penckofer, S., Gulanick, M., Velsor-Friedrich, B., & Bryant, F. (2009). The relationships among self-esteem, stress, coping, eating behavior, and depressive mood in adolescents. *Research in Nursing & Health 2009, 32*, 96–109.	Descriptive, correlational cross-sectional design
Chapter 3	
Hsieh, C., Sprod, L., Hydock, D., Carter, S., Hayward, R., and Schneider, C. (2008). Effects of a supervised exercise intervention on recovery from treatment regimens in breast cancer survivors. *Oncology Nursing Forum, 35–36*, 909–915.	Quasi-experimental
Chapters 4 and 5	
Ostwald, S., Godwin, K., & Cron, S. (2009). Predictors of life satisfaction in stroke survivors and spousal caregivers after inpatient rehabilitation. *Rehabilitation Nursing, 34*, 160–174.	Quantitative
Chapter 6	
Fraas, M., & Calvert, M. (2009). The use of narratives to identify characteristics leading to a productive life following acquired brain injury. *American Journal of Speech–Language Pathology, 18*, 315–328.	Qualitative; phenomenological with thematic analysis
Chapter 8	
Brown, E., Raue, P., Mlodzianowski, A., Barnett, S., Meyers, B., Greenberg, R., et al. (2006). Transition to home care: Quality of mental health, pharmacy, and medical history information. *International Journal of Psychiatry in Medicine, 36*(3), 339–349.	Quantitative (descriptive statistics)
Chapter 9 (this chapter)	
Carr, J. (2007). Psychological consequences associated with intensive care treatment. *Trauma, 9*(2), 95–102.	Review of numerous studies

programs with homeless women would face great difficulty in randomly assigning home-less women to different programs because homeless people generally do not follow sched-ules or have circumstances that would enable them to attend programs that are not conveniently located. If the researchers tried to implement several different programs in one shelter (randomly assigning the women in the shelter to a program), it is likely that the women would share activities from the different programs, causing the programs to blur and making it impossible to isolate the effects of one compared with the other. Therefore, a researcher testing an HIV program with homeless women would likely use a quasi-experimental design, selecting homeless shelters to either receive or not receive the intervention to be tested. In contrast, if the researchers want to test HIV-prevention programs with high school students, they might more easily randomly assign subjects and create a true experiment. Nevertheless, results with high school students would not be easy to apply to the different lives and experiences of homeless women. Therefore, the very control possible with high school students would preclude the study being as useful for homeless women.

As we move to descriptive and correlational designs, control decreases even further because the researcher no longer controls the independent variable. Selection criteria or random selection, however, can still provide some control. In addition, measurement reliability and validity increase our confidence about the accuracy of the factors being studied. Because descriptive and correlational designs still impose control through sampling and measurement, the richness and diversity of real-life clinical situations is limited. Phenomenologic, ethnographic, and grounded theory designs impose the least control over the process of research and, therefore, capture the greatest detail and depth of real experiences. Yet, they can become so subjective or conceptual that the results also may be difficult to apply to real practice. Qualitative designs are not intended to develop knowledge about predictions; but, we often seek knowledge that will allow us to predict in nursing.

Therefore, the answer to the question "How can one get the wrong design for the right question?" involves feasibility in terms of who or what is being studied, what measures are available, and what is already known about the problem or phenomenon. A study of the process of tobacco addiction cannot ethically manipulate the variable of exposure to tobacco, so it will, by necessity, be nonexperimental. A study of drug efficacy requires careful control of as many extraneous factors as possible, lending itself to experimental design. However, withholding drug treatment in some cases may be unethical, leading to the use of quasi-experimental design. Studies of subjective experiences, such as pain, grief, or satisfaction, require understanding best acquired through seeking the insights of those who have experienced or are experiencing the phenomenon, lending themselves to qualitative designs. Yet, a researcher may not be skilled in qualitative methods and so may choose a cross-sectional descriptive design instead.

What should be evident at this point is that study design shapes the approach taken to sampling, measurement, and data analysis. Understanding the basic language of design will allow you to understand many of the decisions made by the researcher(s) regarding the study, clarifying the approaches taken to acquiring subjects or participants and to the data collection itself. Recognizing that the terms used in quantitative design are combined differently to specify the function, control, and time factor in a design will help you to better understand the types of designs described in published research.

In addition to terms that reflect the function of and the use of control and time in a design, some designs are described as mixed methods. Mixed methods refer to some combination of methods in relation to function, time, or control. A study that collects retrospective data by asking parents to complete a questionnaire about family history of heart disease, their children's level of physical activity, and the parents' smoking behavior is an example of collecting data about how things were, thinking back in time. In addition, if this study then collects data of cholesterol level, blood pressure, and HgA_1, this could be classified as a longitudinal study because it links data from the past about activity, history, and smoking with data from the present about blood pressure, cholesterol, and HgA_1.

Another use of the term *mixed methods* is to refer to a combination of qualitative and quantitative methods. The fictional article from Appendix B about nursing students' choices of clinical practice uses a somewhat mixed method because it includes data collection by use of a pen-and-paper quantifiable questionnaire and a written open-ended question that was analyzed using methods associated with qualitative research. As nursing research develops, more and more researchers are recognizing the value of both qualitative and quantitative methods to more fully answer questions of interest to nursing. This has led to increased use of a combination of qualitative and quantitative designs in single studies.

Before beginning this chapter, you were asked to consider how you might best conduct a study of the effects of nursing school attendance on well-being. Now that we have examined various research designs and some of the advantages and disadvantages of each, let us consider some choices you would need to make if you were going to conduct such a study.

First, you could approach a study of the effects of nursing school attendance on well-being from a qualitative perspective or a quantitative perspective. The decision would depend partly on what is already known, such as what is known about influences on well-being in college students, how nursing programs differ from other undergraduate programs, and whether nursing students differ from other undergraduate students in some important ways that might affect well-being. If little is known about any of these factors, a qualitative study of the lived experiences of nursing students in terms of sense of well-being while in school might be the research design to use. If little is known about well-being and nursing students, a researcher might implement a grounded theory design to examine interactions that affect well-being.

A researcher also might decide to do a descriptive correlational study measuring well-being and other factors that would logically be relevant, such as general health, age, family commitments, work schedule, and grade-point average, to see how they relate. If implementing a quantitative study, the researcher could decide to do measurements only at one time point and perhaps include students just entering school, those halfway through school, and those preparing to graduate. Such a study would be cross-sectional. To address problems with internal validity, the researcher would need to consider how comparable students in the three different classes were in factors that affect well-being other than nursing school attendance.

Alternatively, a researcher might decide to do a longitudinal study, following a group of nursing students from the time they enter school to graduation. This type of study would take much time and many resources; it also would be open to such threats to internal validity as mortality, testing, and instrumentation. The question of effects of nursing school attendance and well-being probably does not lend itself to or fit with either quasi-experimental or experimental designs, unless something already has been shown to be a factor that could be manipulated to try to change well-being.

This example demonstrates why studies addressing approximately the same question may use different research designs. As an intelligent user of nursing research, you do not have to decide what type of design to use, but it is helpful for you to understand some considerations that go into selecting a design as well as the meaning and strengths and weaknesses of different research designs.

■ COMMON ERRORS IN PUBLISHED REPORTS OF RESEARCH DESIGNS

As you read published studies, there may be problems with the amount of information provided about the study design. One common problem is lack of detail about the design, leaving the reader uncertain concerning the methods used. In some cases, the only thing we are told is that a particular method or design was used. This happens more in published reports of qualitative studies than in reports of quantitative studies and may occur partly because qualitative methods were less well known or used in nursing in past years. A written report of a study design should not simply tell the reader the label for the design; it also should describe enough of the actual process of the research study to assure the reader that the design was implemented appropriately.

For example, a study that states it uses phenomenologic methods also should tell you enough about the subjects to assure you that they were rich and appropriate sources of data and, generally, how data were collected and analyzed. A study that tells you it used an experimental design also should provide specific information about the random assignment process, creation of the control group, and manipulation of the intervention.

As with measurement in research, a study design can be complex. Nevertheless, it is the responsibility of the author(s) to communicate in writing all the essential aspects of the design so that the reader can intelligently read and understand the study. The use of a time line often helps readers to understand a study design, particularly if it is longitudinal. The other aspect that occasionally is lacking in published reports is a rationale for the choice of research design. We have discussed that a researcher has to make several decisions when selecting a design. Occasionally, the rationales for decisions, such as not including a control group, can help the reader to better understand the problems of the study and how they may affect usefulness for clinical practice.

■ PUBLISHED REPORTS—DID DESIGN AFFECT YOUR CONCLUSION?

The RN in our clinical case is trying to understand how D.M.'s psychosocial needs might best be addressed. Additionally, the nurse wonders how to help D.M.'s adolescent son adjust to learning that his father's accident was alcohol related. The RN in our clinical case has begun to understand that nurses do not have much evidence on what interventions facilitate the psychosocial needs of ICU patients. Additionally, the RN is aware that adolescents whose parents have a substance abuse issue represent a unique cultural group. From this perspective, the research designs are beginning to make sense. In the psychological consequences article, the RN had the opportunity to look over evidence representing both qualitative and quantitative design; the researchers whose studies were based in qualitative design were more interested in understanding the experience of patients, while those who used an experimental design were interested in strict outcomes based on interventions. In the adolescents' stress in different cultures article, the ethnographic portion of this mixed-methods study was able to identify culturally sensitive implications to this demographic group. From this perspective, the researchers' method selection seems reasonable and appropriate.

While most evidence-based studies focus on research in the form of clinical trials, this gold standard can be used only when we know enough about a topic to use a true experimental design. Clinical trials refer to studies that test the effectiveness of a clinical treatment, and some researchers would say that a clinical trial must be a true experiment. For many problems in clinical practice, however, there have been only a few true experimental studies, so it is not uncommon to see clinical trials defined more broadly.

Given the nature of the question and the evidence from the studies, the RN concludes that D.M.'s psychosocial need associated with depression and anxiety should be a dominant focus of care planning. Based on reading the adolescents' stress in different cultures article, the RN also is now more comfortable about dealing with the needs of the patient's son and feels that, if possible, identification and enhancement of the son's personal coping mechanism could be helpful.

■ CRITICALLY READING THE DESCRIPTION OF THE STUDY DESIGN IN A RESEARCH REPORT FOR USE IN EVIDENCE-BASED NURSING PRACTICE

In Box 9.4, you will find questions that you can use to critically read about the design of a research study. Often the study design is part of the methods section of a research report, but since we have discussed designs in a separate chapter, we will also address questions to ask

Box 9.4

How to Critically Read the Description of Study Design in a Research Report

Does the report answer the question "How were those people studied—why was the study performed that way?"

1. Did the report include a clearly identified section describing the research design?
2. Does the design make this a quantitative, qualitative, or a mixed method study?
3. Does the report address approaches taken to assure study rigor, internal validity, and/or external validity?
4. Do I think that the researcher(s) should have designed the study differently in order to answer my clinical question?

about designs as a separate component to consider when reading a report of research. The first question asks, "Did the report include a clearly identified section describing the research design?" The RN reading the adolescents' stress in different cultures study did find a clear statement of the study design, particularly as it related to ethnography; however, some research reports may fail to identify the type of design, making it necessary for you as a reader to try to classify that design based on other information in the report. If you read a report and are uncertain about the study design even after reviewing the complete method section, then it may be that the researchers failed to have a systematic plan for their study, and that would affect your trust of the total study.

The second question to ask is "Does the design make this a quantitative, qualitative, or a mixed method study?" The answer to that question allows you as a critical reader to evaluate the fit of the design to the procedures and measures used in the study. A misfit between design and actual measures would suggest that the researcher(s) may have implemented a less-than-consistent and systematic study and would cause you to wonder about the usefulness of the results of that study for practice. For example, if a research report indicates the study design is ethnography and then indicates that data were collected using a series of written scales, we would have to wonder about the quality of the study, as this type of measurement does not fit with a qualitative design.

A third question to ask as you critically read about a study design is "Does the report address approaches taken to assure study rigor, internal validity, and/or external validity?" In order to answer this, you must be familiar with these concepts and will have to critically read the description of the implementation of the study. Finally, you will want to ask yourself "Do I think that the researcher(s) should have designed the study differently in order to answer my clinical question?" For example, the RN in our clinical case wants to assist D.M. in his psychosocial adjustment while in the ICU. While reading the study about psychosocial consequences of patients in the unit, the nurse recognizes that the clinical question is one about patient experiences and perceptions that lead to depression and anxiety, and therefore, the portions of the article that focus on qualitative design used is appropriate and will give the nurse useful evidence on which to base practice.

The RN realizes that without the research findings contained in the article read, the care provided may have been different and perhaps not nearly as effective in improving the patient's health. The results also suggest the importance of the nurse's role in assessment of the patient's feelings of depression and anxiety. The RN wonders why the researchers were so concerned about the psychosocial needs of ICU patients. To answer that question, the nurse plans to read the beginning of the article that describes the background for the study as well as the research problem.

Clearly, then, the type of research design used in a study affects the usefulness and meaningfulness of the results for clinical practice. The language of research design is complex and confusing at times because several terms are used in different ways in different contexts.

Nevertheless, it is possible to acquire a good general understanding of the meaning of most of the terms so that this important aspect of a research study can be understood and interpreted as related to the applicability of the study to clinical practice.

OUT-OF-CLASS EXERCISE

How to Set the Stage for a Study

At the end of Chapter 8, you were asked to develop some ideas for a research design in order to study the effects of nursing school attendance on well-being. We have discussed in this chapter some possible designs that you may have considered and the need to have a better idea of what is already known before you can settle on a design. Chapter 10 discusses the background and statement of the research problem sections of research reports. It is this first part of a research report that provides the rationale for a study as well as information about previous research. Before reading Chapter 10, write one or two paragraphs that describe why a study of nursing students' well-being and the effect of attendance in nursing school are important enough to warrant a research study. If you were going to conduct such a study, what would you need to describe at the beginning to set the stage? After you have written your case for studying the nursing students' well-being, you are ready to begin Chapter 10.

_____

_____

_____

_____

_____

_____

_____

_____

_____

_____

_____

_____

_____

_____

_____

_____

_____

_____

_____

_____

References

Brown, E., Raue, P., Mlodzianowski, A., Barnett, S., Meyers, B., Greenberg, R., et al. (2006). Transition to home care: Quality of mental health, pharmacy, and medical history information. *International Journal of Psychiatry in Medicine, 36*(3), 339–349.

Carr, J. (2007). Psychological consequences associated with intensive care treatment. *Trauma, 9*(2), 95–102.

Colaizzi, P. F. (1973). *Reflection and research in psychology: A phenomenological study of learning.* Dubuque, IA: Kendall/Hunt.

Giorgi, A. (1971). Phenomenology and experimental psychology: II. In A. Giorgi, W. Fischer, & R. von Eckartsberg (Eds.), *Duquesne studies in phenomenological psychology* (Vol. I). Pittsburgh, PA: Duquesne University Press.

Glaser, B. G., & Strauss, A. L. (1967). *The discovery of grounded theory: Strategies for qualitative research.* New York: Aldine.

Leininger, M. (1991). *Culture care diversity and universality: A theory of nursing.* New York: National League for Nursing Press.

Marter, A., & Agruss, J. (2007). Pacifiers: An update on use and misuse. *Journal for Specialists in Pediatric Nursing, 12*(4), 278–285.

Nastasi, B., Hitchcock, J., Burkholder, G., Varjas, K., Sarkar, S., & Asoka, J. (2007). Assessing adolescents' understanding of and reactions to stress in different cultures: Results of a mixed-methods approach. *School Psychology International, 28*(2), 163–178.

Parse, R. R. (2001). *Qualitative inquiry: The path of sciencing.* Sudbury, MA: Jones and Bartlett Publishers and National League for Nursing Press.

Spiegelberg, H. (1976). *The phenomenological movement* (Vols. I and II). The Hague: Martinus Nijhoff.

Spradley, J. P., (1979). *The ethnographic interview.* New York, NY: Holt, Rinehart & Winston.

Strauss, A., & Corbin, J. (1994). Grounded theory methodology: An overview. In N. K. Denzin & Y. S. Lincoln (Eds.), *Handbook of qualitative research* (pp. 273–285). Thousand Oaks, CA: Sage Publications.

van Kaam, A. L. (1966). Application of the phenomenological method. In A. L. van Kaam (Ed.), *Existential foundations of psychology.* Pittsburgh, PA: Duquesne University Press.

Resources

Denzin, N. K., & Lincoln, Y. S. (Eds.). (2007). *Collecting and interpreting qualitative materials* (3rd ed.). Thousand Oaks, CA: Sage Publications.

LoBiondo-Wood, G., Haber, J., & Krainovich-Miller, B. (2009). Overview of the research process. In G. LoBiondo-Wood & J. Haber (Eds.), *Nursing research: Methods, critical appraisal, and utilization* (6th ed.). St. Louis, MO: Mosby.

Pedhazur, E. J., & Schmelkin, L. P. (1991). *Measurement, design, and analysis: An integrated approach.* Hillsdale, NJ: Lawrence Erlbaum Associates Inc.

Polit, D. F., & Beck, C. T. (2007). *Nursing research: Generating and assessing evidence for nursing practice* (8th ed.). Philadelphia, PA: Lippincott Williams & Wilkins.

10

Background and the Research Problem

Why Ask That Question— What Do We Already Know?

LEARNING OBJECTIVE

The student will relate the background and the research problem to the research methods, results, and conclusions.

Sources of Problems for Research

Background Section of Research Reports

Literature Review Sections of Research Reports
  Directional and Nondirectional Hypotheses
  Null and Research Hypotheses

Linking the Literature Review to the Study Design

Published Reports—Has the Case Been Made for the Research Study?

Common Errors in Reports of the Background and Literature Review

Critically Reading Background and Literature Review Sections of a Research Report for Use in Evidence-Based Practice

KEY TERMS

Conceptual framework
Deductive knowledge
Directional hypothesis
Inductive knowledge
Literature review
Nondirectional hypothesis
Peer review
Primary sources

Research hypothesis
Research objective
Research purpose
Research problem
Research question
Secondary sources
Specific aim
Theoretical framework

Clinical Case • The RN from the clinical case in Chapter 9 continues to work with D.M. and, on the third night in the ICU, D.M. becomes very disoriented and tries to get out of bed. While attempting to settle and soothe D.M., the RN is struck in the face by one of D.M.'s flailing arms, and as a result, experiences a broken nose. As the RN recovers at home over the next couple days, a number of feelings emerge, including anxiety about returning to work, anger, and guilt, feeling that more personal attention given to the patient may have prevented any injury. The nurse realizes that no one has ever discussed the impact of physical injury on nurses, neither during nursing school nor since graduation and wonders whether these reactions are common or unusual. The nurse decides to do a literature search to see whether there has been any research about violence by a patient targeted at health care workers. The RN finds a study titled "Aggression Towards Health Care Workers in Spain: A Multi-facility Study to Evaluate the Distribution of Growing Violence Among Professionals, Health Facilities and Departments" (Gascón et al., 2009) (Appendix A.9). The RN questions what kinds of research have been done about this concern and why the researchers decided to do a retrospective study on this topic. Table 10.1 summarizes the RN's clinical question for this clinical case.

■ SOURCES OF PROBLEMS FOR RESEARCH

We started this book by discussing knowing and knowledge and why research is an important source of knowledge. This led us to recognize the need to understand and intelligently use research in nursing practice. As we moved through discussions of the different sections of most reports of research, we ended each chapter with a "why" question: Why did the researcher come to that conclusion? Why did the researcher use those patients and those measures? Why did the researcher plan the study in that way? We are now ready to discuss the beginning of research reports, in which the most important "why" question of all is asked: Why do this study? This is the most important "why" question, because if there is no good rationale or basis for a research problem, then the rest of the study and report is unimportant.

One of the critical answers to "why do this study" can be found in this chapter. Studies are done to provide evidence for practice. Evidence-based practice, thought of as "integrating individual clinical expertise with the best available external clinical evidence from systematic research" (Sackett, Rosenberg, Gray, Haynes, & Richardson, 1996), should guide the way that nurses practice. Without evidence, best practice standards may go unheeded, important assessment information can be missed, decision making can be impaired, and thus, patient outcomes may decline. The reason "why" studies are conducted is to provide the critical evidence from which all nurses should practice; therefore, that should be one of the primary, driving answers for "why to do this study" . . . to improve practice, and thus, positively influence patient outcomes.

Table 10.1

Statement of Clinical Question From the Clinical Case

What is known about the impact on a nurse of physical injury caused by a patient?

The *Who*	Health care workers
The *What*	Violence by patients
The *When*	Over the past 12 months (from time of data collection)
The *Where*	In the workplace (health facilities and departments)
Key search terms to find	Violence
research-based evidence	Aggression
for practice	Health care workers

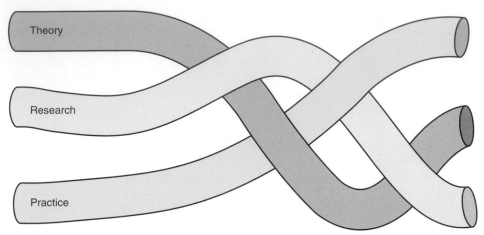

FIGURE 10.1 The woven, or braided, relationships among theory, research, and practice.

A good **research problem** represents a knowledge gap that warrants filling and can be addressed through systematic study. Research problems are derived from several sources, but two general sources of research problems exist. They are (1) problems derived from practice and (2) problems derived from theory. Figure 10.1 illustrates how research, practice, and theory can be viewed as one large braid because they wind together to develop knowledge.

We have focused on research questions that directly relate to practice, and practice is one of the major sources for identification of gaps in knowledge that must be researched. Nursing practice is broad and is a rich source of questions and problems for which we currently do not have answers. Examples of some of the questions that must be answered include the following:

- What are the best ways to support physiologic functioning in acutely ill patients?
- How can we facilitate individual and family growth through the stress of health crises?
- How can we assist patients in making major adjustments associated with chronic illness?
- How can we facilitate and promote positive healthy living, and what makes for a positive and healthy balanced life?
- What allows some people to adapt or cope with illness when some cannot?
- What makes some people more vulnerable to health and illness problems?
- How can we facilitate individuals and families during the transition from life to death?

These questions are broad and cannot be directly tested in a research study, but they do demonstrate the diversity of research areas that arise from nursing practice. Research problems derived from practice may be based on experiences in the practice arena, may be problems derived from mandated evaluation or accrediting requirements, or may reflect social issues as they affect practice.

Theory is another source of research problems. A theory can be defined as an abstract explanation describing how different factors or phenomena relate. In Chapter 8, we discussed theoretical definitions of variables, saying that this type of definition describes a variable conceptually rather than concretely. It is the conceptual or abstract nature of the ideas that, by definition, makes something theoretical. Lazarus's theory of stress, used in several previous examples, provides an abstract explanation for how individuals and their environments interact to lead to stress (Fig. 9.5). Nursing theories, such as those by Sister Calista Roy, Dorothea Orem, Betty Neuman, and others (studied in other courses), provide an abstract explanation of how nursing, persons, environment, and health all interrelate. Any theory can be a source of research problems because theory and research are closely intertwined: Theory is based on and guides research, whereas research tests theory to generate new knowledge.

In general, knowledge can be developed inductively or deductively. **Inductive knowledge** is developed by pulling observations and facts generated through research together to generate theory. Inductive knowledge development starts with pieces to build a whole theory. That theory is then used to suggest further observations that might be expected, which are then used to refine the theory. **Deductive knowledge** is developed by proposing a theory regarding a phenomenon of interest. It starts with the whole and breaks down the parts of the theory, seeking observations and facts to support the abstract relationships proposed in that theory. Observations that support or refute a theory's predictions of relationships are used to revise or refine the theory, which then undergoes further testing. In nursing, many of the observations for either inductive or deductive knowledge development arise from research studies as well as from practice, hence, the intertwining relationships among practice, research, and theory that are illustrated in Figure 10.1.

Although practice and theory are the major sources of research problems, much more is required to develop a specific narrow research problem than just identifying a broad question from either source. In the background section of a research report, we should be able to follow the trail of thinking that has led from a relatively general research problem to a specific, narrowly stated research purpose.

The first sections of most research reports are labeled "Background," "Introduction," "Problem," "Theoretical Framework," "Literature Review," or some combination of these. In all cases, these first sections of a research report should (1) provide the broad context or rationale for the problem, (2) define the problem, and (3) summarize what is already known about the problem. These three purposes are not always discrete and distinct because one purpose also may relate to another purpose. Therefore, information about what is known about a problem also may help to define it, or the context or rationale for a problem also may include what is or is not known about it. However, after reading the introductory sections of a research report, we should have a general understanding of these purposes. The purposes of context and definition are often discussed in the introduction or background section of a research report, whereas a section titled "Literature Review" often specifically describes the current state of knowledge about a problem, based upon a thorough review of the information that is already available. Our discussion will follow this division.

■ BACKGROUND SECTION OF RESEARCH REPORTS

To provide a context for a research problem, most study reports start with a broad and general description of a health concern derived from theory or practice. This description of the concern can be based on national health statistics; the costs of an important health problem; the goals or agenda of an organization that supports health, such as the American Nurses Association (ANA); or an emerging health crisis. For example, the beginning of the report of the study "Sleep, Hunger, Satiety, Food Cravings, and Caloric Intake in Adolescents" (Landis, Parker, & Dunbar, 2009) (Appendix A.1) states that the prevalence of obesity in adolescents has increased worldwide. It goes on to point out that the purpose of the study conducted was to examine the associations among total sleep time, hunger, satiety, food cravings, and caloric intake. The "Psychological consequences associated with intensive care treatment" article (Carr, 2007) (Appendix A.7) starts in the "Introduction" section by pointing out that most existing research studies about patients in the intensive care environment have focused on their physical states of health. Carr (2007) goes on to state that quality of life has emerged in recent years as an area requiring scientific understanding, and therefore, lays the foundation for the purpose of this article. In both of these research reports, however, the authors set the stage by providing the context for the specific problem that they are going to discuss and the reason why they believe it matters.

Providing the context for a specific research problem also often establishes the relevancy of the problem for health care, in general and, possibly, nursing specifically. That sleep, hunger, satiety, food cravings, and caloric intake may correlate with obesity give us a clear idea of why a study should be aimed at understanding the implications of these factors in association with adolescents. This particular study does not directly connect the problem to nursing. Some research reports include a subsection at the beginning that specifically addresses the relationship between the research problem and the nursing, but most will not, as research can be utilized by many different members of the interdisciplinary health care team. Because of this, more often, the potential nursing implications of the problem are addressed indirectly as the research problem is framed and refined.

The RN in our clinical case wants to understand what led the researchers to do a systematic review about patient aggression toward health care workers. The nurse knows that this is a problem that had not been experienced personally until now, nor had been taught anything about it during nursing school. Surprisingly, the nurse discovers that patient violence is considered to be a long-standing problem in some clinical settings and also learns that in recent years, this type of aggression has been on the rise (Gascón et al., 2009). Both of these pieces of information provide the nurse with an initial understanding of why the researchers implemented a systematic review of research in this area.

In addition to setting a broad context for a research problem that may also define the clinical relevancy of that problem, the background section of a report should narrow and refine the research problem. General problems, such as low birth weight and differences in vulnerability in rural and urban settings, are not specific enough to be easily examined using research. Even with qualitative research methods, a specific phenomenon, an aspect of a cultural group, or social interaction must be refined and delineated as the focus of the study to guide data collection and analysis.

Research problems are usually refined either through reference to the existing literature about the problem or through theoretical frameworks. Existing literature used to refine a research problem may include scholarly papers, research studies, or clinical case studies. The focus of the literature when refining the research problem is on the aspects of the problem that have been recognized, what is known about these aspects, and how they may relate. Although the background section refers to existing literature, that literature will be relatively general and address the overall research problem. Often, a background section is followed by a literature review section, in which the literature referenced is usually more focused on the particular research problem than the literature in the background section, which usually differs from the more extensive literature review because the former is relatively general and addresses the overall research problem. The literature review section often addresses the research problem after it has been refined. The background and literature review sections of a research report, then, might fit together to develop a story. The background gives us the general scene and characters, perhaps including the relationships among the characters, and it ends by presenting a specific conflict or problem among selected characters. The literature review continues the story and gives us a much more complete description of the central characters specifically relevant to that problem.

Another approach that may be used to refine a research problem, either by itself or in combination with literature, is application of a theory, theoretical framework, or conceptual framework to the research problem. A **theoretical framework** is an underlying structure that describes how abstract aspects of the research problem interrelate based on developed theories. A **conceptual framework** also is an underlying structure, but it comprises concepts and the relationships among them. We have said that a theory is an abstract explanation describing how different factors or phenomena relate. In the purest sense, these three different terms have different meanings, but understanding those meanings is not essential to intelligently use research because they all describe proposed relationships among abstract concepts.

CORE CONCEPT 10.1

Theory, theoretical frameworks, and conceptual frameworks all provide a description of the proposed relationships among abstract components that are aspects of the research problem of interest.

We must be clear that we are not talking about theoretical definitions of specific variables at this point. As shown in Figure 10.2, abstractions such as theory and theoretical definitions of variables are connected with different sections of the research report. The word *theory* does refer to something that is abstract, so theoretical definitions of variables are abstract definitions of specific variables to be studied and may derive from a specific theory or framework. However, before we can narrow in on specific variables, we must refine the research problem to a point that it can be systematically studied. As Figure 10.2 indicates by the hourglass shape, in the background section of a report, we expect that a broad and general concern, such as the health of incarcerated women, will be narrowed to a specific research purpose. The research purpose is a clear statement of factors that are going to be studied to shed knowledge on the research problem. These factors may also be referred to as the variables to be studied. In general, we expect the research purpose to identify the major variables. Abstract descriptions of these more narrow concepts are then included in the methods section. The discussion and conclusion sections once again use broad and more general abstractions as the results of a study are connected back to the original theory or conceptual framework.

In the study "Sleep, Hunger, Satiety, Food Cravings, and Caloric Intake in Adolescents" (Landis et al., 2009) (Appendix A.1), a conceptual framework was used to develop the intervention. The authors describe a biobehavioral–ecologic framework, which was constructed by

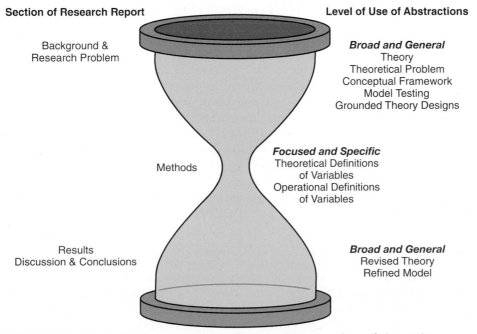

FIGURE 10.2   Relationship between sections of a research report and use of abstract language.

the researchers from a melding of existing scientific and theoretical literature, including domains such as "adolescent risk factors for decreased total sleep time," "consequences of decreased total sleep time," and "increase in body mass index" (Landis et al., 2009, p. 116) (Appendix A.1). The use of this conceptual framework provides a rationale and support for the components of the intervention that the researchers plan to test. This study does not actually test that model or framework directly; rather, it helps to identify research questions for the researchers to address in the course of the study. However, upon conclusion of the study, the authors, in their discussion of the results, comment that these results support the initial construction of the conceptual framework that was the foundation of the intervention and indicate that this is enough evidence to warrant continued study in this area (Landis et al., 2009).

In some studies, you will see terms that are referred to a *study aim* and a *research question*. These terms and several others refer to the specific focus of the research study that is being reported. Two other terms also used refer to the specific focus of a research study are *research purpose(s)* and *research objective(s)*. All of these terms mean essentially the same thing: They refer to a statement of purpose of the research and identify the variables that will be studied.

Often, the research purpose (or question, specific aim, or research objective) also will include language that defines the type of question being asked in the research—whether the question is descriptive, relational, or predictive. The research purpose for the psychological consequences article used the phrase *associated with* in the title (Carr, 2007) (Appendix A.6), thus clearly identifying that it is asking a question about associations or connections. The aggression toward health care workers study uses the term *distribution*, clearly indicating that we are looking for expanse in this trend (Gascón et al., 2009) (Appendix A.9), whereas the transition to home care article utilizes the term *quality*, implying that we are looking for distinctive characteristics to emerge as we read.

CORE CONCEPT 10.2

The terms research purpose, research question, study, or specific aim(s) or research objective(s) all refer to the statement of the variables to be studied that are related to the broad research problem.

In summary, the background section of a research report has two major purposes: (1) to establish the context for the research problem and (2) to refine that problem to a specific research purpose. The section of the report that we are referring to as *background* may simply be the beginning of the report without any title, may be titled "Introduction," or may be titled "Background." Information that provides the broad context for the research problem may include issues from either practice or theory and may reflect societal concerns, health care policy changes, or major health concerns. Refining the research problem may be accomplished using literature, theory, or both. In either case, the goal is to move from the general problem to a specific purpose or question that identifies the variables to be included in the study and often the type of question being asked.

■ LITERATURE REVIEW SECTIONS OF RESEARCH REPORTS

We said earlier that the use of literature to refine the research problem is not necessarily the same as the formal literature review. A literature review is a synthesis of the literature that describes what is known or has been studied regarding the particular research question or purpose.

Much of the literature review consists of a synthesis of existing published research, but some scholarly and theoretical work that is not actual research may also be included in

> **Box 10.1**
>
> **Specific Purposes of the Literature Review**
>
> - Description of what is known about the variables for the study
> - Description of how the variables have been studied in the past
> - Description of with whom the variables have been studied

the review. The literature review is more than a listing or summary of relevant research; it entails the combination of several elements or studies to provide a different or new focus on the research problem. For example, the literature review—titled "Review of the Literature"— in the predictors of life satisfaction article from Chapter 4 (Appendix A.4) points out that data from studies show that depression and poor life satisfaction in stroke survivors correlates to a decrease in life satisfaction in caregivers. This point is made by summarizing the focus of research of a number of studies and summarizing them in this short section. A recitation of all of them would be monotonous and useless. Box 10.1 summarizes the purposes for literature reviews.

CORE CONCEPT 10.3

The literature review is guided by the variables that have been identified in the research purpose and aims to give the reader an overview of what is known about those variables, how those variables have been studied in the past, and with whom they have been studied.

The RN in our clinical case has found a study in which the authors do not specifically identify their review of existing literature as a "literature review" (Gascón et al., 2009) (Appendix A.9), but rather incorporate this information into the introductory section of the study, right before the "methods" section. In this case, the purpose of the authors' research is to review existing information in order to establish that there is a gap in knowledge, which guides future research. We mentioned earlier that authors use other literature to establish and support their specific aim. However, they do not provide a formal review of the literature because that is what they have identified as the gap in knowledge that must be addressed to develop further understanding about an expanding distribution of violence against health care workers.

To assure us that the literature review reflects the state of the science, the author must include current or recent studies. Usually, we would expect that most of the literature cited in a literature review has been published within 3 to 5 years of the date of the study or the publication of the report. However, sometimes little research has been conducted on selected variables, there has been a gap in time since the problem was addressed, or some important or classic studies may have been done more than 5 years ago. In these cases, we may appropriately see literature cited that was published more than 5 years ago. We care about how current the literature cited is because we want to know that the researcher is building on the most current knowledge related to the problem of interest.

Another way of ensuring that a study, either proposed or reported, is based on current knowledge is its use of primary sources. Primary sources are the sources of information as originally written. To be accurate and current, it is important that the researcher has read and synthesized the actual research reports or scholarly papers that are relevant to the study. A secondary source is someone else's description or interpretation of a primary source. For example, Landis et al. (2009), in the sleep and hunger in adolescents study (Appendix A.1), state that Johnson-Taylor and Everhart (2006) found that "previously tested interventions aimed at adolescent diet and physical activity patterns have had limited success [in decreasing obesity in adolescents]" (p. 116). This is an example of using a primary source because Landis et al. must have read Johnson-Taylor's and Everhart's study and reported on what they read. However, suppose that another researcher named "Smith" wanted to study factors associated with adolescent obesity, had read Landis et al.'s research report, and then stated in the literature "Johnson-Taylor and Everhart (2006) found that 'previously tested interventions aimed at adolescent diet and physical activity patterns have had limited success [in decreasing obesity in adolescents]'" (p. 116) (Landis et al., 2009, p. 116) (Appendix A.1). In this case, Smith would be citing a secondary source: Smith has not read the Johnson-Taylor and Everhart study, only Landis et al.'s description of it. We know this because Smith tells us the names of the authors who reported the original study, then references different authors, in this case, Landis et al., as the source of the information.

One problem with secondary sources is the potential for inadvertent error or distortion of the findings of a study. Think about the childhood game of telephone, in which six or seven children sit in a circle, and one child starts a message around the circle by whispering it into the ear of the child next to him or her. That child then whispers the message that he or she heard into the next child's ear. As we all know, by the time the message gets around the circle, it is likely to have changed significantly from what was originally stated. The same problem can occur with reports of research or other scholarly work. The greater the number of times that the work is interpreted beyond the original, the greater the possibility that the actual results will be distorted or changed.

The second reason that we expect a researcher to use primary sources is because the researcher must carefully choose quality sources to support his or her current research study. If we depend on Landis et al.'s sentence about Johnson-Taylor's and Everhart's study, we are also depending on Landis et al.'s judgment about the quality of that study related to the recovery from abdominal surgery study. Once we read the report of Johnson-Taylor's and Everhart's study, we might decide that it is not relevant to the proposed study of health behaviors in pregnant women.

In addition to the use of current and primary sources, the RN in the clinical case should expect to see literature that has been published in referred or peer-reviewed journals. We mentioned in Chapter 1 that the quality of information acquired on the World Wide Web must be carefully evaluated because anyone can create a Web site and claim to be an authority on a subject. Similarly, there is variety in the quality of published literature. A standard that ensures a published report has been carefully scrutinized for quality is the use of peer review. Peer review means that the manuscript for the published report has been read and critiqued by two or more peers before being accepted for publication. *Refereed* is another term that means that there was critical review of manuscripts before being accepted for publication. Manuscripts that are peer reviewed are intentionally sent to individuals who have expertise in the manuscript's topic. Therefore, the reviewers' comments are likely to reflect current and well-established knowledge. Not all sources of reports on research are peer reviewed or refereed. You can find out whether a particular publication is refereed by checking the author's guidelines for a journal— often available on a Web site, and always in the journal itself.

All of the studies used as examples in this chapter are from peer-reviewed journals. However, not all of the citations listed when doing a search using search programs such as CINAHL will be from peer-reviewed publications. As an intelligent user of research for clinical practice, you should consider not only the content of the research study, but also the type of publication. When you read research published in refereed journals, you know that the published report has been reviewed by several individuals with expertise in the research area, giving you some assurance about the quality of the study before you read it.

Part of what assures us of the quality of a literature review and, therefore, the knowledge on which the study was based, is that the literature cited was from refereed publications. Therefore, the RN in our clinical case will read the background literature and the systematic review expecting that recent literature, from primary sources and peer-reviewed journals, will provide information about what is known about patient violence toward health care workers.

The predictors of life satisfaction study (Ostwald, Godwin, & Cron, 2009) (Appendix A.4) used in Chapter 4 provides a good example of a review of the literature. If we look at the literature cited, we see a range of publication dates from 1981 to 2008. Most of the literature was published in 2003 and after, and when we look at the 1981 citation, we see that it is part of a description of the historical development of understanding of life satisfaction. This is an example of a "classic" or an important historical element related to the topic. Further, the references cited are all studies published in major nursing journals that are peer reviewed.

As the RN in our clinical case reads the background literature review that is the basis for the systematic review regarding aggression toward health care workers, an increased understanding is gained about the problem and about what has been studied in depth in the past. The authors use this background to support the need for a systematic review of literature. Because limited studies of this specificity were uncovered, the author mentions this, again alluding to the need for this particular type of study to be done.

Therefore, the literature review should provide focused information about the specific variable(s) to be examined in a study. The review should provide some understanding of what is known about the variables, how they have been studied in the past, and with whom they have been studied. This should logically support the design and methods for the research study reported. Returning to our earlier analogy, by the time the literature review is completed, the major plot and subplots for the story should be clear. For those plots to make sense, we must understand the characters and their past "relationships" or stories.

After the literature review, some research reports include detailed research questions or hypotheses. Not all reports do so because not all research studies have detailed questions or hypotheses. In particular, we do not expect such information in a study using a qualitative approach because the emphasis should be on understanding the whole of an experience or a phenomenon, rather than breaking it down and studying its discrete parts. We also do not expect detailed research questions or hypotheses from quantitative studies whose purpose is general description. However, studies that test theory and predictions from theory or attempt to test the effect of manipulation usually have focused detailed research questions or hypotheses.

The language of research can be confusing at this point. We said earlier that a research problem is broad and general, while a research purpose is narrowly stated, may also be called a research question, and will specify the factor(s) or variable(s) to be examined. Now, we are talking about "detailed" research questions. Another way to think about these questions is as subquestions to the narrow and specific question or purpose of the study. For example, the home care study from Chapter 8 (Appendix A.6) states, "establishing a process where local pharmacists provide consultation for medication reconciliation is promising and delivery models should be developed and evaluated" (Brown et al., 2006, p. 347) (Appendix A.6). This sentence clearly identifies the independent variable of a new study as the consultation for medication reconciliation, and the dependent variable is implied as the result of how patients take those medications, based on the consultation.

Questions like these can break down the larger research purpose into more detailed and specific questions. The questions include not only the specific variables of interest in the study but also the specific relationship to be tested and the time frame for that testing. As an intelligent reader and user of research, you should understand that it is important to know that most reports of research studies start with a general problem, move to a more refined research purpose or question, and then, if appropriate, develop specific measurable questions or hypotheses, as illustrated in Figure 10.3. The research problem, purpose, and question are descriptions of the knowledge sought by the study that differ in their depth and

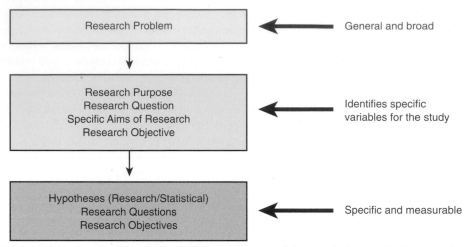

FIGURE 10.3   Levels of development of the statements of the knowledge sought by the study.

specificity, but content from one may overlap with another at times. They also may differ in the actual terms used, such as the research purpose being called a specific aim or the research questions being written as objectives. However, a research report should include at least two, and often three, levels of depth and specificity of statements about the knowledge being sought in the study. These levels are differentiated by the specificity of the statements, with the problem being general, the purpose stating the variables for the study, and the questions or hypotheses stating specific measurable predictions or relationships.

In Chapters 2 and 5, we defined a hypothesis as a prediction regarding the relationships or effects of selected factors on other factors. We now know that the factors in a study are called *variables*. A research question and a research hypothesis are often opposite sides of the same coin because they both state predictions about relationships among variables. A research question puts the predictions in the form of a question, whereas a hypothesis puts the predictions in the form of a statement. There are two types of research hypotheses and questions: directional and nondirectional.

Directional and Nondirectional Hypotheses

A hypothesis may predict whether there will be a relationship between two variables, or it may state the nature of the relationship between them. When we speak about the nature of a relationship, we are referring to whether the relationship is positive or negative; another word for this is the *direction* of the relationship. We talked about negative and positive relationships in Chapter 5, when we discussed correlations. A positive relationship exists between two variables if one increases as the other increases and vice versa. A negative relationship exists if one variable increases as the other variable decreases. Figure 10.4 illustrates a positive relationship between number of freckles and sun exposure and a negative relationship between hours of work and ability to concentrate. A directional hypothesis predicts that two variables will be related and as well predicts the direction of that relationship. It will predict, for example, that as the score for one variable increases, the score for a second variable will increase. A nondirectional hypothesis predicts that two variables will be related but does not predict the direction of that relationship.

Research questions can also be directional and nondirectional. If a researcher asks "Is there a relationship between sun exposure and number of freckles?" this would be a nondirectional question. If a researcher asks "Do the number of freckles increase as the amount of sun exposure increases?" this would be a directional research question. Whether a hypothesis or research question is directional or not depends on the current level of knowledge about the variables of interest or the extent to which theory has been developed about the

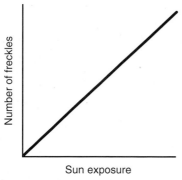
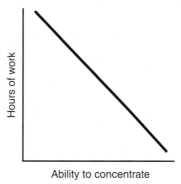

FIGURE 10.4   Graphs depicting positive and negative relationships among variables.

variables. A well-developed theory proposes not only relationships among factors but also the direction of those relationships. Therefore, a study using such a theory would be more likely to have directional hypotheses.

If we look at the predictors of life satisfaction study (Ostwald et al., 2009) (Appendix A.4), we find that the authors had one specific question. This is logical because they were hoping to understand, based on more current therapeutic regimens, the life satisfaction implications of a couple after stroke. This question was nondirectional, asking simply what life satisfaction was in couples after stroke, rather than predicting that one type of couple in which a partner had experienced a stroke would have better outcomes than another couple. An example of a directional research question might have been "Do current therapeutic regimens increase the life satisfaction of couples after one partner experiences a stroke?" This question includes a proposed direction for the effect of the intervention—that is, the intervention is proposed to positively affect life satisfaction.

Null and Research Hypotheses

In addition to hypotheses being directional or nondirectional, there are two forms for hypotheses: the null and research forms. We described research and null hypotheses in Chapter 5. The research hypothesis predicts relationships or differences in variables, whereas the null hypothesis states that there will be no relationship or differences among variables. Remember that the null hypothesis is developed for statistical purposes and represents the assumption made in inferential statistics that most relationships or differences that may be found in any particular sample might have occurred by chance alone. Only when a difference or relationship among variables found in a sample is so large that it would only occur by chance in fewer than 5% of samples can the null hypothesis or statistical hypothesis be rejected. Usually, when a study has a null hypothesis, an alternate hypothesis also is stated, and that alternate hypothesis will predict both a relationship and a direction to that relationship. The idea of a "null" form is not applied to research questions, only to predictions in the form of statements.

Because we did not have any examples of use of null hypotheses in the studies that we have read for the previous chapters, let us think about a study examining pregnancy behaviors to predict pregnancy outcomes using statistical hypotheses. Suppose that the purpose of the study was "to describe and compare the patterns of health-related behaviors, including smoking, alcohol use, use of prenatal care, exercise, and nutrition among women in rural and urban settings, and to test the relationship among these behaviors and the outcomes of low birth weight and premature birth." Two sets of possible hypotheses could be stated:

H_0: There will be no differences in the pattern of tobacco use among pregnant women from urban and rural settings.

H_1: Women from rural settings will use tobacco more when pregnant than will women from urban settings.

H_0: Timing and regularity of use of prenatal care will not be related to birth weight among rural and urban samples.

H_1: Earlier and more regular use of prenatal care will decrease the incidence of low-birth-weight infants in both the rural and urban samples.

The symbol "H_0" represents the null hypothesis, and "H_1" represents the alternate hypothesis. You can see that the null hypothesis is a neutral or negative prediction, written primarily to support the assumptions of inferential statistics. A study that is using research hypotheses without null hypotheses also may use the symbol of an uppercase "H," but they will be numbered consecutively as H_1, H_2, H_3, and so on. A researcher should only include hypotheses at the beginning of a study if there is some basis for the predictions from either previous research or theory, and the literature review should include the information from theory or research that supports the hypotheses.

■ LINKING THE LITERATURE REVIEW TO THE STUDY DESIGN

When we first discussed the literature review, we said that it should give us an overview of what is known about the study variables, how they have been previously studied, and with whom they have been studied. We have discussed the quality of the literature review and mentioned that the research questions or hypotheses are specific predictions that should be supported by the literature review. The final aspect of the literature review that is important is the support it should provide for the study design.

The literature review should provide a synthesis of what is known but also should synthesize the approaches that have been taken to develop knowledge in this area. In this way, a literature review not only synthesizes but also critiques existing research about a problem. A true critique identifies strengths and weaknesses, and this is what we should expect to see in the literature review section of a research report. The strengths and weaknesses of previous research should serve as the basis for the study currently being described. The researcher should tell us at the beginning of the report how the results of this study will fit within the overall structure of knowledge about the problem. For example, the predictors of life satisfaction study (Ostwald et al., 2009) (Appendix A.4) identifies in the literature review most studies that have been conducted report lower life satisfaction in stroke survivors and their spousal caregivers than in the general population (Ostwald et al., 2009). They go on to note that instrumentation variation, settings, and recovery time in studies have also led to inconsistent findings. They summarize by saying that few studies at all have focused on the caregiving spouse. This information supports a descriptive design because it identifies that we lack knowledge about the complexity of the multiple needs of this population. The authors also state that the results of this study are intended to provide rehabilitative nurses with important knowledge for how to assess and care for this population. Thus, the authors indicate how the findings from their study could fit with and increase existing knowledge.

A literature review may specifically address problems in study design from previous research or limitations of past samples. The literature review also may synthesize and critique the existing literature without directly addressing design and sampling issues. However, in either case, one of the purposes of the literature review is to identify the rationale for the design used in the study. Like a well-written story, each section or chapter should build a foundation for the next section or chapter. Choices of research design should be based on approaches taken in the past, with the goal of improving on or expanding on previous knowledge.

In summary, the background and literature review sections of a research report set the stage for the remainder of the study. The background gives the broad context for the research problem and an overview of factors relevant to that problem. This overview may present an abstract set of concepts and their relationships to one another called a *theory, conceptual framework,* or *theoretical framework*. The background usually ends with a statement of a research purpose or questions that specify the variables to be studied. The literature review starts with the purpose and describes the current state of the science in relation to the study variables. To do so, the literature review must be current and use mostly primary sources from peer-reviewed journals. The literature review should include what is known about the variables and how and with whom they have been studied. It establishes the basis for the design of the study and may end in specific research questions or hypotheses.

■ PUBLISHED REPORTS—HAS THE CASE BEEN MADE FOR THE RESEARCH STUDY?

We began this study wondering why the authors of the violence against health care workers study (Gascón et al., 2009) chose to do a review. If we examine the literature review, we find that few studies in the past have focused on this issue. The authors' critique of these past studies is that they have focused on the behaviors of clients within psychiatric settings, although violence like this can occur in any health care environment. The information about findings from previous studies and the limitations of previous studies set the stage for the authors' review, using clearly identified inclusion and exclusion criteria in order to organize and categorize findings about nonphysical effects.

After reading the introduction of the Gascón et al.'s report, the RN in our clinical case has more information to use in understanding the findings from the review, understanding the general problem that the study is attempting to address as well as the specific aim of the review. The nurse now recognizes that these types of occurrences are not isolate and that what has happened in the nurse's professional environment has indeed happened to others working in similar situations.

At the end of Chapter 9, you were asked to make a case for why a study of nursing students' well-being should be implemented. After reading this chapter, you should have a clearer idea about how you might have developed that rationale and why it can be an important part of a research report. The background and literature review set the stage for the rest of the research report by giving us a general setting for the study in terms of the problem; the specific purpose of the study, including the study variables; and an understanding of how this study will fit with current theory and research-based knowledge.

■ COMMON ERRORS IN REPORTS OF THE BACKGROUND AND LITERATURE REVIEW

One of the first errors that may occur in the background and literature review sections of a research report is a failure to develop a consistent link among the research problem, the research purpose, and any specific hypotheses or questions. The fictional article that describes the study of nursing students' choices of practice after graduation (Appendix B) gives a good example of a background that does not directly link the problem, purpose, and research questions. The introduction to that report discusses the general problem of the nursing shortage and the need for workforce planning. It then states that in addition to the sheer number of students, we must consider choice of practice in workforce planning, indicating that specific sites for practice will have greater needs for nurses in the future. International differences are mentioned, but there is no further mention of international aspects through the rest of the report. The next section, titled "Background," continues with the thread that students who will choose the most severe shortage sites should be targeted for recruitment to schools of nursing and concludes with a research purpose to "examine the relationships among nursing students' demographic characteristics and their choices for practice following graduation." At this point, the connections become weak. After the research purpose, the author lists three specific questions, the first of which addresses specific demographic variables (age, gender, race, and marital status), but the second and third introduce new variables, students' well-being and students' experiences that relate to their choices of practice, that have not been mentioned at any point in the preceding section. This is like an author of fiction placing an entirely new character into the middle of a story without connecting that character to anything or anyone in the previous part of the story.

The example in the fictional article is somewhat extreme, and what makes it an even poorer example is that no literature review is included. Consequently, we have no idea of what research has been done with students and choice of practice, what methods were used to conduct the research, or what types of students were studied. Published research reports vary in the consistency and links that they draw among the research problem, the purpose, and specific measurable questions. If, as an intelligent reader of research, you finish the background and literature review section and still do not know what is going to be studied and why, one explanation may be that connections among the problem, the purpose, and the research questions have not been clearly or consistently identified in this section of the report.

A second problem that can occur is a failure to provide the information needed to fulfill the important purposes for these sections. For example, a literature review may provide a thoughtful synthesis of what is known about the variables of interest in the study but may fail to connect it to the purpose of the study being reported. This can leave us uncertain concerning the basis for the researcher's selection of research design and approach to measurement or how the study will fit with current knowledge.

Another problem that can occur is a failure to adequately reference statements. If the author of a research report makes a statement about the variables of interest that reflects knowledge that is not common and does not provide a reference, then we are left wondering how much we can trust the statement. We must wonder whether the statement is simply the opinion of the researcher, some stray fact that was found on the World Wide Web, or a well-documented research-based piece of knowledge. Occasionally, the number of references imbedded in a sentence in a literature review can almost be distracting from the meaning of the sentence, but those references assure us that the information is well founded and accurate.

The last potential problems with background and literature review sections of research reports are those we have discussed: the use of secondary sources and out-of-date references. The point of these beginning sections is to give us a clear and accurate picture of the state of knowledge about the research problem and to develop a coherent set of connections between that knowledge and the specific research purpose and questions. Secondary sources and references that are all more than 5 years older than the date of publication of the study do not give us much confidence that the study will fit well with current levels of knowledge.

■ CRITICALLY READING BACKGROUND AND LITERATURE REVIEW SECTIONS OF A RESEARCH REPORT FOR USE IN EVIDENCE-BASED PRACTICE

There are seven questions that you can ask yourself as you read the background and literature review sections of a research report, and these are listed in Box 10.2. We will take these one by one and examine each more closely. First, and most obvious, is "Does the report include a clearly identified background and/or literature review section?" Several of the reports that we have read in previous chapters do not clearly identify the background or literature review; they simply start with a statement of a problem or concern and then describe literature relevant to that problem, eventually concluding with a research question or purpose. The lack of specific headings may or may not interfere with your understanding about why a study was implemented. You will have to judge whether this is a problem.

A second question is "Do I think the background discusses aspects of my clinical question?" The RN in our clinical case selected this article to gain a better understanding of the scope of violence in the health care environment. If the background had focused on the workforce impact of patient aggression, the nurse might have quickly decided that the study was not going to be relevant to the clinical question being posed. A third question that is related is "Does the literature help me understand why the research question is important to nursing?" In all but this last clinical

Box 10.2

How to Critically Read the Background Section of a Research Report?

Does the report answer the question "Why ask that question—what do we know?"

1. Does the report include a clearly identified background and/or literature review section?
2. Do I think the background discusses aspects of my clinical question?
3. Does the literature help me understand why the research question is important to nursing?
4. Is the majority of the literature cited current (less than 5 years old) or very important to understanding the research question?
5. If a nursing or other theory was presented, does it connect to my clinical question?
6. Is the specific research question/problem/hypothesis connected logically to the literature and/or theory presented in the background section?
7. Is the specific research question/problem/hypothesis relevant or related to my clinical question?

case, we have asked patient care questions relevant to direct nursing care, and even in the last clinical case, we are asking a question that will affect a nurse's ability to deliver patient care. So, one aspect that we would expect to find in the literature review, sometimes explicitly and at other times implicitly, is identification of the relevance of the research question to nursing.

The next question to ask yourself is "Is the majority of the literature cited current (less than 5 years old) or very important to understanding the research question?" Some reports may include literature that is dated and neither seems relevant nor addresses the stated problem for the research. For example, although most of the report of the review by Gascón et al. is logical and connected (Appendix A.9), the last sentence in the introduction seems to be giving us information that is not immediately relevant to the research aim that follows. Specifically, the researchers indicate that "the study was focused solely on that violence which the California Occupational Safety and Health Administration (CalOSHA) classifies as Type II (exercised by customers, users, or patients), excluding other types of aggressions which might coexist in the work environment" (Gascón et al., 2009, p. 31) (Appendix A.9). Yet, in no place before or after this do the authors discuss the different types of aggressions that coexist. Therefore, after critically reading this introduction, we might conclude at least that this last statement does not seem that important to our understanding of the research aim.

The fifth question, "If nursing or other theory was presented, does it connect to my clinical question?" also addresses congruency and logical building of content in a background and literature review. If you read any research report and find in it a description of a theory that is not later connected to the purpose or question addressed in the research, you should wonder why it was included at all. As we stated earlier, theory can be a very important source of research problems, and often a background section describes a theoretical framework or conceptual model to support the approach taken to a clinical problem. But if that theoretical framework or conceptual model does not seem to be relevant to your clinical question and is not used in a specific manner to establish the research study, then it is superfluous and detracts from the reader's understanding of a study.

The sixth and seventh questions are related—"Is the specific research question/problem/hypothesis connected logically to the literature and/or theory presented in the background section?" and "Is the specific research question/problem/hypothesis relevant or related to my clinical question?" Thus, these questions critically examine the specific research purpose or question or hypotheses and ask whether these flowed from the background and literature review, providing a specific focus for the research study that addresses the clinical question of interest. Remember the analogy of these sections resembling a story. If this story concludes with an unrelated ending, we clearly recognize that it is not a very good story. Similarly, if the specific research question, problem, or hypothesis is not connected to the background and literature review "story" that has preceded it, the quality of those sections have to be questioned. Moreover, if the specific research question, problem, or hypothesis does not seem relevant to the clinical question of interest, then reading and understanding the rest of the report will not be particularly useful.

OUT-OF-CLASS EXERCISE

Pulling It All Together

We have now completed the second section of this book. We have looked at the entire research report, starting with the conclusions and moving forward to the background and literature review. As we discussed the sections, we also focused on selected aspects of the research process. The last two chapters return to the traditional approach to discussing research: starting at the beginning of a study or report and moving to the end. We discuss how the research process is related to the published research report and to the nursing process itself. We also examine the history of nursing research and how evidence-based practice and quality improvement relate to the research process. To prepare you for these chapters and to help you pull together the different sections of a research report, write an abstract that describes a research problem addressed by the in-class exercise. Decide on one question that you think could have been answered by that study. Then, in approximately 250 words (one page, double spaced), write an abstract that includes (1) background, (2) objective or purpose, (3) methods, (4) results, and (5) conclusions. If you have had the opportunity, you may be able to use real results generated in your class. If not, make up the results. The point of the exercise is to write a concise description of a research study using the specific language of research. Go back and read some of the abstracts of the research reports that we have used in this book or find some published research of interest to you to serve as examples of what your abstract should look like. Remember that abstracts are organized differently in different journals, but for this exercise, try to use the five headings listed in this paragraph.

If you did not have an in-class study, you may want to take the fictional article from Appendix B and think of another question that might be addressed, given the variables in that study, or at least rewrite the abstract for the study using the headings listed in the previous paragraph. After you have completed this exercise, you are ready to move on to Chapter 11.

References

Brown, E., Raue, P., Mlodzianowski, A., Barnett, S., Meyers, B., Greenberg, R., et al. (2006). Transition to home care: Quality of mental health, pharmacy, and medical history information. *International Journal of Psychiatry in Medicine, 36*(3), 339–349.

Carr, J. (2007). Psychological consequences associated with intensive care treatment. *Trauma, 9*(2), 95–102.

Gascón, S., Martínez-Jarreta, B., González-Andrade, J., Santed, M., Casalod, Y., & Rueda, M. (2009). Aggression towards health care workers in Spain: a multi-facility study to evaluate the distribution of growing violence among professionals, health facilities and departments. *International Journal of Occupational and Environmental Health, 15*(1), 29–35. Retrieved November 25, 2009, from Research Library. (Document ID: 1650113891).

Landis, A., Parker, K., & Dunbar, S. (2009). Sleep, hunger, satiety, food cravings, and caloric intake in adolescents. *Journal of Nursing Scholarship, 41*(2), 115–123.

Ostwald, S., Godwin, K., & Cron, S. (2009). Predictors of life satisfaction in stroke survivors and spousal caregivers after inpatient rehabilitation. *Rehabilitation Nursing, 34*, 160–174.

Sackett, D. L., Rosenberg, W. M. C., Gray, J. A. M., Haynes, R. B., & Richardson, W. S. (1996). Evidence based medicine: What it is and what it isn't. *British Medical Journal, 312*(7023), 71–72.

Resources

LoBiondo-Wood, G., Haber, J., & Krainovich-Miller, B. (2009). Overview of the research process. In G. LoBiondo-Wood & J. Haber (Eds.), *Nursing research: Methods, critical appraisal, and utilization* (6th ed.). St. Louis, MO: Mosby.

Polit, D. F., & Beck, C. T. (2007). *Nursing research: Principles and methods* (8th ed.). Philadelphia, PA: Lippincott Williams & Wilkins.

11

The Research Process

How Is the Research Process Related to a Published Research Report?

KEY TERMS

Aggregated data
Assumptions
Codebook

Dissemination
Pilot study

Clinical Case • In Chapter 8, our clinical case concerned an RN who worked in home health and cared for patients who had short-stay breast cancer surgeries. Shortly after altering care based on the evidence from research, the RN was invited to participate in a new research group. The goal of the group is to develop and implement a study of patient and staff relationships as a predictor of rehospitalization of women who have had surgery for breast cancer. The RN is considering returning to school to earn a master's degree and decides that this group will provide a good opportunity to increase knowledge about the research process. The research group is being led by a professor from the school of nursing affiliated with the RN's hospital and an oncology clinical nurse specialist (CNS) who has a joint appointment with the RN's hospital and the school of nursing.

In previous chapters, we learned about the different sections of a research report and discussed the process of doing research, but we have not yet focused on the research process itself. Now that we are comfortable with much of the language of research and with some fundamental elements of the aspects of the research process that are reflected in a research report, it is time to look at the research process as a whole. This chapter describes the research process from beginning to end, links that process to the research report, and discusses the relationship between the research process and the nursing process.

■ THE RESEARCH PROCESS

In Chapter 2, we briefly described the five steps of the research process:

1. Define and describe the knowledge gap or problem.
2. Develop a detailed plan to gather information to address the problem or gap in knowledge.
3. Implement the study.
4. Analyze and interpret the results of the study.
5. Disseminate the findings of the study.

A process, whether it is the research process, the nursing process, or the critical thinking process, is, by definition, fluid and flexible. All of these processes refer to steps because certain parts of the process are necessary before one can successfully move to the next part. However, the steps do not always follow one another in a step-by-step manner: At times, the results of a step in the process leads to returning to the preceding step, or possibly two steps occur at the same time.

CORE CONCEPT 11.1

The steps of the research process are not always linear: They may overlap or be revisited during the research process.

For example, a refined research purpose is necessary before beginning to develop a detailed research plan, but it is possible that as a plan is developed, the research purpose may be revisited and refined further. Similarly, a research plan is needed before a study is implemented, but it is possible that as the study is implemented, the plan will be revised. In fact, in most qualitative methods, the methods are expected to change as the study progresses. Therefore, although this chapter discusses the steps of the research process in order, the process may be more fluid and flexible in action.

Define and Describe the Knowledge Gap or Problem

The RN in our clinical case, who is beginning to participate in a research group, finds that by attending the first meeting of the group, this is the start of the first step in the research process. The CNS begins by describing a question that has been developed based on the CNS's work on the surgical unit. The CNS has noticed that in some patient cases, the ICU staff and the patients and family develop warm and interactive relationships, whereas in other cases, the patient–staff relationship is poorly developed, with limited communication and contact. The CNS wonders why this difference occurs and how the differences in relationships may affect patients. Another member of the research group states their belief that when the staff has better communication with patients and their families, the patients have shorter hospitalizations and are rehospitalized less frequently. Other members of the group begin talking about reasons why they believe that relationships between patients and staff differ. Some focus on characteristics of patients, some on nursing staff, and some on medical staff. Then, another member of the group suggests that length of hospitalization itself is an important factor in both what kind of relationship is established between staff and patients and rehospitalization. The RN in our clinical case suggests that the staff:patient ratio and whether a woman is admitted on the weekend also affect nurse–patient relationships and hospital outcomes.

It is obvious to the RN that at this point in the group's process, there is no agreement about the knowledge gap that must be addressed. Each nurse's input about the factors influencing relationships and hospital outcomes is different, and based on their own personal experience and care. Creating a flowchart of all the ideas that have been discussed is suggested. Figure 11.1 illustrates the results that might have come from this effort. Once the group sees all its ideas in a flowchart, it begins to identify some of the areas that it must explore further. For example, the group identifies that it must find out what is known about staff–patient relationships. Relationships and communication are recognized as two separate, yet connected, concepts. The group agrees that it will focus on the relationships between nursing staff and patients, since nurses spend more focused time with the patients, but will consider how physician–patient relationships may also be a factor in the nurse–patient relationships. Beyond looking for information about nurse–patient relationships within surgical units, the group agrees that it needs to look for information about the effects of relationships on health care outcomes as well as information about factors that may affect relationships, such as staff:patient ratio and nurse and patient characteristics. The members of the group divide the list of various ideas they have discussed and agree to conduct a literature review focusing on a particular subset of ideas, returning in 2 weeks to share what they have found. The process described in this hypothetical situation illustrates aspects of the first step in the research process.

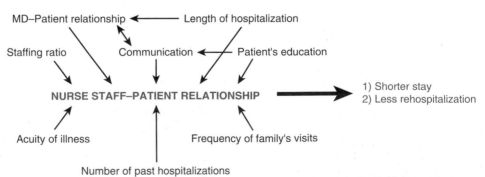

FIGURE 11.1   Possible flowchart developed during brainstorming about a research problem.

The information required for this first step will be acquired from existing theory and research to identify what is known about the problem and the relevant factors related to the problem. This step also requires thoughtful analysis because rarely does theory or past research easily blend into an obvious research purpose. At this point in the research process, often what is needed is an explosion of ideas and information, all of which then must be thoughtfully analyzed and synthesized to develop a refined purpose. The brainstorming session that our RN experienced may be the first of several sessions in which many ideas are explored, validation and information about those ideas are sought and digested, and new ideas are generated. This step can be both exciting and frustrating: exciting because of the amount to be discovered about a problem of interest and frustrating because of the amount to digest and integrate to develop a refined research purpose.

For example, our hypothetical research group may find a great deal of information about nurse–patient communication, primarily with adult patients. However, perhaps little has been done examining nurse–parent communication in short-term surgical settings with patients who have cancer. Perhaps the focus primarily has been on communication rather than on the broader concept of relationships. The group does find theory about the concept of relationship formation in general, which certainly includes the concept of communication as well as characteristics of the participants in a relationship. The group recognizes that several of the nurse theorists have focused on nurse–patient relationships and have identified a range of concepts that are important to their development. They also found several studies that conclude by recognizing the importance of the relationship between staff and patients of breast cancer patients. Yet, they find few research studies that link nurse–patient communication or relationships to long-term outcomes, such as length of hospitalization or rehospitalization. Finally, nothing exists in either theory or literature about structural factors, such as overall staff:patient ratio or timing of admissions during weekends versus weekdays and nurse–patient relationships. Despite this lack of literature, the RN believes, from personal experience, that when patients are admitted on the weekends, they and their families often do not establish as good a relationship with the weekend staff as do patients who come in during the week with the regular weekday staff.

All of these findings leave the group with even more information than they compiled when they brainstormed and with no immediately obvious connections between all the possible factors that it might consider. This is what was meant by an "explosion of information": As ideas are analyzed in this step of the research process, they sometimes explode into multiple new ideas to explore.

Despite the potential explosion of information, notice that our hypothetical group has now acquired a foundation of knowledge about what is known, has been theoretically considered, or has been studied in the past. Developing that foundation of knowledge is the goal of the first step of the research process. That foundation of existing knowledge should include existing research, practice experience, and any appropriate and relevant theory. The challenge then becomes synthesizing the existing knowledge; critically examining practice experience, theory, and past research; and identifying a research purpose that includes specific factors or variables to be studied. Notice also that the foundation of knowledge found strongly supports the relevancy of the problem that this group has identified for nursing practice.

In addition to establishing a foundation of knowledge about the research problem, another part of this first step entails identifying assumptions that are imbedded in the approach to the problem and the purposes being considered. Assumptions are ideas that are taken for granted or viewed as truth without conscious or explicit testing. Assumptions can be difficult to identify because they are ideas that we "just know" or "all understand" and are usually unspoken. However, assumptions can sometimes color how a research problem is viewed so that the approach to knowledge development is limited in some way. Several assumptions are often made in nursing research, and one researcher studied reports of research to describe some of these. Williams (1980) identified 13 assumptions that are commonly present in nursing studies. Included were assumptions that stress is something to avoid, that health is a priority for most people, and that people operate on the basis of cognitive information. Identifying the assumptions imbedded in a study can be helpful because we may realize that the assumptions must be researched and confirmed before we can move forward in knowledge development.

In the hypothetical study that we are discussing, there is an assumption that relationships between patients and staff can be viewed as "good" or "bad." There is a second assumption that patients' experiences in the surgical unit will affect their health afterward. Because of these assumptions, the research group is not considering exploring whether the terms *good* and *bad* apply to relationships; it is beginning with looking at factors that make relationships good or bad. Perhaps this approach is too simplistic and there are only different types of relationships, some of which are more or less helpful in promoting positive health outcomes for the patients. If so, the study of factors that make relationships good or bad may miss some important types of relationships.

As the research problem is refined into a specific purpose, the types of questions that will be addressed and the approach likely to be taken are often beginning to be identified. We previously discussed how research questions that address prediction or examine the effects of manipulation of a variable require a relatively large amount of background or foundational knowledge. It becomes increasingly clear to our hypothetical research group that not enough research or theory about factors affecting nurse–patient relationships or the effects of these relationships on outcomes exists to make predictions or to plan to manipulate any factor. Because the researchers cannot find studies and theory that convince them to predict that a certain variable will have a desired outcome, they realize that they must consider questions about relationships between variables in the nurse–patient relationship or questions that describe the nurse–patient relationship.

The group also begins to consider whether a qualitative, quantitative, or mixed method approach is most logical as it begins to refine the general problem of nurse–patient relationships. Some of the group argues that because so little has been studied regarding the patients' experiences in their interactions with nursing staff, the first study should be phenomenological. Others suggest that a grounded theory approach might be taken, broadly based on Peplau's theory of interpersonal relations (1952). A grounded theory approach based on Peplau's theory would aim to develop concepts and links that are grounded in nurses' and patients' experiences of developing and maintaining relationships. Others believe that nursing theory and existing theory about relationships in general as well as past research about nurse–patient communication provide a set of relevant factors that can be measured and tested to see how they affect nurse–patient relationships in women having short-stay breast cancer surgery. These members think that a correlational study is what is needed. Everyone agrees about the need to discover whether staff–patient relationships can be linked to outcomes, such as a shorter total hospitalization or fewer rehospitalizations.

It is not uncommon that during the first step of the research process several potential research studies are identified that are relevant to the problem. Refining a problem clarifies the nature of the gaps in knowledge as well as the factors relevant to the problem. In many cases, the problems of interest to nursing are too complex to address in a single study. Let us assume for now that after several meetings, substantial discussion, and review of theory and the literature, the hypothetical group in our clinical case agrees on a tentative purpose: to identify and examine factors that affect nurse–patient relationships in the short-stay surgical settings and the role that these relationships have in patient outcomes. This purpose tells us that the variables in this study will be unspecific "factors," nurse–parent relationships, and patient outcomes. This purpose will probably need further refining, which will occur as the group moves into the second step of the research process. In this next step, the group takes the purpose it has identified and develops a specific research plan that includes the research design and methods of measurement and sampling.

Develop a Plan to Gather Information

As the purpose for a study is refined, ideas about gathering information about the problem being studied also begin to generate. As researchers review past research studies regarding the problem, they consider not only the findings from that research but also the methods and samples used. This helps to clarify gaps in knowledge and identifies measures and approaches that previously have been successful in addressing the problem. For example, our hypothetical research group has found that most studies of nurse–patient communication have been conducted with adults who were the primary medical care recipients rather than with adults who have just had a major surgery and are being discharged home within 48 hours. They also found that many of the communication studies have used videotaping as a method of data collection, with analysis of discrete episodes of communication as the focus of study. Because this group is interested in more than isolated episodes of communication, it knows that it needs a different research method, since videotaping of episodic communication will not provide the information they need.

The second step of the research process is complex and involves many considerations and decisions. This step includes deciding on the general approach to be taken to the study and a specific research design; identifying and developing plans for the study sample or participants; and planning the measurement process, including specific techniques, measures, and timing. Finally, at the end of this step, an institutional review board (IRB) proposal must be written and submitted in preparation for implementation of the study.

The group in our clinical case intentionally left its preliminary statement of a research purpose broad because it had not reached an agreement about whether this research needed to develop further knowledge about nurse–patient relationships or describe how factors that it has found in the literature and from practice affect that relationship. The group eventually decides that a mixed method approach makes the most sense, beginning with a grounded theory study of the relationships between nursing staff and breast cancer patients in the short-stay surgical unit. It plans to follow this with a descriptive correlational study about how the factors they have identified from research and practice affect the length of hospitalization and rehospitalization within the following month. These factors include history of hospitalization, stage of cancer, educational level, timing of initial admission, and average staff:patient ratio during hospitalization as well as any factors that are identified from the grounded theory study that can reasonably be included. Following this overall decision about the study, the group is able to refine their purpose: to describe the perceptions of nurses and patients of their relationship during the hospitalization for short-stay breast cancer surgery, including their perceptions of how that relationship does or does not impact health outcomes, and to describe how nurse, patient, and hospital unit factors impact length of hospitalization and need for rehospitalization within a month after discharge.

The refined purpose described reflects several decisions that have been made by the research group. It has decided that a grounded theory method is a better design for its purpose than a phenomenological design because it is examining interactions, has a general theory in Peplau's psychodynamic nursing theory, and will help develop knowledge about relationships. The group has ruled out doing a true longitudinal study, as it did not find strong research evidence about factors relevant to staff–patient relationships or the effect of factors on the outcomes of interest. A longitudinal study requires more time and resources than a cross-sectional correlational study, and the group members believe that they do not have the knowledge base to justify that effort at this time. The group has also settled on two outcomes—length of hospitalization and occurrence of rehospitalization within a month of discharge—partly for pragmatic reasons. They know that administration and insurance companies are interested in shortened hospitalization and avoiding unnecessary rehospital-ization, so they expect that they may be able to get support for this study from the hospital. Also, these two outcomes are easily measured. Other outcomes that the group discussed included patients' sense of control and efficacy, rate of recovery, and rate of complications. These are all still considered relevant by the group, but it agreed that potential difficulties with measurement precluded examining them in this study.

Thus, the second step of the research process requires critical thinking and decision making. Researchers must consider what is known, what has been shown to work, and what is feasible. The last consideration includes issues of time, cost, established measures or approaches, and other resources, such as space or access to samples. We will discuss these further when we discuss factors that affect research.

Decisions about the best possible methods for implementing the chosen study designs must also be made during this part of the research process. In the case of the grounded the-ory phase of the hypothetical study, for example, researchers must make decisions about methods of data collection, such as interviews, observations, or use of journaling, as well as the timing for the data collection. Similarly, to implement the descriptive correlational phase of the study, researchers will have to make decisions about measures, such as chart audits, and the use of a questionnaire or a structured interview. The issues of rigor, validity, and reli-ability that we discussed in Chapters 8 and 9 are central to making these decisions about methods and measurement.

Another important part of the second step is deciding on the sample for the study and approaches to the process of sampling, as discussed in Chapter 6. For example, the surgi-cal unit sees patients at different stages in their breast cancer treatment. Although the group plans to measure severity of illness during the second phase of the study, it recognizes that the stage of cancer, whether or not this is the first admission for the cancer, and individual physician practices all also will affect the length of hospitalization. The grounded theory phase of the study will benefit from researchers' talking with several patients, including those who have experience with the surgical unit and those who do not. After some discus-sion of normal patient census and the most common types of patients seen, the research group decides to limit the study to women newly diagnosed with breast cancer. This deci-sion is based on the experience of our RN and several other group members who suggest that patients who have already had treatment such as chemotherapy for their cancer have dif-ferent needs and outcomes than those who have just been diagnosed and the surgery is their first treatment.

In addition to deciding who will participate in the study, the group in our clinical case must consider how comfortable patients will be when talking about their relationships with nursing staff, and how the care provided by the nursing staff, as well as their behaviors, might change regarding their relationships with patients when they know there is a study in progress. This would be an example of the Hawthorne effect described in Chapter 9. Patients might be concerned about repercussions on their care if they express any negative feelings, and staff might be concerned about negative effect on their performance evaluations. These issues could lead to a threat to internal validity from testing and to researcher effects threat-ening external validity. The research group decides to use individuals who are not associ-ated with the surgical unit in any way as data collectors and to put extra effort into ensuring anonymity of participants and subjects to address this concern.

The hypothetical group in our clinical case will make other specific decisions as it moves through the second step, and the details of these decisions could probably fill several chapters. Overall, this process is based on a further exploration of the past research to iden-tify research designs and methods that have been used, measures that are available, and sampling considerations. This research literature, along with the realities of the specific set-ting for the research, the knowledge and experience of the researchers, and resources such as time and money, all will be considered in developing a detailed plan to gather information

Box 11.1

Considerations Affecting the Development of the Detailed Research Plan

- Methods and samples used in previous research
- Potential setting(s) for the study
- Experience and knowledge of the researcher(s)
- Resources available, such as time and money
- Subject safety and rights
- Rigor, reliability, and validity.

about the research purpose. Box 11.1 summarizes these and other considerations affecting the development of the research plan.

Once a detailed plan is developed, the last part of this second step is to ensure the protection of human subjects and to acquire the resources needed for the study. We discussed informed consent and the role of IRBs in Chapter 7. The type of study we are discussing in this chapter would likely have to receive IRB approval from the hospital board as well as from the university board. This will require two written proposals describing the study background, purpose, literature review, design, and measures and how the rights of subjects will be assured. Developing this type of IRB proposal often helps a researcher or research group to tighten the details of their plan of study but also takes time and must be considered when planning a time line for a research study. In addition, many studies cannot be implemented without acquiring some outside resources to support the time and materials needed. Depending on the complexity of the proposed study and the resources inherent in the study site, researchers often must write and submit proposals for funding before they can implement it. Again, the writing, review, and receipt of funding can take weeks to months. However, both the review of IRB proposals and the funding proposals provide outside input into the plans for a research study and often significantly improve those plans before the study is implemented.

Implement the Study

The third step in the research process is to implement the study. This is when the advance planning and decisions can pay off and when unexpected issues can arise. One of the biggest responsibilities of the researcher during implementation is to maintain meticulous documentation of the sampling and data collection process. This documentation allows the researcher to later clearly identify any points in the study at which plans were changed and the rationale for decisions made during the implementation process. Areas that may need to be addressed and documented during this step include data about numbers and characteristics of those who were approached to be in the study but declined or later dropped out, any revisions in sampling criteria, any changes in the timing or the measurement process, and any anecdotal or incidental data that become relevant during the study implementation.

In Chapters 6 and 8, we discussed things that can go wrong with sampling and measurement and how important it is to consider those aspects when deciding on the usefulness of research for practice. The careful documentation kept by researchers during the study implementation is the basis for reporting information that will allow us to evaluate the sampling and measurement process. In addition, incidents or occurrences that are unexpected may have a big effect on the meaning of results of a study. For example, suppose that patients who had one particular physician all declined to be in our hypothetical study.

Or, suppose that as the study is implemented, patients start approaching the research staff and ask to participate before they have been recruited. Either of these observations suggests that there may be some underlying factor at work during the process of study implementation. In the first case, that factor may be a physician who has told parents not to participate, because the physician is unhappy about the study, thus eliminating data about relationships with a provider who is controlling. In the second case, the underlying factor might be that patients have a strong need to talk about their experiences, which this study is meeting. This unmet need may be important to consider when gaining understanding about staff–patient relationships. One could speculate about the meaning of either observation, but what is important is to document the observation for future consideration as the results of the study are analyzed.

During the study implementation, the steps of the research process may be particularly fluid, moving back and forth between this step and the previous step of planning or to the next step of analysis and interpretation. As we discussed in Chapter 8, in the implementation step, qualitative methods depend on a spiraling process of data collection followed by data analysis and interpretation that informs the next round of data collection. Sometimes during the study implementation, the plans for sampling prove to be unrealistic, perhaps because criteria are too strict or because the desired subjects for the study are not willing to participate. The researchers will then have to revise their sampling plan to implement the study. Or perhaps data collectors note that all subjects are confused and have difficulty answering some part of a questionnaire. The researchers will have to use this information to decide whether to change their measures in the middle of their study or to continue with a measure that may have problems with reliability. These are just a few examples of the many kinds of problems that can be encountered during the study implementation. The process requires time, care, consistency, and ongoing monitoring.

Analyze and Interpret the Results

The fourth step of the research process involves the analysis and interpretation of study results. As we indicated, this step may be interwoven with the step of implementation in a qualitative study. In contrast, most of the data analysis in a quantitative study is usually reserved until the entire data collection process is complete. This difference reflects the differences in philosophy behind the two types of approaches. A qualitative method uses data as it is generated to build additional data, with the goal of arriving at information that is dense and thick to inform our understanding of a phenomenon. Quantitative methods strive to control and isolate phenomena to understand each discrete element. Therefore, quantitative methods defer analysis of most of the data until the collection process is complete to avoid contaminating the data collection process with ideas generated from the analysis. The exception to this is in analysis of sample characteristics. A purposive sample or a matched sample, as discussed in Chapter 6, requires the analysis of subject characteristics during the study implementation to effectively implement the sampling plan.

Data analysis, whether carried out in a qualitative or quantitative study, requires the same level of meticulous care and documentation that is needed during the implementation step of the research process. In qualitative research, this is accomplished through the audit trail and notations within the software programs that are often used during data analysis. In quantitative research, decisions about data analysis are often documented in a codebook. In research, a codebook is a record of the categorization, labeling, and manipulation of data about variables in a quantitative study. It includes information about how each of the variables in the study was measured; how the data from the study were reviewed and transferred into computer files; and all decisions made regarding the management of problems, such as incomplete responses or confusing responses. Like an audit trail, a codebook provides a detailed description of how the data from a study were managed.

Qualitative data are often collected in an interview, so the first thing that must be done is to transcribe the data into a word-processing program. Once transcribed, the data can be either loaded into a qualitative analysis program or printed and analyzed on hard copy. In either case, data management often includes careful reading and listening to interviews that have been transcribed to ensure that the transcription is accurate and complete. Similarly, quantitative data have to be entered into computer software programs to be analyzed. This can be done in several ways, including direct entry of numbers from quantitative measurement into a data file or use of an optical scanner that reads and records numbers off a data collection measure into a data file. In either case, once it is in a data file, the data must be carefully examined for accuracy. Human error in keying numbers into a file or computer error in scanning answer sheets can significantly affect and even invalidate study results.

The researcher can proceed with the analysis and interpretation of the results once data have been put into a form that allows that process. As discussed in Chapters 4 and 5, data analysis is complex and challenging. It also is an exciting time in the research process because the researchers begin to find out what their study says about the research problem that started this whole process. In addition to information about data management, codebooks in quantitative data analysis often include information about decisions regarding analysis approaches and the mathematical manipulation of the data. For example, a researcher can decide to use a mean score of items from a measure of a variable in the analysis or to use a score that is just the sum of all the items. Alternatively, a researcher may decide to study all subjects as one large group in which members have differences on a variable of interest or to divide subjects into two groups that clearly differ on that variable. All of these types of decisions are usually documented in the codebook so that as the research progresses, the researcher can recall those decisions and the rationale behind them. Thus, both the audit trail and the codebook reflect documentation of data management and analysis, which are important aspects of the fourth step of the research process.

Interpretation is the last part of this step. Interpretation of the results of a study entails pulling the whole process together into a meaningful whole. The theory and research literature that served as a foundation for the study, the decisions made in the planning step of the process, and the decisions and observations that were made during the implementation step all must be considered and tied into the results of a study. At this point, the expertise of the researchers and their personal knowledge and experience are also used in interpreting results. For example, suppose that during the implementation of the hypothetical study of staff–patient relationships, patients started hearing about the study and asking staff to be included. The research team will have to decide why this occurred and how it affected the data collected. The RN and research team in our clinical case may decide that this interest in participating in the study reflected a strong need on the patients' part to feel included in their care. Or they might conclude that patients needed an avenue for expressing their feelings about the nursing staff and the care they receive. These are different interpretations and would have different meanings for the results of the study. It is important to remember that these subjective interpretations do not necessarily represent the reality of the findings; a different study would need to be done to accurately understand the true meaning of the actions of the patients who asked to be included in the study.

Disseminate the Findings

The last step of the research process brings us back to where we started in this book—to the research report. Dissemination of research findings refers to the spreading of knowledge and is an essential step in the research process because knowledge development is wasted unless it becomes known so that it can be used. The dissemination of research findings may be accomplished in several ways. Findings may be disseminated through a report of the research to the agency or organization that funded or hosted the study. This type of dissemination is targeted at the specific groups that were closely involved in the study. Often, the results of a research study also are reported back to participants in that study. In addition, findings from a study may be verbally reported in the form of presentations to agencies or funding groups or at scholarly and professional meetings. Findings from research are reported in published journals in both print and online formats. Finally, research findings are sometimes disseminated to the public through the lay press, television, or other medium. Each of these types of approaches to dissemination of findings targets different groups of potential users of the research, with the report to those closely involved in the study clearly reaching a much smaller group than a published article in a major professional journal.

Because research dissemination targets different groups, the depth and detail of the dissemination vary. However, in all cases, the goal of dissemination is to accurately share the knowledge gained from the research so that it is useful and meaningful to the targeted recipients of that knowledge. For example, a summary of a research study that is being sent out in a regional newsletter will probably focus on a brief description of the problem, the sample, and one or two key findings. A presentation of a paper reporting the findings of a study at a professional meeting will usually be limited to 15 or 20 minutes, allowing inclusion of more detail than a newsletter column but less than what would be included in a published report in a research journal. A published report in a practice-focused journal will probably include fewer specifics about the research process than a report appearing in a research journal. However, in all cases, the researcher must be sure that the findings of a study are clearly and accurately stated.

The other consideration that is important for all types of dissemination is ensuring the anonymity of subjects or participants in a study. This requires that data primarily are reported in the aggregate and that there is careful scrutiny of that data. Aggregated data means that the results from the study are reported for the entire sample rather than for individual members in the group. Usually, when data are aggregated, no specific result from the study can be attributed to any participant in the study. However, with a small sample, it is possible that even with aggregated data and elimination of any traditional identifiers, the anonymity of individual subjects might be lost.

For example, suppose that the hypothetical study of staff–patient relationships acquired a sample of 50 subjects in the descriptive correlational phase. One characteristic of subjects that will be reported is race, and perhaps only three subjects in the study were from a certain culture. Further, suppose that there was one finding stating a difference in patients' perceptions of staff by race, with Asian patients reporting much more negative experiences with staff. The staff on the surgical unit could read those results and likely know immediately which patients reported negative experiences because they have so few Asian patients, thus eliminating the anonymity of those patients. In this type of circumstance, it is possible that a result may have to be withheld from dissemination to protect the rights of the subjects in the study. Given that the reason the results may breech anonymity is because the numbers of Asian patients was so small and, therefore, that the results may have happened by chance alone and must be confirmed with a larger sample, the withholding of such a result does not jeopardize knowledge development.

It should be noted that even at this last step in the research process, a researcher might revisit an earlier step. Sometimes only when writing up the findings of a study does a researcher discover the need to consider and report a specific descriptive result or conduct a particular statistical test. Sometimes after sharing findings from a study with others, suggestions are made for additional analysis that may shed further light on the research problem. Of course, the findings from a study often raise new questions or suggest new research problems, taking us back to the first step.

It should be clear from this description of the research process that it is complex, exacting, and challenging (Box 11.2). The dissemination product of that research often does not

---

Box 11.2

Characteristics of the Research Process

- Systematic
- Complex
- Exacting
- Challenging

---

provide a full picture of all the thought and work that went into a research study. Throughout this book, we have discussed common errors that can occur in a research report. However, any report of research deserves to be read with respect because of the effort and risk taken by the researcher to implement the research process and then make public the results of his or her efforts. Few research studies are perfect, and research reports certainly vary in their completeness and usefulness to practice. However, reports of research reflect a substantial time commitment of one or more individuals to address a gap in knowledge through the use of the complex and often strenuous process of research. The next section looks more closely at how and why publications of research do not always fully reflect the research process.

RESEARCH PROCESS CONTRASTED TO THE RESEARCH REPORT

In Chapter 2, we discussed the relationship between the research process and the sections of a research report. This relationship is illustrated in Figure 11.2. Now that we have discussed the research process in more detail, a fuller comparison of the process to the research report is possible.

The first step of the research process of describing and defining the knowledge gap or problem is summarized in the background and literature review sections of a research report. These sections give us the context for a research problem and tell us about relevant theory and research regarding aspects of the problem. The information included in the report is a synopsis of the much more extensive information that was gathered and synthesized during the first step in the research process. The research purpose and specific questions or hypotheses that conclude the first sections of a report reflect the final refinement of the research problem into specific variables and a specific type of research question.

The second step of the research process is reflected in the methods section of a research report. The methods section tells us the study design, sampling plan, methods of measurement, and procedures. Again, all of the previous research, practicalities, and experience that enter into the decisions about settings for a study, the sample, and the measurement are distilled into a few paragraphs describing the final decisions that were reached about the study plan.

The third step of implementing the study is usually reflected in the results section of a research report because it is there that we learn who participated in the study. We may also see part of the implementation of the study reflected in the methods section if what occurred during the implementation process changed the sampling or measurement approaches taken. In either case, the information included in a report rarely reflects all of the details of a study's implementation.

The fourth step of analysis and interpretation of the results of a study are reflected in both the results and conclusions sections of a research report. Of all the steps of the research process, probably this one is most fully described in the report. However, even with this step, a great deal more goes into the process than is reflected in the results and conclusion sections of most reports.

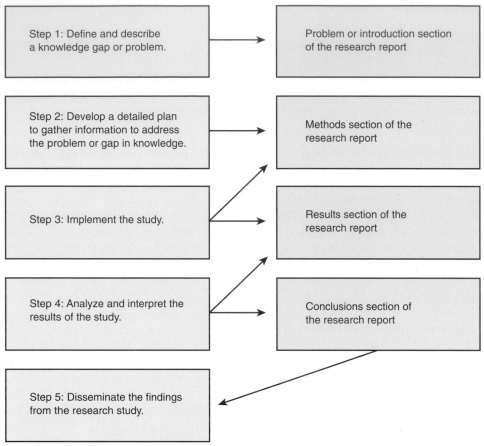

FIGURE 11.2   The relationship between the research process and the sections of a research report.

Finally, the fifth step in the research process is the research report itself. However, developing and publishing a research study report also requires more effort than may be obvious when looking at the final product. The publication of a research study depends on several factors. These include the fit between the purpose of the study and the emphasis of journals that publish research, the relevance and quality of the research study, and the ability of the researcher to express clearly and succinctly all the pertinent elements that are needed to fully understand and use the research. The first two factors primarily affect the user of research because they affect what research is available through journals and online. Some research journals publish all types of research in each issue; others develop themes for different issues, limiting the types of studies that they will publish at any particular time. Other journals reflect specialties, such as obstetric nursing, and are only interested in research that is relevant to that specialty. Some journals do not want to publish research that is highly theoretical because they target readers who want practical and practice-focused information. To disseminate the study findings, a researcher first has to find journals that fit with the purpose of the completed study.

We mentioned in Chapter 10 that research reports from refereed or peer-reviewed journals are more respected because they have been reviewed and critiqued by experts in the area of the research. Some research is not published because problems with the quality of the research are identified during the review process that decreases the meaningfulness or validity of the study's results. This does not mean that the research was bad, but simply that some flaw or aspect of the study creates enough doubt about the findings or meaning of the results to preclude warranting publication.

Another factor that affects publication of research studies is the ability of the researcher to express in writing adequate information to accurately describe the entire research process. As you will recall, many of the common errors in research reports discussed throughout this book were errors of omission or lack of complete information. We have now seen how much more thought and work goes into the research process than can go into a research report. The challenge for a researcher, then, and for the reviewers and editors who contribute to the final publication, is to describe clearly and completely all the aspects of the research process that were relevant to the particular study. The goal is to provide the readers with enough information to allow them to fully understand the study and to make intelligent decisions about the usefulness and meaning of the research for practice. One way that this is accomplished is by using the language of research to limit the need to fully explain each study aspect. Yet, that very language of research may interfere with using research in practice because the practitioner may not be familiar with or understand that language.

■ FACTORS THAT AFFECT THE RESEARCH PROCESS

In the previous section, we discussed factors that affect the publication of research studies. What about factors that affect whether a research study is implemented? Potential barriers to the implementation of research include lack of knowledge; lack of resources, such as money, time, or both; and lack of methods or measures.

Occasionally, research is not implemented because those who see a problem do not have the knowledge or skill to carry out the research process. For example, an RN in practice may see an important problem but be unable to find others who have a similar interest with the skills to implement the research. The RN also might not be experienced enough to know that the problem they have identified could qualify as a research study. Similarly, a community or a group of patients may see a problem that is not recognized as important by providers or by those who are prepared to implement research.

Research requires time and effort and is not without expense. Some research is not implemented because there are no resources to support the particular study. Expenses in research range from routine small costs, such as copying expenses and paper, to potentially huge costs for sophisticated measures, such as ultrasounds or specialized laboratory testing. Costs are associated with the researcher's time and the time of others, such as data collectors or workers who enter data. Costs are associated with providing space and equipment needed for some research. As well, costs may be directly associated with subjects in the study, such as incentive payments, or reimbursement for travel or lodging.

Financial support for research can come from numerous sources, including individuals; local, regional, or national foundations or organizations; or the government. In almost every case, to receive financial support for a study, a researcher must prepare a proposal describing the study and identifying how the study will help to meet the goals of the funding source. Herein lies another limit or potential barrier to some research.

Sources of financial support for research usually have goals or initiatives that relate to the purpose of the group providing the support. Occasionally, these goals are specific, such as those of the National Alzheimer's Association, which are to support research into the mechanisms and treatment of Alzheimer's disease. Sometimes these goals are broad, such as the goal of the National Institute for Nursing Research (NINR) to support knowledge development in nursing. However, even the NINR, with its broad goal, has research priorities and target areas for research, such as studies with vulnerable populations, which may influence the success of a particular study in receiving funding. The Web site of a professional organization, such as Sigma Theta Tau or the NINR, usually publishes its research priorities. When developing a proposal for a research study, decisions about the study purpose, sample, or methods may be based, at least in part, on the goals and priorities of the potential funding source.

In addition to direct financial support for research, sources of indirect support also may affect the types of research implemented. In nursing, large health care organizations and nursing colleges in universities often employ individuals with the expectation that they will implement research as part of their role. These organizations pay for part of the time a researcher spends on research because the results of research fit with the mission of the organization. A nurse researcher in a large metropolitan medical center, for example, may not need to find financial support for his or her time but may need to limit the types of research implemented to problems directly relevant to delivery of tertiary health care.

Another factor that affects the implementation of research is the availability of safe and tested methods and measures to study what we are interested in studying. For example, we may be interested in predictors of pancreatic cancer because it is so lethal but have no effective way to identify the dependent variable of interest—pancreatic cancer—until an individual is so ill that it is no longer feasible to implement measurement of selected biologic or psychosocial parameters. Or a researcher may be interested in a concept, such as empathy, but finds that no instruments have been developed that can be used to measure empathy. Sometimes it is unethical to implement a study using what might be the best design validity because of the need to protect the rights of human subjects, as discussed in Chapter 7.

One approach that researchers can take to address some of the limits related to measures and methods is to implement a pilot study. A pilot study is a small research study that develops and demonstrates the effectiveness of selected measures and methods. Occasionally, this type of study is used to demonstrate the potential importance of a selected factor to a research problem. At other times, it is used to demonstrate the reliability or validity of selected measures in a unique situation or sample. A pilot study also may be used to demonstrate the ability of the researcher(s) to implement a study. Because knowledge development regarding any particular gap in knowledge is a process that takes time and usually requires multiple studies, pilot studies can be an important first step in building a research program.

■ GENERATING KNOWLEDGE THROUGH RESEARCH CAN BE FUN!

We started this book by stating that the goal was not to make you a researcher but to give you the knowledge and tools needed to understand and use research intelligently. However, we do not want to end this chapter, or this book, with an emphasis on how complex and arduous the research process can be or the many potential barriers there can be to both implementing and publishing research. The research process is a wonderful and exciting challenge. It is like a giant interactive puzzle because as each piece is solved and fit into place, the rest of the pieces change and must be addressed in their new form, given what has already been completed. Fitting each piece into the puzzle can be extremely satisfying, and finishing small sections of the puzzle through completion of a research study can be rewarding.

Part of the reason the research process is fun is because it is a continuous learning experience for those involved. When one is trying to develop new knowledge, the challenges of planning and implementing a valid and meaningful study always require problem solving and creative solutions, so the opportunity to learn and create can be immense. More and more, we are recognizing that most research is best approached by using teams with members from different backgrounds and disciplines. This allows the knowledge brought to bear on a research problem to be wide ranging and to enhance the potential for a high-quality product.

We started this chapter with the RN joining a newly formed group seeking to address a research problem. We talked about the process employed by this group and how that process relates to the research report. As we discussed the research process, you may have noticed some similarities between it and the nursing process. For one thing, both are processes, and both have been broken down into steps. In the broadest sense, the nursing and research processes are similar because they are used to solve problems. Both a research problem and a patient care problem (whether the patient is an individual, family, or community) can be viewed as a complicated puzzle, where often only some of the pieces are available at any time point.

Both types of problems are initially addressed through gathering information. In the nursing process, this gathering of information is referred to as assessment, and in the research process, it is referred to as describing and refining the knowledge gap or problem. However, in both cases, we are collecting information to guide us in understanding the problem and formulating a plan.

The second, third, and fourth steps of the nursing and research processes also initially may appear similar, although they differ in some major ways. Although the second step of the nursing process is planning and the second step of the research process is developing a detailed plan, the two processes differ because they have fundamentally different purposes. The purpose of the nursing process is to provide informed, scientifically based nursing care for human responses to potential or actual health problems. The purpose of the research process is to develop or validate knowledge. The goal of the nursing process is action to promote the established outcome of improved health. The goal of the research process is to acquire new knowledge, and the outcomes for that new knowledge cannot be known until the knowledge is established. Therefore, the second and third steps of the nursing process address planning and implementing care, whereas the second and third steps of the research process address planning and implementing acquisition of new information. As a result, the fourth steps of these two processes have different focuses because evaluation in the nursing process is concerned with outcomes, whereas data analysis and interpretation are concerned with understanding. Table 11.1 summarizes the similarities and differences between the two processes. We discuss the roles of nursing in research more in the next chapter.

Although there are some similarities and differences in the processes of nursing and research, it is essential that there be a strong relationship between the two. The research process should provide knowledge that is the basis for the nursing process. This is why this entire book focuses on understanding and intelligently using research in practice. In addition, the nursing process will often be the source of problems that need to be addressed using the research process. As we plan, implement, and evaluate nursing care, we often find problems or face questions about the best ways to achieve our outcome of improved health. The nursing and research processes differ in purpose, but they are closely linked and together ensure the growth and development of nursing as a profession.

Table 11.1

Comparison of the Research Process and the Nursing Process		
	RESEARCH PROCESS	**NURSING PROCESS**
Similarities	A process with steps A form of problem solving Complex "puzzle"	A process with steps A form of problem solving Complex "puzzle"
Differences	Purpose is to develop knowledge	Purpose is to provide scientifically based care
	Plans and implements knowledge acquisition	Plans and implements delivery of care
	Analysis and interpretation concerned with knowing	Evaluation concerned with outcomes

CORE CONCEPT 11.2

While different in purpose, the nursing process shares several steps and skills with the research process.

■ PUBLISHED REPORTS—WHAT DO YOU CONCLUDE NOW?

We have used numerous research study reports in this book as examples of how research can be used and related to clinical practice. In several cases, the studies examined a research problem from the two different approaches of qualitative and quantitative methods. None of the studies that we examined could be called perfect, and to expect them to be so is unreasonable, but each made a meaningful contribution to our knowledge about patients and patient care. No one study, however, gave us the full answer to our clinical questions and often had clear limitations in trying to apply the findings to our RN's clinical case. This is often a frustration for nurses in practice. With a better understanding of the research process, it should be clearer now why usually no one study fully answers a clinical question. Clinical questions are usually too complex, and too many variables and factors must be considered and examined for any one study to provide a complete answer. However, as research studies about a particular clinical problem accumulate, we should see answers begin to unfold. This is the essence of evidence-based practice, which explicitly recognizes the need for an accumulation of knowledge regarding a problem to ensure the best and safest delivery of health care. Excellence in delivery of evidence-based care is one of the qualities recognized and valued by the Magnet Recognition Program, a program developed by the American Nurses Credentialing Center (ANCC). "Recognizing quality patient care, nursing excellence, and innovations in professional nursing practice, the Magnet Recognition Program provides consumers with the ultimate benchmark to measure the quality of care that they can expect to receive. When *U.S. News & World Report* publishes its annual showcase of 'America's Best Hospitals,' being an ANCC Magnet organization contributes to the total score for quality of inpatient care" (ANCC, 2009).

Therefore, what do you conclude now about the needs of the RN from Chapter 1, who is facing complex planning for the 17-year-old adolescent patient who is struggling with physiologic and psychological issues related to her weight? What do you conclude about how the RN from Chapter 3 is taking care of C.T. following a mastectomy, and how the nurse should intervene with the patient's needs regarding activities of daily living? What should the RN in Chapter 4 do differently in caring for the stroke patient and her husband? How should the RN plan protocols that increase patient life satisfaction following stroke and also address the spousal caregiver needs? You should now be able to accomplish the following tasks and answer five questions as you read the research we have reviewed. As you look at these questions, realize how much you have learned and how much you now know regarding research.

- You can read and understand the background and literature review of a report to find out "Why was the research question asked—what do we already know?"
- You can read the design and methods sections of a research report to find out "How were those people studied—why was the study performed that way?"
- You can read the sampling section of the research report to find out "To what types of patients do these research conclusions apply?"

- You can read the results and conclusions sections of the report to find out "Why the authors reached their conclusions—what did they actually find?"
- Finally, you can use the answers from the above four questions to decide "What is the answer to the question—what did the study conclude?"

You also now know that finding the "answer" to your question will only be the beginning, and that it may give you new knowledge and insight into patient care but may also leave you asking even more questions.

■ CONCLUSION

It is the authors' hope that as you read and use research, you will develop an interest in and excitement about the process of research as well as for the problems that it addresses. Although the baccalaureate nurse is not expected to plan and implement research, there are several roles for nurses in the research process, such as participation in planning a study or in subject recruitment and data collection. If you have come away from this book with an understanding of how to better read, understand, and utilize research, then you are well on your way to providing even more competent patient care through this process. Just as research is a process of constant movement toward better understanding how we can provide patient care, so is the journey of lifelong learning to incorporate into nursing care. We hope that the information contained in this book will be a most useful part of *your* journey.

References

ANCC. (2009). Magnet Recognition Program overview. Retrieved January 8, 2010 from http://www.nursecredentialing.org/Magnet/ProgramOverview.aspx

Peplau, H. E. (1952). *Interpersonal relations in nursing: A conceptual frame of reference for psychodynamic nursing.* New York, NY: G. P. Putnams' Sons. [Reprinted 1991, New York, NY: Springer].

Williams, M. A. (1980). Editorial: Assumptions in research. *Research in Nursing & Health, 3*(2), 47–48.

Resources

LoBiondo-Wood, G., Haber, J., & Krainovich-Miller, B. (2009). Overview of the research process. In G. LoBiondo-Wood & J. Haber (Eds.), *Nursing research: Methods and critical appraisal for evidence-based practice* (7th ed.). St. Louis, MO: Mosby.

Locke, L. F., Silverman, S. J., & Spirduso, W. W. (2009). *Reading and understanding research* (3rd ed.). Thousand Oaks, CA: Sage Publications.

Polit, D. F., & Beck, C. T. (2007). *Nursing research: Principles and methods* (8th ed.). Philadelphia, PA: Lippincott Williams & Wilkins.

Tomey, A. M., & Alligood, M. R. (2009). *Nursing theorists and their work* (7th ed.). St. Louis, MO: Mosby.

APPENDIX A

Research Articles

The nine articles contained in this appendix are referred to and discussed in various chapters throughout the text. While articles may be mentioned in several chapters, they normally correspond to topics specific to one or two chapters.

The following table will help link the articles to the chapters in which they are discussed:

ARTICLE	CORRESPONDING CHAPTER(S)
A.1. Sleep, Hunger, Satiety, Food Cravings, and Caloric Intake in Adolescents	1. Evidence-Based Nursing: Using Research in Practice 2. The Research Process: Components and Language of Research Reports
A.2. The Relationships Among Self-Esteem, Stress, Coping, Eating Behavior, and Depressive Mood in Adolescents	1. Evidence-Based Nursing: Using Research in Practice 2. The Research Process: Components and Language of Research Reports
A.3. Effects of a Supervised Exercise Intervention on Recovery From Treatment Regimens in Breast Cancer Survivors	3. Discussions and Conclusions
A.4. Predictors of Life Satisfaction in Stroke Survivors and Spousal Caregivers After Inpatient Rehabilitation	4. Descriptive Results
A.5. The Use of Narratives to Identify Characteristics Leading to a Productive Life Following Acquired Brain Injury	6. Samples
A.6. Transition to Home Care: Quality of Mental Health, Pharmacy, and Medical History Information	8. Data Collection Methods
A.7. Psychological Consequences Associated with Intensive Care Treatment	9. Research Designs: Planning the Study
A.8. Mixed Methods in Intervention Research: Theory to Adaptation	9. Research Designs: Planning the Study
A.9. Aggression Towards Health Care Workers in Spain: A Multi-facility Study to Evaluate the Distribution of Growing Violence Among Professionals, Health Facilities and Departments	10. Background and the Research Problem

Sleep, Hunger, Satiety, Food Cravings, and Caloric Intake in Adolescents

Andrea M. Landis, RN, PhD[1]; Kathy P. Parker, RN, PhD, FAAN[2]; Sandra B. Dunbar, RN, DSN, FAAN[3]

Abstract

Background and Purpose: *Prevalence of adolescent obesity has increased world-wide. Although diet and exercise patterns are major determinants of weight, recent studies with adults and children have shown that total amount of sleep is inversely associated with body mass index (BMI). The purpose of this study was to examine associations among total sleep time (TST), hunger, satiety, food cravings, and caloric intake in a sample of healthy adolescents.*

Design Methods: *Participants were recruited from the community and a local high school. Demographic data such as sleeping habits, pubertal status, food cravings, caloric intake, physical activity, height, and weight were collected between October 2006 and April 2007. Participants also completed a 7-day sleep-hunger-satiety diary. Descriptive and parametric procedures were used for data analyses ($\alpha = .05$).*

Findings: *The sample (N = 85) included 56% females (n = 48), 76% African American (n = 65) adolescents. Mean age was 15.6 ± 1.4 years and mean BMI was 24.3 ± 5.4 kg/m². Mean reported 7-day cumulative nocturnal sleep was 52.9 (±6.0) hours; mean reported cumulative daytime sleep (or napping) was 3.7 (±3.4) hours. Multiple regression analyses showed age, gender, and race were associated with feelings of hunger, satiety, total food cravings, and caloric intake. A greater total food cravings score was associated with increased daytime sleep.*

Conclusions: *These findings indicate an unexpected association between increased daytime sleep and eating behaviors that potentially lead to obesity. Longitudinal studies using objective measures of sleep, appetite regulation, and caloric intake are needed to better understand relationships between appetite and sleep in adolescents from varying racial and gender groups.*

Clinical Relevance: *By carefully considering adolescent sleep (especially daytime sleep), race, and gender, clinicians and school health nurses in the US and other countries are in a unique position to develop novel approaches to prevent and reduce obesity.*

Obesity is a significant problem and is increasing world-wide (Popkin & Gordon-Larsen, 2004). Increases in obesity rates are noted in both developed and developing countries (Kosti & Panagiotakos, 2006). In 2004, 17.4% of U.S. adolescents aged 12–19 years

[1]*Psi-at-Large*, Postdoctoral Fellow, University of Washington School of Nursing, Seattle, WA

[2]Dean of Nursing, University of Rochester School of Nursing, Rochester, NY

[3]*Alpha Epsilon*, Professor, Department of Adult and Elder Health Nursing, Nell Hodgson Woodruff School of Nursing, Emory University, Atlanta, GA

Source: Journal of Nursing Scholarship, 2009, Vol. 41, No. 2, 115–123. Copyright 2009 Sigma Theta Tau International.

were overweight as compared to 5% in 1980 (Ogden et al., 2006). An array of nonmodifiable (e.g., genetic disorder) and modifiable (e.g., diet, physical activity) risk factors for adolescent obesity compounds this problem globally (Centers for Disease Control [CDC], 2007).

Keywords: *sleep, adolescent health, obesity, food cravings.*

One modifiable risk factor that has received little attention is quantity of sleep. Adolescents typically require more sleep than they obtain and are at high risk for the consequences of sleep deprivation (Carskadon, 2002). Recent studies in children and adults have shown that TST is inversely associated with body mass index (BMI), but similar studies are needed in adolescents (Gangwisch, Malaspina, Boden-Albala, & Heymsfield, 2005; Reilly et al., 2005). Sleep-deprivation-related changes are believed to adversely affect selected endocrine system function and metabolic pathways, leading to decreased satiety and energy expenditure, and increased hunger, food cravings, and caloric intake in adults (Spiegel, Tasali, Penev, & Van Cauter, 2004; Taheri, Lin, Austin, Young, & Mignot, 2004).

The adolescent developmental period may be an optimal time to address modifiable risk factors, since obesity in adolescence is a strong predictor of obesity in adulthood (Gordon-Larsen, Adair, Nelson, & Popkin, 2004). Previously tested interventions aimed at adolescent diet, and physical activity patterns have had limited success (Johnson-Taylor & Everhart, 2006), possibly because of failure to appreciate an association between TST and appetite regulation. Thus, the purpose of this study was to examine associations between TST (daytime and nocturnal sleep) and outcomes of hunger, satiety, food cravings, and caloric intake in a sample of otherwise healthy adolescents.

■ CONCEPTUAL FRAMEWORK

The theoretical context for this study was a biobehavioral-ecological framework, derived by the researcher from a synthesis of scientific and theoretical literature (see Fig. A1.1). The framework, which is not fully tested, is focused on demographic, biologic, and behavioral-environmental risk factors for and consequences of decreased TST that could ultimately contribute to increased BMI.

Demographic Factors. That contribute to decreased TST in adolescents include age, race, and gender. Longitudinal sleep studies show that older teenagers sleep less than do younger teens, delay bedtime, and increase weekend TST to compensate for sleep deprivation accumulated during the school week (Carskadon, 2002). Gender and race are associated with differences in reported sleeping and waking patterns in children (Crosby, LeBourgeois, & Harsh, 2005; Giannotti & Cortesi, 2002).

Biological changes in sleep also contribute to decreased TST. Well-controlled studies have indicated that a marked linear decline in slow-wave sleep (NREM sleep stages 3 and 4) occurs as teens age (Carskadon, 2002). In addition, adolescents experience a significant increase in sleep tendency during the daytime (greater sleepiness) at higher maturation levels (Carskadon, 1990). They also experience a shift in circadian rhythm in which they tend to stay up later at night and to sleep later in the morning, delaying the timing or phase of their nocturnal sleep period. This pattern has been reported in numerous studies from a variety of countries (Gau & Soong, 2003; Giannotti & Cortesi, 2002; Wolfson & Carskadon, 1998).

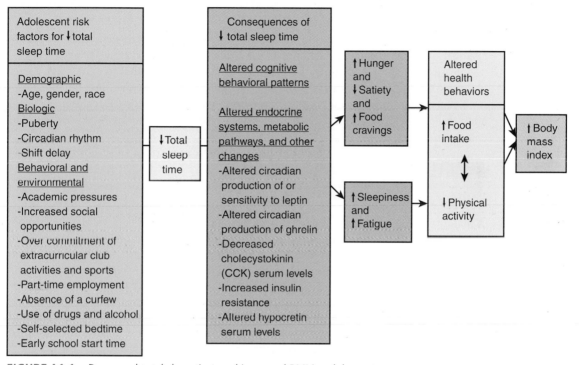

FIGURE A1.1 Decreased total sleep time and increased BMI in adolescents.

TST can be influenced by behavioral and environmental factors, including decreased parental control over curfews and volitional behaviors such as socializing with peers, increased TV viewing and computer use, and evening social activities (Carskadon, 2002). Adolescents also have increased academic obligations, often over-commit to extracurricular activities and part-time employment, and tend to experiment with drugs (including nicotine) and alcohol, which can interfere with TST. Also, adolescents in the US must often rise early in the morning because of school start times, which typically become progressively earlier as students progress from middle to high school (Wolfson & Carskadon, 1998).

Consequences of Decreased TST.   Only 9% of 9th to 12th graders sleep optimal amounts (>9 hours) on school nights (Summary of Findings, 2006). Inadequate amount of sleep can lead to a variety of cognitive changes and alterations in endocrine system function and metabolic pathways. Cognitive consequences of decreased TST include sleepiness (inability to maintain the awake state) (Wolfson & Carskadon, 1998). Fatigue (mental or physical exhaustion) may occur in response to decreased TST, but the relationship of fatigue to daytime sleepiness and TST is unclear (Ancoli-Israel, 2005). Both sleepiness and fatigue may decrease the motivation to maintain a healthy balance between energy consumption and expenditure.

Many hormones (e.g., insulin, hypocretin) may mediate interactions between decreased TST and increased BMI. A decrease in TST has been associated with reduction of the normal nocturnal secretion of leptin (a hunger-suppressing hormone) and reduced suppression of ghrelin (a hunger-stimulating hormone) in young adults, leading to alterations in appetite and energy balance (Spiegel, Leproult, & Van Cauter, 1999; Taheri et al., 2004).

In summary, evidence links decreased TST and increased BMI in adults and young children. Adolescents are known to have reduced TST. Demographic, biological, behavioral, and environmental factors contribute to their risk for sleep loss. Decreased TST and adolescence could, in turn, be associated with altered hunger, satiety, food cravings, and caloric intake.

■ METHODS

Population and Sample

A majority of the sample was recruited from the community and a large public high school (grades 9–12), with a predominantly African American (>90%) racial profile. In order to participate in the study, participants had to be: (a) age 14–18 years old, (b) able to speak and read English, (c) enrolled full-time in school, and (d) reachable by telephone. Exclusion criteria included: (a) a history of chronic or underlying conditions associated with sleep disturbances, (b) routinely taking medications that may adversely affect sleep, and (c) a BMI < 5th percentile. Because of limited numbers of prospective Asian and Hispanic participants, only African American and Caucasian students were included in the study. The final sample consisted of 85 healthy adolescents.

Measures

Participant Screening Form, School Sleep Habits Survey, and Pubertal Status. The participant screening form included demographic data such as age, gender, race, and exclusion criteria. Descriptive data on certain sleeping and waking behaviors (such as part-time employment) during the previous 2 weeks were assessed using a previously validated School Sleep Habits Survey (Wolfson & Carskadon, 1998). Pubertal status was assessed using the Self-Rating Scale for Pubertal Development (Carskadon & Acebo, 1993), on which participants report growth in height and body hair, skin changes, and facial-hair growth (boys only) and breast development and menarche (girls only). For each item, scores range from 1 (prepubertal) to 4 (full maturation). Coefficient alphas for the pubertal scale were .67 (boys) and .58 (girls).

Body Mass Index. BMI (kg/m^2) was calculated from measures of height and weight. BMI is accepted as a reliable and valid index of relative adiposity in adolescents (Mei et al., 2002). Height was measured using a portable stadiometer (Seca Portable Stadiometer Model 214) and weight with a calibrated scale (Tanita Electronic Scale BWB-800S). BMI was transformed into age- and sex-specific percentiles and classifications (normal, at risk for overweight, overweight) as defined per Centers for Disease Control and Prevention guidelines (CDC, 2008).

Caloric Intake and Energy Expenditure (From Physical and Sedentary Activity). Caloric intake and energy expenditure were measured using standardized-format interviews. For caloric intake, the researcher used standardized probe questions to elicit specific details of all foods, including cooking methods and brand names, and beverages consumed in the previous 24 hours. Empty containers (e.g., 20 oz. plastic soda bottle), a set of measuring cups, household items, and unused cafeteria dishes were used to quantify portion sizes. The list of food and beverages was entered into Nutritionist Pro™ (Axxya Systems LLC; Stafford, TX), a nutrition-analysis software program to calculate total energy consumption (kilocalories [kcal]). A previous study comparing the 24-hour diet recall with the Block Kids Questionnaire of adolescents aged 12–17 years resulted in a modest correlation for caloric intake ($r = 0.58$; Cullen, Watson, & Zakeri, 2008). For energy expenditure (i.e., kcal expended), physical and sedentary activity were assessed using the interviewer-administered Physical Activity Checklist Interview (PACI; Sallis et al., 1996), then the metabolic equivalent (MET) value and duration (hours) of each activity were multiplied by body weight in kilograms. The PACI allows measuring a student's participation in various physical and selected sedentary activities (television viewing, computer use, and playing video games) during one 24-hour period. All activities were summed to determine the total estimated minutes spent doing physical activity and the physical activity MET scores. Previous reports on the PACI indicating self reported and interviewer-administered activity recall found intraclass correlations ranging from .64 to .79 (Sallis et al., 1996).

Food Cravings. Food cravings of a participant were measured using the Food Craving Inventory (FCI-II; White, Whisenhunt, Williamson, Greenway, & Netemeyer, 2002). The FCI-II is a 28-item self-report measure of specific food cravings during the past month, scored on a Likert scale (1 = *never* to 5 = *always*, almost every day). It has four subscales: sweets, carbohydrates starches, high-fat foods, and fast-food fats (e.g., pizza). The responses were averaged to obtain a "Total Food Cravings Score." Reported internal consistency for the four subscales ranges from .76 to .93 (White et al., 2002), and for this sample, coefficient alphas ranged from .68 to .83.

Seven-Day Sleep, Hunger, and Satiety Diary. Participants were asked to complete a sleep diary beginning on a Monday for 7 consecutive nights. They recorded their bedtime and awake time each day, and the number and duration of naps. "Cumulative nocturnal sleep" was the sum of the number of hours recorded between bedtime and wake-up time for all 7 nights. "Cumulative daytime sleep" (or naps) was the sum of the number of hours of sleep recorded from awake time to bedtime for all 7 days. "Cumulative nocturnal–daytime sleep" was the sum of nocturnal and daytime sleep. Sleep diaries have shown satisfactory validity ($r = 0.97$) in comparison to objective measures (actigraphy) in the adolescent population (Gaina, Sekine, Chen, Hamanishi, & Kagamimori, 2004).

Hunger and satiety were also measured based on sleep diary methodology using a 7-day diary. Participants responded to the following questions each day: "How hungry were you when you woke up?" "How hungry were you after school (or mid-day)?" and "How hungry do you feel right now, before bed?" Responses were rated on an 11-point horizontal scale with 0 = *not hungry at all* to *extremely hungry*. Higher scores represent greater perceived hunger. Cumulative hunger scores for waking up, after school (mid-day), and before bed were calculated as the sum of the hunger scores for all 7 days. Participants also responded to questions about how full they felt 30 minutes after breakfast, lunch, and dinner on an 11-point scale with 0 = *not full at all* to 10 = *extremely full*. Higher scores indicate greater perceived satiety or fullness. If a participant skipped a meal, "Did not eat" was noted. Cumulative satiety scores for breakfast, lunch, and dinner were calculated as the sum of the satiety scores for all 7 days.

Procedures

The study was conducted from October 2006 to April 2007, excluding school breaks, standardized testing periods, and the week following the transition to daylight savings time. The Institutional Review Board for Protection of Human Subjects at Emory University and the county school district approved the study. Potential high school participants were recruited at the beginning of class; the researcher gave a short presentation describing the study. Forms were distributed to assess student interest, obtain contact information, and request permission to call parents-guardians. For all prospective participants, parents-guardians were contacted to request a meeting at their home or a designated school office with their child. Those volunteering to participate gave written informed consent and assent. Immediately after obtaining consent, interviews on physical activity and diet were conducted, surveys administered, height and weight measured, and a 7-day sleep-hunger-satiety diary initiated. Participants were given verbal and written instructions on how to complete and return the diary and received phone or e-mail prompts during the week reminding them to complete the diary.

Data Analysis

All analyses were performed using SPSS software version 15.0. A mean cumulative bedtime, wake-up time, or hunger score was entered for any missing data in the participant's sleep diary ($<1.0\%$ missing data for each variable). Participants who reported skipping a specific meal on the satiety diary were excluded from regression analyses predicting satiety for that specific meal. We used descriptive statistics to summarize sample demographic and clinical features. The variables kilocalories and hunger before bed were transformed to correct for moderate skewness of the data. Cumulative daytime sleep was recoded into a categorical variable with three levels (no daytime sleep, between 0–2.9 hours, >2.9 hours per week; the latter two categories were based on a median split), yielding groups of approximately equal sample size. This variable was transformed into two dummy variables for inclusion in the regression analysis. Separate backward multiple linear regression analyses were performed to determine which independent variables from the conceptual framework (TST [daytime and nocturnal sleep], age, gender, race, puberty category, energy expenditure [from physical and sedentary activity]) explained the greatest amount of variance in each dependent variable (satiety, hunger, food cravings, and caloric intake) separately. Effect sizes for the multiple regressions were measured using Cohen's f^2. Effect sizes of .02, .15, and .35 are considered small, medium, and large, respectively (Cohen, 1988). A significance level of $\alpha = .05$ was selected for all analyses.

■ RESULTS

Sample demographic features are shown in Table A1.1. Over 40% of the sample was overweight (>85th percentile). The sample spent more time participating in sedentary than in physical activities. Sleep, hunger, satiety, food cravings, caloric intake, and energy expenditure variables are shown in Tables A1.2 and A1.3. The mean reported school night

Table A1.1

Demographic, Biological, and Behavioral/Environmental Features of the Sample ($N = 85$)

VARIABLE	MEAN (SD)	MINIMUM	MAXIMUM
Demographic variables			
Age (years)	15.6 (1.4)	14.0	18.0
Females (n/%)	48/56.5%		
African American (n/%)	65/76.5%		
BMI (kg/m²)	24.3 (5.4)	16.6	43.4
Behavioral-environmental variables			
Total minutes physical activity (24-hr period)	128.3 (85.4)		
Total minutes sedentary activity (24-hr period)	197.2 (137.4)		
School-night bedtime (SD in minutes)	11:40 pm (61)		
School-day wake time (SD in minutes)	6:30 am (32)		
Weekend bedtime (SD in minutes)	11:55 pm (77)		
Weekend wake time (SD in minutes)	9:02 am (98)		
Part-time job (n/%)	12/14.1%		
Extra-curricular activities (n/%)	33/38.8%		
Sports (n/%)	40/47.1%		
Tobacco use—once or twice per day (n/%)	1/1.2%		
Illicit drug use—once or twice per day (n/%)	3/3.5%		
Alcohol use—once or twice per day (n/%)	3/3.5%		

Table A1.2

Nocturnal, Daytime, Nocturnal-Daytime Sleep Variables of the Sample ($N = 85$)

VARIABLE	MEAN (SD)
Nocturnal sleep (hours)	
Cumulative nocturnal sleep	52.9 (6.0)
Mean school-night nocturnal sleep	7.37 (.9)
Mean weekend nocturnal sleep	8.04 (1.3)
Daytime sleep (hours)	
Cumulative daytime sleep	3.7 (3.4)
Mean school daytime sleep	1.23 (.8)
Mean weekend daytime sleep	1.73 (1.4)
Daytime sleep categories (%)	
No daytime sleep	38.8%
Between 0–2.9 hours	29.4%
>2.9 hours	31.8%
Nocturnal-daytime sleep (hours)	
Cumulative nocturnal-daytime sleep	55.1 (6.4)

Note. Cumulative Nocturnal, Daytime, and Nocturnal-Daytime Sleep are the sum of the number of reported hours of sleep for all 7 days. Mean School Night and Weekend Nocturnal Sleep and Mean School and Weekend Daytime Sleep are the number of reported hours of sleep per day. Cumulative daytime sleep was recoded into a categorical variable with three levels (no daytime sleep, between 0–2.9 hours, and >2.9 hours per week).

Table A1.3

Hunger, Satiety, Food Cravings, Caloric Intake, and Energy Expenditure of the Sample ($N = 85$)

VARIABLE	MEAN (SD)	MINIMUM	MAXIMUM
Hunger			
Upon awakening	27.9 (15.2)	0.0	62.0
After school mid-day	39.1 (12.7)	6.3	65.0
Before bed	18.7 (13.0)	0.0	52.0
Satiety			
After breakfast[a]	39.4 (13.2)	12.8	70.0
After lunch[b]	43.9 (10.9)	14.0	69.0
After dinner[c]	50.4 (12.9)	19.8	70.0
Food cravings			
High fats	2.1 (.7)	1.0	4.1
Sweets	2.9 (.9)	1.0	4.6
Carbohydrates-starches	2.3 (.7)	1.0	3.8
Fast foods	2.9 (1.0)	1.0	4.5
Total score	2.5 (.7)	1.1	3.9
Caloric intake	2194.2 (820.7)	642.0	4398.1
Energy expenditure	916.6 (451.3)	234.0	2298.3

Note. Upon Awakening, After School/Mid-day, Before Bed, After Breakfast, After Lunch, and After Dinner are the sum of the hunger and satiety scores for all 7 days. Possible scores range from 0 to 77. Higher scale values indicate greater perceived hunger or satiety. Food-craving scores range from 1 to 5, with 1 indicating *Never* and 5 indicating *Always-Almost every day.* Caloric Intake and Energy Expenditure are in kilocalories per 24 hours. [a]$N = 48$ because of excluding those who did not eat breakfast. [b]$N = 75$ because of excluding those who did not eat lunch. [c]$N = 83$ because of excluding those who did not eat dinner.

nocturnal sleep for the sample was approximately 7.5 hours; this is much less than the optimal 9 hours of sleep per school night (Summary of Findings, 2006). Cumulative nocturnal sleep did not significantly differ between race and gender. Mean reported school night and weekend nocturnal sleep were statistically different ($t = -7.73$, $df = 84$, $p < .01$) and indicates participants accumulated a "sleep debt" over the week. Independent t-tests showed that mean nocturnal sleep for those who napped was significantly lower than for those who did not nap ($t = 2.03$, $df = 83$, $p = .05$).

Results of the multiple regression analyses are shown in Table A1.4. Race was an independent predictor for the hunger and satiety regression models indicating that African American adolescents had decreased hunger upon awakening and decreased feelings of satiety (or fullness) after breakfast and lunch compared to Caucasian adolescents. Race and daytime sleep were the only significant predictors in the regression model indicating that perceived total food cravings were greater in younger African American adolescents than in other adolescents in the sample and were associated with increased daytime sleep. Age and gender were the only significant predictors in the model indicating that caloric intake was higher in younger male adolescents. There were no significant predictive models for satiety after

Table A1.4

Results of Multiple Regressions to Predict Hunger, Satiety, Food Cravings, and Caloric Intake ($N = 85$)

VARIABLE	B	SE	t	p-VALUE	MODEL	f^2
Variables to predict hunger upon awakening	-7.59	3.81	—	.05*	$R^2 = .05$, $F_{(1,83)} = 3.97$, $p = .05$	.05[a]
Race			1.99			
Variables to predict satiety after breakfast	—	3.69	—	.01*	$R^2 = .16$, $F_{(1,46)}$[c] $= 8.78$, $p < .01$	.19[b]
Race	10.94	2.72	2.96			
Variables to predict satiety after lunch	-8.26		—	<.01*	$R^2 = .11$, $F_{(1,73)}$[d] $= 9.24$, $p < .01$	.13[a]
Race			3.04			
Variables to predict total food cravings	-0.09	0.05	—	.06	$R^2 = .13$, $F_{(3,81)} = 5.89$, $p < .01$	.22[b]
Age	0.43	0.16	1.89	.01*		
Race	0.31	0.15	2.60	.04*		
Daytime sleep (>2.9 hours)			2.10			
Variables to predict caloric intake	-1.39	0.64	—	.03*	$R^2 = .14$, $F_{(3,81)} = 4.31$, $p = .007$	.16[b]
Age	-5.76	1.92	2.18	<.01*		
Gender	3.97	2.04	3.00	.06		
Daytime sleep (>2.9 hours)			1.94			

Note. Race (Caucasian = 0, African American = 1). Gender (Male = 0, Female = 1). B = unstandardized beta coefficient. f^2 = Cohen's f^2, [a]small effect size, [b]medium effect size. [c]N = 48 because of excluding those who did not eat breakfast. [d]N = 75 because of excluding those who did not eat lunch.

*p = .05.

dinner or hunger after school and before bed. The models resulted in "medium" effect sizes for satiety after breakfast, total food cravings, and caloric intake.

■ DISCUSSION

Our findings are similar to those of other studies of sleep in adolescents in terms of reported decreased TST, late school-night bedtimes, late rising times on weekends, and early school times (Carskadon, 1990; Wolfson & Carskadon, 1998). One outcome of this lifestyle for certain adolescents is insufficient nighttime sleep, possibly manifesting as compensatory napping (or daytime sleep). In this study, increased daytime sleep was associated with decreased nocturnal sleep; it significantly predicted total food cravings. The findings support an unexpected association between daytime sleep and eating behaviors that potentially lead to obesity. Nonetheless, many adolescents have too little sleep at the incorrect circadian phase (Carskadon, Acebo, & Jenni, 2004). This pattern is associated with increased risk for daytime sleep and may disrupt the diurnal rhythm of appetite-regulating hormones. Future studies including appetite markers such as serum leptin may help explain these unexpected results.

Our understanding of the role of sleep in the regulation of appetite is relatively limited, especially in adolescents. Leptin, a hormone released by the adipocytes in adipose tissue, provides information about energy status to hypothalamic regulatory centers (Ahima, Saper, Flier, & Elmquist, 2000). Leptin levels are reciprocally related to changes in hunger and typically fluctuate in a diurnal pattern with lower levels during the day in relation to periods of increased hunger and higher levels during the night in relation to normally low hunger levels (Chin-Chance, Polonsky, & Schoeller, 2000). In contrast to the anorexigenic effects of leptin, ghrelin is a peptide produced predominantly in the stomach that stimulates appetite (van der Lely, Tschop, Heiman, & Ghigo, 2004). Ghrelin concentrations also follow a diurnal rhythm with higher levels during the day in association with increased hunger and lower levels during the night when hunger is normally low (Muccioli et al., 2002). Thus, leptin and ghrelin have a reciprocal relationship, and sleep loss seems to alter these hormones in a way that could promote food intake and the development of obesity (Mullington et al., 2003).

A leading study in adults exhibited decreased levels of leptin, increased levels of ghrelin, and an increase in reported hunger and appetite for calorie-dense foods with high carbohydrate content after a 2-night sleep restriction (Spiegel et al., 2004). In this study, further analysis of the total food cravings score subscales showed similar findings. Cravings for carbohydrate-starch and high fat foods were greater in those with increased daytime sleep. Thus, the amount of daytime sleep observed in this study may alter normal endocrine and metabolic processes, thus affecting certain food cravings.

Results of this study suggest possible racial and gender differences in hunger, satiety, caloric intake, and food cravings, which may predispose a certain race or gender to risk of obesity. Although racial and gender differences in sleep among adolescents are not well described in the literature, such differences in appetite regulation are striking. A recent study of African American youth aged 7- to 12-years-old indicated lower ghrelin suppression after eating a meal when compared to Caucasian youth (Bacha & Arslanian, 2006). Alteration in meal-induced ghrelin suppression could account for the hunger and satiety differences between African American and Caucasian adolescents. In addition, an earlier study indicated significantly higher serum leptin levels in female participants compared to male participants during pubertal development (Blum et al., 1997). In addition, the most recent U.S. National Health and Nutritional Examination Survey (NHANES) data (2003–2004) indicates continuing significant differences in obesity prevalence by racial group for both sexes. For adolescents aged 12–19 years, the prevalence rate of overweight was highest among non Hispanic Caucasian male participants (19.1%) and non-Hispanic African American female participants (25.4% females; Ogden, et al., 2006). Thus, race and gender might be considered significant predictors of appetite regulation and BMI indicating direction for further research.

Several intrinsic limitations to this study are noted. Sleep data were reported subjectively. Self-report sleep diaries are subject to recall biases and missing data, as well as imprecision with respect to reporting bed and wake times. Likewise, use of a single 24-hour diet recall may not have sufficiently described an individual's usual caloric intake; multiple pass 24-hour recalls on the same individual over several days are required to increase reliability (Gibson, 2005). Similarly, in this study, we did not measure socioeconomic and physiological variables in association with appetite regulation and BMI. In addition, this study is a cross-sectional analysis using a non-random sampling procedure that means only associations are presented and generalizability of the results is limited. Nonetheless, the study indicates preliminary support for future studies to understand the causal pathway of how TST of adolescents may foster weight gain and possibly obesity by affecting appetite regulation, food cravings, and caloric intake.

■ CONCLUSIONS

These data show an unexpected association between daytime sleep (which may reflect an increased need for nocturnal sleep) and behaviors, such as greater food cravings that can potentially lead to obesity. They also indicate that targeted attention could be given to age, racial, and gender differences that may influence hunger, satiety, food cravings, and caloric intake and put adolescents from different racial and gender groups at greater risk for obesity. The regression models indicate that daytime sleep was a significant predictor of total food cravings after controlling for age, gender, race, puberty status, and energy expenditure. Future studies that incorporate longitudinal design, random selection sampling to assure external validity, and objective measures of sleep, appetite regulation, and caloric intake are required to better understand how daytime sleep may affect appetite regulation.

The conceptual framework used in this study indicated demographic, biologic, and behavioral–environmental risk factors for and consequences of decreased TST in the sample; it also showed which variables (TST, age, gender, race, puberty category, energy expenditure) explained the greatest amount of variance in satiety, hunger, food cravings, and caloric intake. While the conceptual model was not fully tested, support for its continued study is warranted to determine if changes in satiety, hunger, food cravings, and caloric intake can ultimately contribute to an increase in BMI. The rising epidemic worldwide in overweight and obese adolescents requires urgent attention. Clinicians and school health nurses in the US and other countries are in a unique position to develop novel approaches to preventing and reducing obesity.

■ ACKNOWLEDGMENTS

This study was supported by Grant F31NR009897 from the National Institute of Nursing Research and Sigma Theta Tau Internationl, Alpha Epsilon Chapter, Small Research Grant Award. The authors acknowledge the contribution and adolescent sleep expertise of Mary Carskadon, PhD.

■ CLINICAL RESOURCES

Web site for International Obesity Taskforce: http://www.iotf.org

Web site about teens and sleep from National Sleep Foundation: http://www.sleepfoundation.org

Teen obesity Web site from CDC: http://www.cdc.gov/nccdphp/dnpa/obesity/childhood/index.htm

References

Ahima, R., Saper, C., Flier, J., & Elmquist, J. (2000). Leptin regulation of neuroendocrine systems. *Frontiers in Neuroendocrinology, 21*, 263–307.

Ancoli-Israel, S. (2005). Sleep and fatigue in cancer patients. In M. Kryger, T. Roth, & W. C. Dement (Eds.), *Principles and practice of sleep medicine* (4th ed., pp. 1218–1224). Philadelphia, PA: Elsevier Saunders.

Bacha, F., & Arslanian, S. (2006). Ghrelin and peptide YY in youth: Are there race-related differences? *Journal of Clinical Endocrinology & Metabolism, 91*, 3117–3122.

Blum, W. F., Englaro, P., Hanitsch, S., Juul, A., Hertel, N., Muller, J., et al. (1997). Plasma leptin levels in healthy children and adolescents: Dependence on body mass index, body fat mass, gender, pubertal stage, and testosterone. *Journal of Clinical Endocrinology and Metabolism, 82*, 2904–2910.

Carskadon, M. A. (1990). Patterns of sleep and sleepiness in adolescents. *Pediatrician, 17*, 5–12.

Carskadon, M. A. (2002). Factors influencing sleep patterns of adolescents. In M. Carskadon (Ed.), *Adolescent sleep patterns: Biological, social, and psychological influences* (pp. 4–26). Cambridge, UK: Cambridge University Press.

Carskadon, M. A., & Acebo, C. (1993). A self-administered rating scale for pubertal development. *Journal of Adolescent Health, 14*, 190–195.

Carskadon, M. A., Acebo, C., & Jenni, O. G. (2004). Regulation of adolescent sleep: Implications of behavior. *Annals of the New York Academy of Sciences, 1021*, 276–291.

Centers for Disease Control. (2007). *Contributing factors.* Retrieved January 15, 2008, from http://cdc.gov/nccdphp/dnpa/obesity/contributing factors.htm

Centers for Disease Control. (2008). *About BMI for children and teens.* Retrieved September 5, 2008, from http://www.cdc.gov/nccdphp/dnpa/healthyweight/assessing/bmi/childrens BMI/aboutchildrensBMI.htm

Chin-Chance, C., Polonsky, K., & Schoeller, D. (2000). Twenty-four-hour leptin levels respond to cumulative short-term energy imbalance and predict subsequent intake. *Journal of Clinical Endocrinology & Metabolism, 85*, 2685–2691.

Cohen, J. (1988). *Statistical power analysis for the behavioral sciences* (2nd ed.). Hillsdale, NJ: Erlbaum.

Crosby, B., LeBourgeois, M., & Harsh, J. (2005). Racial differences in reported napping and nocturnal sleep in 2- to 8-year-old children. *Pediatrics, 115*, 225–232.

Cullen, K., Watson, K., & Zakeri, I. (2008). Relative reliability and validity of the block kids questionnaire among youth aged 10 to 17 years. *Journal of the American Dietetic Association, 108*, 862–866.

Gaina, A., Sekine, M., Chen, X., Hamanishi, S., & Kagamimori, S. (2004). Validity of child sleep diary questionnaire among junior high school children. *Journal of Epidemiology, 14*, 1–4.

Gangwisch, J., Malaspina, D., Boden-Albala, B., & Heymsfield, S. (2005). Inadequate sleep as a risk factor for obesity: Analyses of NHANES 1. *Sleep, 28*, 1289–1296.

Gau, S., & Soong, W. (2003). The transition of sleep-wake patterns in early adolescence. *Sleep, 26*, 449–454.

Giannotti, F., & Cortesi, F. (2002). Sleep patterns and daytime functioning in adolescence: An epidemiological survey of an Italian high school student sample. In M. Carskadon (Ed.), *Adolescent sleep patterns: Biological, social, and psychological influences* (pp. 132–147). Cambridge, UK: Cambridge University Press.

Gibson, R. S. (2005). *Measuring food consumption of individuals: Principles of nutritional assessment* (2nd ed.). New York, NY: Oxford University Press.

Gordon-Larsen, P., Adair, L., Nelson, M., & Popkin, B. (2004). Five-year obesity incidence in the transition period between adolescence and adulthood: The National Longitudinal Study of Adolescent Health. *American Journal of Clinical Nutrition, 80*, 569–575.

Johnson-Taylor, W., & Everhart, J. (2006). Modifiable environmental and behavioral determinants of overweight among children and adolescents: Report of a workshop. *Obesity, 14*, 929–966.

Kosti, R., & Panagiotakos, D. (2006). The epidemic of obesity in children and adolescents in the world. *Central European Journal of Public Health, 14*, 151–159.

Mei, Z., Grummer-Strawn, L., Pietrobelli, A., Goulding, A., Goran, M., & Dietz, W. (2002). Validity of body mass index compared with other body-composition screening indexes for the assessment of body fatness in children and adolescents. *American Journal of Clinical Nutrition, 75*, 978–985.

Muccioli, G., Tschop, M., Papotti, M., Deghenghi, R., Heiman, M., & Ghigo, E. (2002). Neuroendocrine and peripheral activities of ghrelin: Implications in metabolism and obesity. *European Journal of Pharmacology, 440*, 235–254.

Mullington, J., Chan, J., Van Dongen, H., Samaras, J., Price, N., Meier-Ewert, H., et al. (2003). Sleep loss reduces diurnal rhythm amplitude of leptin in healthy men. *Journal of Neuroendocrinology, 15*, 851–854.

National Sleep Foundation. (2006). 2006 sleep in America poll: Summary of findings. Washington, DC: National Sleep Foundation.

Ogden, C., Carroll, M., Curtin, L., McDowell, M., Tabak, C., & Flegal, K. (2006). Prevalence of overweight and obesity in the United States, 1999–2004. *JAMA, 295*, 1549–1555.

Popkin, B., & Gordon-Larsen, P. (2004). The nutrition transition: Worldwide obesity dynamics and their determinants. *International Journal of Obesity & Related Metabolic Disorders, 28*(Suppl. 3), S2–S9.

Reilly, J., Armstrong, J., Dorosty, A., Emmett, P., Ness, A., Rogers, I., et al. (2005). Early life risk factors for obesity in childhood: Cohort study. *British Medical Journal, 330*, 1–7.

Sallis, J. F., Strikmiller, P., Harsha, D., Feldman, H., Ehlinger, S., Stone, E., et al. (1996). Validation of interviewer- and self-administered physical activity checklists for fifth grade students. *Medicine & Science in Sports & Exercise, 28*, 840–851.

Spiegel, K., Leproult, B. S., & Van Cauter, E. (1999). Impact of sleep debt on metabolic and endocrine function. *The Lancet, 354*, 1435–1439.

Spiegel, K., Tasali, E., Penev, P., & Van Cauter, E. (2004). Sleep curtailment in healthy young men is associated with decreased leptin levels, elevated ghrelin levels, and increased hunger and appetite. *Annals of Internal Medicine, 141*, 846–850.

Taheri, S., Lin, L., Austin, D., Young, T., & Mignot, E. (2004). Short sleep duration is associated with reduced leptin, elevated ghrelin, and increased body mass index. *PLoS Medicine, 1*, 210–217.

van der Lely, A., Tschop, M., Heiman, M., & Ghigo, E. (2004). Biological, physiological, pathophysiological, and pharmacological aspects of ghrelin. *Endocrine Reviews, 25*, 426–457.

White, M., Whisenhunt, B., Williamson, D., Greenway, F., & Netemeyer, R. (2002). Development and validation of the food craving inventory. *Obesity Research, 10*, 107–114.

Wolfson, A., & Carskadon, M. (1998). Sleep schedules and daytime functioning in adolescents. *Child Development, 69*, 875–887.

The Relationships Among Self-Esteem, Stress, Coping, Eating Behavior, and Depressive Mood in Adolescents

Pamela Martyn-Nemeth,[1][*] Sue Penckofer,[2][**] Meg Gulanick,[2][**] Barbara Velsor-Friedrich,[2][**] Fred B. Bryant[3][**]

Abstract: *The prevalence of adolescent overweight is significant, almost 25% in some minorities, and often is associated with depressive symptoms. Psychological and psychosocial factors as well as poor coping skills have been correlated with unhealthy eating and obesity. The purpose of this study was to examine relationships among self-esteem, stress, social support, and coping; and to test a model of their effects on eating behavior and depressive mood in a sample of 102 high school students (87% minority). Results indicate that (a) stress and low self-esteem were related to avoidant coping and depressive mood, and that (b) low self-esteem and avoidant coping were related to unhealthy eating behavior. Results suggest that teaching adolescents skills to reduce stress, build self-esteem, and use more positive approaches to coping may prevent unhealthy eating and subsequent obesity, and lower risk of depressive symptoms (2008 Wiley Periodicals, Inc. Res Nurs Health 32:96–109, 2009).*

Keywords: *self-esteem, stress, coping, eating behavior, depressive mood, adolescent.*

The prevalence of adolescent overweight has increased from 5% to 17% over the past 30 years in the United States. In some ethnic minorities the prevalence can reach as high as 25% (Centers for Disease Control [CDC], 2007a). There are serious long-term health consequences for adolescents who are overweight. For example, the prevalence of Type 2 diabetes is increasing among children and adolescents and is greater among minority than majority groups, primarily due to excess body weight (Bloomgarden, 2004). In addition, all overweight adolescents are at increased risk for depressive mood and clinical depression (Goodman & Whitaker, 2002; Sjöberg, Nilsson, & Leppert, 2005). Overweight adolescents tend to remain overweight as adults, with an increased risk of diabetes, cardiovascular disease, and cancer (Freedman et al., 2005). The overall estimated economic burden of obesity in the nation for the year 2002 was 93 billion dollars (Finkelstein, Fiebelkorn, & Wang, 2003). These expenses are projected to rise as today's young people reach adulthood.

Unhealthy eating behavior has been proposed as a contributing factor to the etiology of overweight in both adolescents and adults (Budd & Hayman, 2006). In adults, obesity has been linked to stress-induced eating, low levels of social support, and inadequate coping

[1]College of Nursing, University of Illinois, Chicago, IL
[2]School of Nursing, Loyola University Chicago, Chicago, IL
[3]Department of Psychology, Loyola University Chicago, Chicago, IL
[*]Postdoctoral student.
[**]Professor.

Source: Research in Nursing & Health, 2009, Vol. 32, 96–109.

skills (Laitinen, Ek, & Sovio, 2002). In adolescents, low self-esteem, stress, and poor coping have been associated with unhealthy eating attitudes related to eating disorders (Fryer, Waller, & Kroese, 1997). The teen years are associated with changes in self-esteem and stress related to school, family, friends, self, and one's future. Low self-esteem, stress, low levels of social support, and avoidant coping have been related to unhealthy eating behaviors as well as depressive mood in adolescents (Cartwright et al., 2003; Falkner et al., 2001; Sjöberg et al., 2005; Wadsworth & Compas, 2002). Most of these relationships have been explored primarily in females, in European-American populations, and from an eating disorders perspective.

It has been suggested that coping may serve as a mediator between stress and health outcomes, including eating behavior and psychological health (Fryer et al., 1997; Southall & Roberts, 2002). The relationships among self-esteem, stress, social support, coping, eating behavior, and depressive mood have not been examined simultaneously, nor has coping been examined as a mediator of this process. The purpose of this study was to investigate relationships among self-esteem, stress, social support, and coping and to test a model of their effects on unhealthy eating behavior and depressive mood in adolescents.

Low self-esteem has been associated with adolescent overweight and overeating, even after controlling for body mass index (Ackard, Neumark-Sztainer, Story, & Perry, 2003). In addition, ethnic and racial differences have been identified for their relationship with self-esteem and eating behavior. For White and Hispanic girls, low self-esteem has been associated with being overweight to a greater degree than among Black girls (Brown et al., 1998; Strauss, 2000). Thus, there is evidence that unhealthy eating behavior is associated with low self-esteem and that this may vary among ethnic and racial groups.

Stress has been proposed as a factor that leads to increased food consumption in vulnerable adults, including dieters and self-described emotional eaters (Greeno & Wing, 1994). Youth (aged 8–11 years) with high levels of dietary restraint (an index of control over eating), consumed more total calories and snacks when experiencing higher levels of stress (Roemmich, Wright, & Epstein, 2002). Increased stress also has been associated with high fatty food consumption, decreased fruit and vegetable intake, and decreased breakfast consumption among adolescents (Cartwright et al., 2003).

The role of social support in adolescent eating behavior is supported by evidence that it buffers stressful experiences (Yarcheski & Mahon, 1999), by enhancing positive coping strategies (Brissette, Scheier, & Carver, 2002). Social support has been shown to have a direct impact on health behavior (Mahon, Yarcheski, & Yarcheski, 2004), including dietary practices (Kubik, Lytle, & Fulkerson, 2005). Overweight adolescents have lower levels of social support and participate in fewer health promoting behaviors than adolescents with normal body weight (Chen, Wang, & Chang, 2006). The lower levels of social support may be related to the stigmatization of being overweight, which may limit social networks and thus contribute to social isolation (Falkner et al., 2001).

In adolescence, coping might serve as a mediator between stress and health outcomes, including dietary intake and psychological wellbeing (Dinsmore & Stormshak, 2003; Laitinen et al., 2002). Avoidant coping has been correlated with overeating and unhealthy eating attitudes and behavior in adolescents (Fryer et al., 1997). The avoidant strategies most closely linked to unhealthy eating are tension-reducing strategies such as crying, shouting, or taking drugs (Garcia-Grau, Fuste, Miro Saldana, & Bados, 2002). Eating itself has been identified as a maladaptive coping mechanism used to abate stress (Lee-Tarver, 1999; Solomon, 2001). Although several investigators have studied the relationship between coping and eating patterns in adolescents, samples have included mostly White females, with minorities and males underrepresented. In addition, dietary patterns have been explored from an eating disorder perspective, and the focus was not on obesity (Fryer et al., 1997; Garcia-Grau et al., 2002; Lesk, 1996).

Although avoidant coping patterns have been related to unhealthy eating behaviors, approach coping has been associated with health promoting behaviors and fewer risk-taking behaviors such as sexual activity and substance abuse (Steiner, Erickson, Hernandez, & Pavelski, 2002). The relationship between approach coping and healthy behavior has provided support for interventions that use coping skills training in disease management and weight loss programs for adolescents (Grey, Boland, Davidson, Li, & Tamborlane, 2000). In a prospective randomized trial of coping skills training in a school-based weight loss program targeted to pre-diabetic middle school minority students, those receiving a coping skills training intervention demonstrated lower blood glucose and insulin levels and decreased central adiposity compared to students who did not receive the coping skills training (Grey et al., 2004). These researchers suggested that coping may play an important role in health promotion and body weight regulation among ethnic minority school children.

Healthy nutritional status promotes physical, intellectual, and emotional health (Grodner, Long, & DeYoung, 2004), and eating behavior is a significant contributor to nutritional status through its influence on body weight (Grodner et al., 2004). Certain eating behaviors that are associated with a healthy diet and body weight include eating at regular mealtimes, eating breakfast, and eating meals with the family (Taveras et al., 2005; Videon & Manning, 2003). Conversely, skipping meals, snacking, eating at fast food restaurants, and eating while watching television have been associated with increased fat and total calorie consumption, increased body weight, and a lower intake of fruits, vegetables, vitamins, and minerals (Francis, Lee, & Birch, 2003; Stockman, Schenkel, Brown, & Duncan, 2005). In addition, the disparities in body weight between Whites and other ethnic groups are in part due to cultural eating patterns, such as a greater preference for high fat food among Black girls (Crawford, Story, Wang, Ritchie, & Sabry, 2001). The factors related to the regulation of eating behavior and body weight are complex and interrelated, thus needing further study. One of the weaknesses in the conceptualization of eating behavior is that it has either encompassed eating pathology, or has described healthy versus unhealthy eating activities without a synthesized construct of normative eating behavior.

Depressive mood has been related to eating and dietary problems, as well as to low self-esteem, stress, low levels of social support, and avoidant coping skills. Low self-esteem and increased stress are independently associated with depressive mood (Southall & Roberts, 2002), with daily hassles associated with poorer psychological adjustment than to major life events (Seiffge-Krenke & Klesslinger, 2000). Higher levels of social support are related to fewer depressive symptoms (Brissette et al., 2002) and lack of social support has been identified as a correlate of depressive mood among overweight adolescents (Sjöberg et al., 2005). In longitudinal studies, avoidant coping styles have been shown to predate the onset of depressive symptoms, suggesting that depressive mood is an outcome of avoidant coping styles (Seiffge-Krenke, 2000; Seiffge-Krenke & Klesslinger, 2000).

In summary, it is known that low self-esteem is associated with overeating and weight gain in adolescents, and stress-induced eating and inadequate coping skills have been related to overeating and obesity in adults. Avoidant coping has been proposed as a mediator of unhealthy eating behavior and depressive mood (Seiffge-Krenke, 1995; Steiner et al., 2002). However, important questions remain about the relationship of self-esteem, stress, social support, and coping to eating patterns and depressive mood in racially/ethnically diverse male and female adolescents. A better understanding of the interrelationships among these factors would facilitate the development of nursing strategies to promote healthy coping and eating patterns and reduce depressive symptoms in ethnically diverse adolescents.

This study was guided by the theoretical framework developed by Seiffge-Krenke (1995) for adolescent coping, which was derived from Lazarus and Folkman's (1984) conceptualization of adult coping. Adolescent coping processes are thought to differ from those of adults (Compas, Connor-Smith, Saltzman, Thomsen, & Wadsworth, 2001), therefore, a framework specific to adolescents was chosen. Consistent with the conception of Lazarus and Folkman, the individual is said to engage in a cognitive appraisal of the perceived stressor. Cognitive appraisal of the stressor is affected by (a) the nature of the stressor, (b) internal coping resources, and (c) external social resources. Coping entails cognitive or behavioral response(s), which have been grouped as approach or avoidant strategies. Approach strategies entail active problem-solving coping responses to manage or solve the problem; avoidant strategies comprise passive responses to withdraw from or ignore the problem (Seiffge-Krenke, 1995). The Seiffge-Krenke framework differs from Lazarus and Folkman in that social support, through relationships with parents, family, and peers, is viewed as an important external social resource for adolescents. Developmental factors are also considered in the framework, as coping strategies change with maturation and personal experience. Coping strategies increase in early adolescence, reflecting the increase in stressors encountered with puberty, then stabilize during middle adolescence, reflecting advances in cognitive development and social maturity (Seiffge-Krenke, 1995).

The variables for the current study were organized in a directional model as shown in Figure A2.1. Self-esteem, stress, and social support were conceptualized as antecedents to the coping process. Self-esteem is a key internal resource; social support represents an external coping resource. In adolescence, stressors primarily include relationships with family and peers, academic demands, and issues with self and the future (Lewis & Frydenberg, 2002; Seiffge-Krenke, 1995). Coping was conceptualized as a mediator of the effects of self-esteem, stress, and social support on the outcomes of eating behavior and depressive mood. It was hypothesized that adolescents with low self-esteem, increased stress, and decreased social support would use a predominance of avoidant coping strategies. The predominance of avoidant coping strategies would then mediate the negative outcomes of unhealthy eating behavior and depressive mood. The research questions were:

1. Are self-esteem, stress, social support, and coping related to unhealthy eating behavior and depressive mood in adolescents?

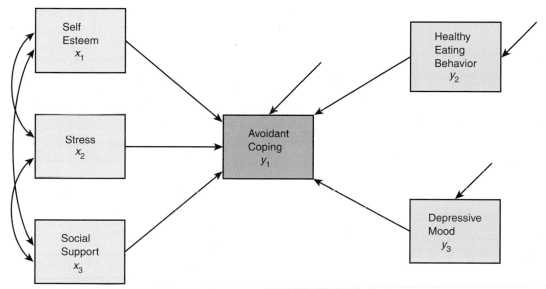

Controlled variables: age, gender, ethnicity, SES

FIGURE A2.1   Study model.

2. Does the use of food as a coping mechanism relate to being overweight?
3. Does coping mediate the relationship of low self-esteem, increased stress, and decreased social support with the outcomes of unhealthy eating behavior and depressive mood?

■ METHODS

Design and Setting

A descriptive, correlational cross-sectional design was used. Two public high schools (School A = 2,068 and School B = 1,563 students) in a suburban metropolitan area of the Midwest were sites for data collection from February through May 2005. The communities in which the students lived were predominantly residential, consisting of families with children. The community crime rates of both communities exceeded the national average (State Crime Statistics, 2002). Approximately one-third of the adults living in the communities had a high school diploma, and the median income was $46,500, which was slightly lower than the national average. The ethnic/racial distributions of the communities were primarily Black (82.7% and 52.9%), Hispanic (10.5% and 10.9%), and White (9.7% and 38.7%), as reported by the U.S. Census Bureau (2000).

Sample

The inclusion criteria were adolescents currently enrolled in high school, who were able to read and write English (in order to complete a 45-minute questionnaire). Both sexes and all racial and ethnic groups were included. To determine the sample size, moderate effect sizes of .2–.3 were estimated using the published literature. The path model with 14 parameters (3 y-variables, 3 x-variable covariates, 5 paths, and 3 residual terms for y-variables; Fig. A2.1) required a sample size of 100 to achieve 80% power to detect a .224 effect size (Hintze, 2001). In addition, other sources report a sample size of at least 100 is needed when conducting path analysis (Thompson, 2000). A convenience sample of 119 high school students from the two sites was recruited through school announcements, flyers, and school staff. Once missing data and outliers were examined, there were 102 usable surveys for this study. The high school students ($N = 102$) who participated were largely minority (65.7% Black, 21.6% Hispanic, 12.7% White) and female (79%), with a mean age of 16.8 years (Table A2.1).

Measured Variables

Self-Esteem.   Self-esteem was measured with the Rosenberg Self-Esteem short-form (Rosenberg, 1965), a self-administered 6-item, 4-point Likert-type instrument (1 = *strongly disagree* to 4 = *strongly agree*) developed to measure global self-esteem in adolescents.

Table A2.1

Health and Demographic Characteristics ($N = 102$)		
CHARACTERISTIC	n	(%)
Sex		
Female	81	79.4
Male	21	20.6
Age		
14	5	4.9
15	10	9.8
16	21	20.6
17	32	31.4
18	34	33.3
Race/ethnicity		
Black/African American	67	65.7
Hispanic/Latino	22	21.6
White	13	12.7
Socioeconomic status		
Low	10	9.8
Low-middle	29	28.4
Middle	35	34.3
Upper-middle	20	19.6
High	8	7.8
Body mass index percentile		
Underweight	2	2.0
Normal weight	48	47.1
Risk for overweight	20	19.6
Overweight	28	27.5
Missing data	4	3.9

The possible scores range from 6 to 24; higher scores indicate higher levels of self-esteem. The instrument is concise and has a 5th grade reading level. Reliability using Cronbach alpha of .78 has been reported in ethnically diverse adolescents (Ackard et al., 2003). Construct validity has been determined through factor analysis (Rosenberg, Schooler, Schoenbach, & Rosenberg, 1995; Shevlin, Bunting, & Lewis, 1995). The Cronbach alpha coefficient was .75 in this study.

Stress. Using the six major adolescent stressors identified in the Coping Across Situations Questionnaire (CASQ; Seiffge-Krenke, 1995; school, parents, friends, romantic interests, self, and future), a 6-item stressor scale assessing level of stress in each of these respective domains (1 = *not at all* to 4 = *very much*), was constructed for the study. This instrument paralleled previously validated stress measures, equivalent in focus and content to these six items studied (Compas, Davis, Forsythe, & Wagner, 1987; Connor-Smith & Compas, 2002), thus providing evidence of construct validity for the measure. In addition, higher stress scores were significantly correlated with a higher frequency of all coping strategies ($r = .30$, $p = .002$) in the major domains that are associated with stress in the literature (Seiffge-Krenke, 1995). Scores ranged from 6 to 24, with higher scores indicating more stress. The Cronbach alpha in our study was .70.

Social Support. Social support was measured with the Medical Outcomes Survey (MOS; Sherbourne & Stewart, 1991). The scale has 19 items using a Likert-type scale (1 = *none of the time*, 5 = *all of the time*). Higher scores are reflective of more social support. The tool measures functional aspects of support. Cronbach alphas ranged from .91 to .97 and validity was ascertained using multitrait scaling and factor analysis (Sherbourne & Stewart). The MOS has demonstrated reliability with minority adolescents (Allen et al., 2004; Bachanas et al., 2002). Two items were eliminated as they did not relate to adolescents. The Cronbach alpha reliability coefficient for the remaining 17 items was .94 for this sample.

Coping. Coping was measured with the Coping Across Situations Questionnaire (CASQ) (Seiffge-Krenke, 1995). This scale is specific to adolescents and measures approach and avoidant coping. Participants select from a list of 20 coping strategies across six problem situations that coincide with major adolescent stressors (school, parents, peers, romantic interests, self, and future). The respondents are able to choose as many of the coping strategies as they typically use when problems occur in each situation. The proportion of avoidant coping use was computed for each adolescent using the total number of coping strategies as the denominator, and the sum of avoidant coping strategies as the numerator. The range for the proportion of avoidant coping was .00 to .55, indicating that some adolescents used no avoidant coping, and others used up to 55% avoidant coping. The proportion of avoidant coping was a better representation than frequency of avoidant coping because the former approach controls for the total numbers of coping strategies each individual employs, whereas the latter approach does not. The use of proportion for coping has previously been reported (Seiffge-Krenke, Weidemann, Fentner, Aegenheister, & Poeblau, 2001). The Cronbach alpha for this instrument has ranged from .73 to .88; construct validity has been established through factor analysis (Seiffge-Krenke, 1995). The Cronbach alpha was .94 for this study. One additional coping strategy, *I try to forget the problem with food*, was added at the end of the CASQ with the author's permission (I. Seiffge-Krenke, personal communication, May 2004). The additional item was used for descriptive analysis and was not calculated into the overall coping scores.

Eating Behavior. Eating behavior was measured using a modification of the Project EAT Survey (2004), a self-report instrument that measures a range of variables related to nutritional health and normative eating patterns among ethnically and socioeconomically diverse adolescents. Stability and internal consistency of the tool has been demonstrated (M. Eisenberg, personal communication, June 2004). For this study, a factor analysis using principal axis factor method was performed on the eating behaviors from the scale. A single dominant factor emerged with eight items representing normative eating behaviors. The presence of healthy behaviors (e.g., regularity of meals, frequency of eating meals with the family) and the absence of unhealthy behaviors (e.g., skipping meals, watching television while eating), were complementary and represented one dominant factor for eating behavior. The items were scored by summing the Likert-style scale ratings (e.g., 1 = *never*, 4 = *everyday*) to obtain a single sum score. The possible range of scores was from 8 to 36 with higher scores reflecting unhealthy (or *less* healthy) eating behavior and lower scores reflecting healthy (or less unhealthy) eating behavior. This score is a composite index of the frequency of unhealthy eating behaviors. The Cronbach alpha was .62.

Depressive Mood. Depressive mood was measured as an affective indicator of psychological well-being using the Kandel Depressive Mood Scale for adolescents (Kandel & Davies, 1982). This 6-item, 3-point Likert-style (1 = *not at all* to 3 = *very often*) mood assessment scale measures depressive mood. Higher scores on the tool are reflective of depressive mood. The instrument has been used with large samples of ethnically, racially, and socioeconomically diverse adolescents. The Cronbach alpha was reported as .79 and construct validity was determined with factor analysis (Kandel & Davies, 1982). The Cronbach alpha for the current sample was .77.

Demographic Data and Health Information. Age (in years), sex, ethnicity/race, and socioeconomic status (SES) were obtained by self-report using the demographic subscale from the Project EAT Survey (Ackard et al., 2003). Ethnicity/race was assessed with the question, "Do you think of yourself as": (a) White, (b) Black or African American, (c) Hispanic or Latino, (d) Asian American, (e) Hawaiian or Pacific Islander, or (f) American Indian or Native American. Participants were allowed to choose more than one group. The parents' highest educational level was used to identify socioeconomic status. This indicator has been shown to correlate well with socioeconomic level (Ackard et al., 2003). Self-reported height and weight were obtained to calculate the body mass index (BMI). For this study, the BMI was converted to a percentile using the CDC Body Mass Index-For-Age Percentile Growth Charts 2000. A BMI < 5th percentile is defined as underweight; 5th percentile to <85th percentile as normal weight; 85th percentile to <95th percentile as at risk for overweight; and ≥95th percentile as overweight (CDC, 2007b). In this sample, 47% were either at risk for overweight or overweight (Table A2.1).

Procedures

Approval was obtained from the University Institutional Review Board for the protection of human subjects. Permission and support for the study were obtained from each respective school. Packets were provided to all interested students along with a verbal description of the study. A written letter to parents describing the study was included in each packet with the investigator's contact information for additional questions. Data were collected after both parents and students agreed to participate, and had signed an informed consent (parents) and informed assent (adolescents). The survey was administered to small groups (up to 10 students) on the school premises, during lunch or after school, by the principal investigator. The survey data were collected anonymously; no identifiers linked the participants to the surveys. Following survey completion, the students received a $10 gift card to a local store for their participation and an information sheet containing contact information for the school health staff and the investigator. All students were made aware that counseling could be received from the school-based health center counseling staff if they felt under stress, were sad or upset, or had any questions regarding their health.

Data Analysis

The data were entered into a database (SPSS 15.0) and screened for missing data and outliers. All cases with missing data and outliers were removed. Screening for normality using histogram plots and the Kilmogorov–Smirnov statistic was completed and revealed that all variables were normally distributed. Differences in the six key variables of self-esteem, stress, social support, coping, eating behavior, and depressive mood were examined by the demographic characteristics of age, gender, ethnicity/race, and socioeconomic status, using multivariate analysis of variance (SPSS). Age was further examined using a t-test of independent means to determine if there were differences for younger adolescents (14–15 years) versus older adolescents (16–18 years). Pearson correlations were computed to determine the relationship of "using food to cope" and body mass index. The proposed model was evaluated with path analytic techniques.

■ RESULTS

No significant differences in demographic characteristics emerged. The range, mean, and standard deviation for the six key variables are reported in Table A2.2.

Table A2.2

Means, Standard Deviations, and Ranges for Self-Esteem, Stress, Social Support, Coping, Eating Behavior, and Depressive Mood

	SELF-ESTEEM	STRESS	SOCIAL SUPPORT	AVOIDANT COPING (%)	EATING BEHAVIOR	DEPRESSIVE MOOD
Mean/*SD*	18.6/3.4	16.0/4.0	77.1/19.9	29.2/9.5	23.1/4.9	20.6/4.9
Possible range	6–24	6–24	0–100	0–100	8–36	10–30
Actual range	11–24	6–24	16.2–100	0–55	13–35	10–30
Normative range	16–18		70–77.7	20–25		17–18

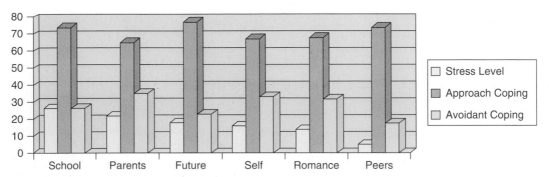

FIGURE A2.2   Percentage of stress level, approach, and avoidant coping used by situation.

Self-Esteem

The level of self-esteem for this sample was moderately high. Overall 68% were satisfied with themselves. Most of the adolescents (94%) felt that they had a number of good qualities, and 93% felt they were able to do things as well as most people.

Stress

Stress levels were normally distributed. Stress levels were greatest for school (26%) and parents (21%). These were also the situations in which the students reported using the greatest number of coping strategies (Fig. A2.2).

Social Support

Social support levels for the group were high. The adolescents reported the greatest support in the area of emotional information, such as having someone to listen to you, help you with problems, and give advice.

Coping

Approach-oriented coping comprised 70.6% of all coping strategies used; avoidant coping comprised 29.4% of coping strategies. The most frequent approach strategies used were discussing the problem with parents or other adults, thinking and trying to find solutions, and talking about the problem with the person concerned. The most frequent avoidant strategies were behaving as if everything is alright, avoiding thinking about the problem, and energy releasing activities. Most approach strategies were used in dealing with problems related to school (74%), most avoidant strategies with problems related to parents (35%), self (33%), and romantic interests (32%; Fig. A2.2).

Responses to the additional item, *I try to forget the problem with food*, added to the end of the CASQ indicated that about one-fourth of adolescents used this strategy to cope with problems related, respectively, to self (26%), romantic interests (26%), parents (25%), and school (22%). Using food to cope was associated with a greater number of avoidant strategies

($r = .47, p = .001$). Adolescents who were above normal weight (>85th percentile BMI) also reported a greater frequency of the use of food to cope (68.8% of risk for overweight teens vs. 37.5% of teens of normal weight; $t(4.39) = -2.08, p = .04$). Using food to cope was positively correlated with a higher BMI percentile ($r = .26, p = .009$).

Eating Behavior

Eating behavior scores ranged from 13 to 35 ($M = 23.1$). Several unhealthy eating behaviors were reported. Breakfast was the least frequently eaten meal, with only 13% of the students reporting eating breakfast every day over the past week. Only 36% reported eating lunch every day, despite having a scheduled lunch period in school. Dinner was the most frequently eaten meal (59%), yet only 16% of students reported eating daily meals with most of the family; and 51% indicated that they were too busy to eat dinner with the family over the past week.

Depressive Mood

The range of scores on the Depressive Mood Scale spanned the full range of the scale, from a level of 10 to 30 (Table A2.2). The mean was higher than that reported in the literature with this instrument ($M = 17-18$; Eisenberg, Olson, Neumark-Sztainer, Story, & Bearinger, 2004; Fulkerson, Sherwood, Perry, Neumark-Sztainer, & Story, 2004). Thirty-five percent scored higher than 23. Scores of 23 or greater have been correlated with the diagnosis of depression (Kandel & Davies, 1982).

Model Testing

A path analysis was used to test a causal model of coping as the mediator between stress, self-esteem, and social support and the outcomes of unhealthy eating behavior and depressive mood. The data were analyzed using Lisrel 8.72 (Jöreskog & Sörbom, 2004). Age, sex, race/ethnicity, and socioeconomic status were controlled by using multivariate regression techniques to partial out the demographic variation in the dependent variables (avoidant coping, unhealthy eating behavior, and depressive mood). The remaining variances in avoidant coping, unhealthy eating behavior, and depressive mood were saved as unstandardized residuals of each of these variables. The unstandardized residuals for avoidant coping, unhealthy eating behavior, and depressive mood were then entered as dependent variables in the path model. One-tailed tests at the .05 level of significance were used. Model fit was evaluated using three absolute and three relative fit indices. The absolute fit indices comprised: the Minimum Fit Function Chi-Square (χ^2), the Goodness of Fit Index (GFI), and the Standardized Root Mean Residual (SRMR). The relative fit indices chosen were the Normed Fit Index (NFI), the Non-Normed Fit Index (NNFI), and the Comparative Fit Index (CFI; Kline, 2005).

The initial model did not demonstrate adequate model fit. To improve the model, two direct effects of self-esteem and stress to depressive mood were added (Fig. A2.3). Self-esteem and stress have been associated with depression in the literature (Seiffge-Krenke, 1995). The model fit was much improved and met recommended target values (Kline, 2005; Table A2.3).

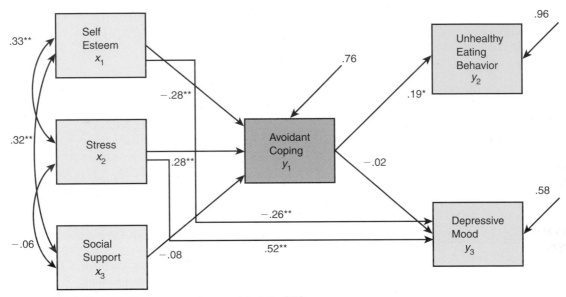

Controlled variables: age, gender, race/ethnicity, SES

* $p < .05$

** $p < .01$

FIGURE A2.3 Revised path model with standardized path coefficients.

In the final model (Fig. A2.3), low self-esteem ($\beta = -.28, p < .002$) and increased stress ($\beta = .28, p < .0014$) were significant predictors of avoidant coping. Low self-esteem and increased stress also had significant direct effects on depressive mood ($\beta = .26, p < .01$ and $\beta = .52, p < .001$, respectively). Avoidant coping had a significant direct effect on unhealthy eating behavior ($\beta = .19, p = .03$), but no significant effect on depressive mood. The methods outlined by Baron and Kenny (1986) were used to test for mediation. The model failed to show that coping was a mediator of eating behavior. The relationship

Table A2.3

Model Fit Indices

FIT INDICES	TARGET VALUE	INITIAL MODEL, $N = 102, df = 7$	REVISED MODEL, $N = 102, df = 5$
x2	$p > .05$	56.0 ($p < .001$)	9.6 ($p = .09$)
GFI	$\geq .90$	.87	.97
SRMR	$\leq .08$	.14	.07
NFI	$\geq .90$	.59	.93
NNFI	$\geq .90$	.14	.88
CFI	$\geq .90$	.60	.96

between avoidant coping and unhealthy eating behavior was not significant when controlling for the effect of self-esteem on eating behavior.

■ DISCUSSION

According to the Seiffge-Krenke framework, internal and external resources interrelate with stress to influence coping styles. Coping styles subsequently have an impact on psychological well-being and health behavior (Seiffge-Krenke, 1995). Results of the current study partially support these propositions. Increased stress was correlated with low self-esteem and avoidant coping, while low self-esteem was associated with avoidant coping, which is consistent with prior research (Byrne & Mazanov, 2001; Wilburn & Smith, 2005). Social support was not significantly related to stress or coping. This finding is inconsistent with findings of earlier studies. One possible explanation is that the social support scale may not have captured the types of social support beneficial to adolescents in managing stress in this sample. Additionally, Meehan, Durlak, and Bryant (1993) found that for adolescents, social support may be more weakly related to coping with negative situations than it is with the promotion of positive experiences. It may be that adolescents associate social support with happiness and entertainment rather than with the management of stress. In the current study, the focus was on negative aspects of the stress and coping relationship, which may have partially accounted for the absence of a relationship with social support.

Adolescents in this study used a greater proportion of avoidant coping strategies than previously reported (Seiffge-Krenke, 1995). There is evidence that avoidant coping can be adaptive in adolescent populations that are facing uncontrollable or chronically high levels of stress (Dempsey, Overstreet, & Moely, 2000; Gonzales, Tein, Sandler, & Friedman, 2001; Grant et al., 2000). Given that the present adolescent sample consisted predominantly of middle to low SES minority adolescents living in neighborhoods having a higher level of crime than surrounding communities, it seems reasonable to assume that most participants were experiencing at least some degree of uncontrollable environmental stress in their life circumstances. This might explain why the present sample had higher levels of depressive mood and avoidant coping than found in past studies.

Twenty-five percent of the adolescents in this sample reported that they used food as a coping mechanism to deal with problems related to parents, self, and romantic interests. This is a concerning number of youth who are eating for non-nutritive purposes. Using food to cope also was associated with increased body weight. Solomon (2001) identified that overweight adult women were more likely to report eating to cope than women of normal weight, but eating to cope has not been well studied in adolescents. The practice of eating to cope may lead to two potential problems. Overeating may lead to unhealthy weight gain (Ackard et al., 2003) and food choices during episodes of stress-induced eating tend to be less healthy (Pelchat, 1997). Foods that are typically craved during episodes of stress-induced eating tend to be sweet or salty snacks and high-fat types of foods (Laitinen et al., 2002). Eating to relieve stress is usually an unplanned activity. Adolescents who plan and eat meals with regularity tend to demonstrate healthier food intake (Dwyer et al., 2001; Rampersaud, Pereira, Girard, Adams, & Metzl, 2005).

Coping did not serve as a mediator between self-esteem and eating behavior as originally proposed. Path analysis revealed a direct effect of self-esteem on coping and an indirect effect of self-esteem on eating behavior through coping. Adolescents with lower self-esteem used more avoidant coping strategies; and those who used more avoidant coping strategies reported less healthy eating behavior. Fryer et al. (1997) used multiple regression analyses to test a causal model of the relationships between stress, coping, self-esteem, and disordered eating in adolescent girls. The sequence of the causal relationships in Fryer's study differed from that in the current study in that stress and poor coping promoted low self-esteem. Self-esteem imperfectly mediated disturbed eating attitudes. Contrary to Fryer et al.'s findings, findings of the current study suggest that low self-esteem promotes avoidant coping. The findings from the two studies may vary because in the current study, normative eating behaviors were measured. Fryer et al., in contrast, focused on disordered eating, which included characteristics such as *feeling that food controls one's life, a preoccupation with thinness, and feeling guilty*. These characteristics suggest an internalization of negative feelings towards the self, which may be an indicator of low self-esteem. Because Fryer et al. used regression analyses to test separate parts of the underlying causal model piecemeal and never tested the model's overall goodness-of-fit, it is unclear how well the underlying casual model actually fit their data, thus poor model fit may well explain the differences noted. Further exploration of the pathways among stress, coping, self-esteem, and eating behavior is needed.

In the current study, stress did not have a direct effect on eating behavior, whereas previous researchers have identified an association between stress and eating patterns (Cartwright et al., 2003). The stress scale used in the current study may have been too general to capture stressors associated with eating. In addition, the stress scale asked respondents to rate their stress levels over the past 3 months. Stressors that lead to stress-induced eating may be more short-term in nature and were not captured using a 3-month period of time.

Low self-esteem and increased stress were directly related to depressive mood, which is consistent with prior research (Southall & Roberts, 2002). Depressive mood emerged as a significant potential health problem in this study. The mean depressive mood score was higher than that reported in prior studies of adolescents (Eisenberg et al., 2004; Fulkerson et al., 2004; Paxton, Valois, Watkins, Huebner, & Drane, 2007). Thirty-five percent of the current sample had levels of depressive mood scores that have been correlated with the diagnosis of depression (Kandel & Davies, 1982). Fifty percent of the current sample was at risk for overweight or overweight by definition, and adiposity has been associated with depression in adolescents (Erermis et al., 2004). This may explain the high levels of depressive mood reported in this sample.

Low self-esteem and avoidant coping were predictors of unhealthy eating behavior in this ethnically/racially diverse sample of male and female adolescents. Although the sample was comprised of primarily Black females, no significant differences in the model variables were noted by demographic variables. This is an important initial finding because previous studies of coping and eating behavior were conducted with White female adolescents. Despite known cultural differences in eating patterns, these psychological factors may influence eating behavior across racial, ethnic, and gender groups and should be considered when designing strategies to promote healthy eating patterns.

Limitations

Because the data were collected at one point in time, using a cross-sectional, correlational design, causation can only be inferred, and stability of variables over time is unknown. The sample size also may have been a limiting factor. Although an adequate sample size was obtained based on the prospective power analysis, observed effect sizes were actually smaller than expected, which reduced the ability to detect mediating effects of avoidant coping. Indeed, mediating effects are often small in magnitude (MacKinnon, Lockwood, Hoffman, West, & Sheets, 2002). In the present study, the six mediating effects of coping through which the antecedent variables of self-esteem, stress, and social support influenced the outcome variables of unhealthy eating behavior and depressive mood ranged in absolute standardized value from .01 to .05 (median absolute value = .015). Assuming a standardized mediation effect size of .015, the present sample of 102 adolescents provided a statistical power of only .33 to detect mediation at two-tailed $p < .05$. This retrospective power analysis reveals that the present study was twice as likely to miss small mediation effects as to detect them.

A large sample of both normal-weight and above-normal-weight adolescents would have been beneficial to more adequately test for associations with body weight. The sample also had a small number of males (21%), even though male recruiters were used in both school sites to help increase the number of male participants. Very little is known about the factors that affect eating behavior in males; therefore, further study of eating behavior in male adolescents is needed. Recruitment strategies and study procedures that will successfully attract males need to be considered in future study designs.

The instruments demonstrated acceptable psychometric properties, although the eating behavior measure had a reliability level that was slightly low. Eating behavior is a diverse and multidimensional construct; thus, scales that measure various dimensions of eating patterns from a normative eating behavior perspective are needed. In addition, a major limitation is that BMI percentile was calculated from self-reported heights and weights; thus, BMI would have been more accurate if actually measured.

Nursing Implications

Low self-esteem and avoidant coping emerged as significant predictors of unhealthy eating behavior and thus may influence the use of emotional eating to cope with stress among adolescents. It may be important for nurses to assess adolescents for this practice and to suggest alternative stress management strategies. Adolescents with low self-esteem and high stress levels also may be at risk for depressive mood. Early identification of these individuals allows for assessment for depression, anxiety, and other signs of psychological maladjustment that may affect eating behavior.

It has been suggested that healthy eating behavior is part of a larger construct of health promoting behavior; and that high self-esteem and approach-oriented coping are associated with healthy behaviors in general. Further investigation is needed into the causal factors of health promoting behaviors in adolescents with the premise that these behaviors do not occur in isolation.

■ ACKNOWLEDGMENTS

This work was supported by the Arthur J. Schmitt Foundation and Sigma Theta Tau, Epsilon Upsilon Chapter.

References

Ackard, D. M., Neumark-Sztainer, D., Story, M., & Perry, C. (2003). Overeating among adolescents: Prevalence and associations with weight-related characteristics and psychological health. *Pediatrics, 111*, 67–74.

Allen, E. C., Manuel, J. C., Legault, C., Naughton, M. J., Pivor, C., & O'Shea, T. M. (2004). Perception of child vulnerability among mothers of former premature infants. *Pediatrics, 113*, 267–273.

Bachanas, P. J., Morris, M. K., Lewis-Gess, J. K., Sarett-Cuasay, E. J., Flores, A. L., Sirl, K. S., et al. (2002). Psychological adjustment, substance use, HIV knowledge, and risky sexual behavior in at-risk minority females: Developmental differences during adolescence. *Journal of Pediatric Psychology, 27*, 373–384.

Baron, R. M., & Kenny, D. A. (1986). The moderator-mediator variable distinction in social psychological research: Conceptual, strategic, and statistical considerations. *Journal of Personality and Social Psychology, 51*, 1173–1182.

Bloomgarden, Z. T. (2004). Type 2 diabetes in the young: The evolving epidemic. *Diabetes Care, 27*, 998–1010.

Brissette, I., Scheier, M. F., & Carver, C. S. (2002). The role of optimism in social network development, coping, and psychological adjustment during a life transition. *Journal of Personality and Social Psychology, 82*, 102–111.

Brown, K. M., McMahon, R. P., Biro, F. M., Crawford, P., Schreiber, G. B., Similo, S. L., et al. (1998). Changes in self-esteem in black and white girls between the ages of 9 and 14 years: The NHLBI Growth and Health Study. *Journal of Adolescent Health, 23*, 7–19.

Budd, G. M., & Hayman, L. L. (2006). Childhood obesity: Determinants, prevention, and treatment. *Journal of Cardiovascular Nursing, 21*, 437–441.

Byrne, D. G., & Mazanov, J. (2001). Self-esteem, stress, and cigarette smoking in adolescents. *Stress and Health, 17*, 105–110.

Cartwright, M., Wardle, J., Steggles, N., Simon, A. E., Croker, H., & Jarvis, M. J. (2003). Stress and dietary practices in adolescents. *Health Psychology, 22*, 362–369.

Centers for Disease Control and Prevention. (2007a). *Overweight prevalence*. Retrieved May 26, 2008, from http://www.cdc.gov/nccdphp/dnpa/obesity/childhood/prevalence.htm

Centers for Disease Control and Prevention. (2007b). *About BMI for children and teens*. Retrieved May 26, 2008, from http://www.cdc.gov/nccdphp/dnpa/bmi/childrens_BMI/about_childrens_BMI.htm

Chen, M. Y., Wang, E. K., & Chang, C. J. (2006). Cross-validation and discriminant validity of an adolescent health promotion scale among overweight and nonoverweight adolescents in Taiwan. *Public Health Nursing, 23*, 555–560.

Compas, B. E., Connor-Smith, J. K., Saltzman, H., Thomsen, A. H., & Wadsworth, M. E. (2001). Coping with stress during childhood and adolescence: Problems, progress, and potential in theory and research. *Psychological Bulletin, 127*, 87–127.

Compas, B. E., Davis, G. E., Forsythe, C. J., & Wagner, B. M. (1987). Assessment of major and daily stressful events during adolescence: The adolescent perceived events scale. *Journal of Consulting and Clinical Psychology, 55*, 534–541.

Connor-Smith, J. K., & Compas, B. E. (2002). Vulnerability to social stress: Coping as a mediator or moderator of sociotropy and symptoms of anxiety and depression. *Cognitive Therapy and Research, 26*, 39–55.

Crawford, P. B., Story, M., Wang, M. C., Ritchie, L. D., & Sabry, Z. I. (2001). Ethnic issues in the epidemiology of childhood obesity. *Pediatric Clinics of North America, 48,* 855–878.

Dempsey, M., Overstreet, S., & Moely, B. (2000). Approach and avoidance coping and PTSD symptoms in inner-city youth. *Current Psychology, 19*, 28–45.

Dinsmore, B. D., & Stormshak, E. A. (2003). Family functioning and eating attitudes and behaviors in at-risk early adolescent girls: The mediating role of intra-personal competencies. *Current Psychology, 22*, 100–116.

Dwyer, J. T., Evans, M., Stone, E. J., Feldman, H. A., Lytle, L., Hoelscher, D., et al. (2001). Adolescents' eating patterns influence their nutrient intakes. *Journal of the American Dietetic Association, 101*, 798–802.

Eisenberg, M. E., Olson, R. E., Neumark-Sztainer, D., Story, M., & Bearinger, L. H. (2004). Correlations between family meals and psychosocial well-being among adolescents. *Archives of Pediatrics and Adolescent Medicine, 158*, 792–796.

Erermis, S., Cetin, N., Tamar, M., Bukusoglu, N., Akdeniz, F., & Goksen, D. (2004). Is obesity a risk factor for psychopathology among adolescents? *Pediatrics International, 46*, 296–301.

Falkner, N. H., Neumark-Sztainer, D., Story, M., Jeffrey, R. W., Beuhring, T., & Resnick, M. D. (2001). Social, educational, and psychological correlates of weight status in adolescents. *Obesity Research, 9*, 32–42.

Finkelstein, E. A., Fiebelkorn, I. C., & Wang, G. (2003). National medical spending attributable to overweight and obesity: How much, and who's paying? *Health Affairs, W3*, 219–226.

Francis, L. A., Lee, Y., & Birch, L. L. (2003). Parental weight status and girls' television viewing, snacking, and body mass indexes. *Obesity Research, 11*, 143–151.

Freedman, D. S., Khan, L. K., Serdula, M. K., Dietz, W. H., Srinivasan, S. R., & Berenson, G. S. (2005). The relation of childhood BMI to adult adiposity: The Bogalusa Heart Study. *Pediatrics, 115*, 22–27.

Fryer, S., Waller, G., & Kroese, B. S. (1997). Stress, coping, and disturbed eating attitudes in teenage girls. *International Journal of Eating Disorders, 22*, 427–436.

Fulkerson, J. A., Sherwood, N. E., Perry, C. L., Neumark-Sztainer, D., & Story, M. (2004). Depressive symptoms and adolescent eating and health behaviors: A multifaceted view in a population-based sample. *Preventive Medicine, 38*, 865–875.

Garcia-Grau, E., Fuste, A., Miro, A., Saldana, C., & Bados, A. (2002). Coping style and disturbed eating attitudes in adolescent girls. *International Journal of Eating Disorders, 32*, 116–120.

Gonzales, N. A., Tein, J. Y., Sandler, I. N., & Friedman, R. J. (2001). On the limits of coping: Interaction between stress and coping for inner-city adolescents. *Journal of Adolescent Research, 16*, 372–395.

Goodman, E., & Whitaker, R. C. (2002). A prospective study of the role of depression in the development and persistence of obesity. *Pediatrics, 110*, 497–504.

Grant, K. E., O'Koon, J. H., Davis, T. H., Roache, N. A., Poindexter, L. M., Armstrong, M. L., et al. (2000). Protective factors affecting low-income urban African American youth exposed to stress. *Journal of Early Adolescence, 20*, 388–417.

Greeno, C. G. & Wing, R. R. (1994). Stress-induced eating. *Psychological Bulletin, 115*, 444–464.

Grey, M., Berry, D., Davidson, M., Galasso, P., Gustafson, E., & Melkus, G. (2004). Preliminary testing of a program to prevent type 2 diabetes among high-risk youth. *Journal of School Health, 74*, 10–15.

Grey, M., Boland, E. A., Davidson, M., Li, J., & Tamborlane, W. V. (2000). Coping skills training for youth with diabetes mellitus has long-lasting effects on metabolic control and quality of life. *The Journal of Pediatrics, 137*, 107–113.

Grodner, M., Long, S., & DeYoung, S. (2004). *Foundations and clinical applications of nutrition.* St. Louis, MO: Mosby.

Hintze, J. (2001). *NCSS and PASS Statistical Software.* Kaysville, UT: NCSS.

Jöreskog, K. G., & Sörbom, D. (2004). *Lisrel 8.72: Structural equation modeling.* Chicago, IL: Scientific Software International.

Kandel, D. B., & Davies, M. (1982). Epidemiology of depressive mood in adolescents: An empirical study. *Archives of General Psychiatry, 39*, 1205–1212.

Kline, R. (2005). *Principles and practice of structural equation modeling.* New York, NY: Guilford Press.

Kubik, M. Y., Lytle, L., & Fulkerson, J. A. (2005). Fruits, vegetables, and football: Findings from focus groups with alternative high school students regarding eating and physical activity. *Journal of Adolescent Health, 36*, 494–500.

Laitinen, J., Ek, E., & Sovio, U. (2002). Stress-related eating and drinking behavior and body mass index and predictors of this behavior. *Preventive Medicine, 34*, 29–39.

Lazarus, R. S., & Folkman, S. (1984). *Stress, appraisal, and coping.* New York, NY: Springer.

Lee-Tarver, A. (1999). Adolescent coping strategies. (Doctoral dissertation, Auburn University, 1999). *Dissertation Abstracts International, 60*, 1462.

Lesk, S. B. (1996). Perceptions of family climate and peer support on female adolescent coping styles and eating behavior (Doctoral dissertation, Hofstra University, 1996). *Dissertation Abstracts International, 57*, 4091.

Lewis, R., & Frydenberg, E. (2002). Concomitants of failure to cope: What we should teach adolescents about coping. *British Journal of Educational Psychology, 72*, 419–431.

MacKinnon, D. P., Lockwood, C. M., Hoffman, J. M., West, S. G., & Sheets, V. (2002). A comparison of methods to test mediation and other intervening variable effects. *Psychological Methods, 7*, 83–104.

Mahon, N. E., Yarcheski, A., & Yarcheski, T. J. (2004). Social support and positive health practices in early adolescents: A test of mediating variables. *Clinical Nursing Research, 13*, 216–236.

Meehan, M. P., Durlak, J. A., & Bryant, F. B. (1993). The relationship of social support to perceived control and subjective mental health in adolescents. *Journal of Community Psychology, 21*, 49–55.

Paxton, R. J., Valois, R. F., Watkins, K. W., Huebner, E. S., & Drane, J. W. (2007). Sociodemographic differences in depressed mood: Results from a nationally representative sample of high school adolescents. *Journal of School Health, 77*, 180–186.

Pelchat, M. L. (1997). Food cravings in young and elderly adults. *Appetite, 28*, 103–113.

Project EAT: Eating Among Teenagers. (2004). Retrieved May 26, 2008, from http://www.epi.umn.edu/research/eat/

Rampersaud, G. C., Pereira, M. A., Girard, B. L., Adams, J., & Metzl, J. D. (2005). Breakfast habits, nutritional status, body weight, and academic performance in children and adolescents. *Journal of the American Dietetic Association, 105*, 743–760.

Roemmich, J. N., Wright, S. M., & Epstein, L. H. (2002). Dietary restraint and stress-induced snacking in youth. *Obesity Research, 10*, 1120–1126.

Rosenberg, M. (1965). *Society and the adolescent self-image.* Princeton, NJ: Princeton University Press.

Rosenberg, M., Schooler, C., Schoenbach, C., & Rosenberg, F. (1995). Global self-esteem and specific self-esteem: Different concepts, different outcomes. *American Sociologic Review, 60*, 141–156.

Seiffge-Krenke, I. (1995). *Stress, coping and relationships in adolescents*. Mahwah, NJ: Erlbaum.

Seiffge-Krenke, I. (2000). Causal links between stressful events, coping style, and adolescent symptomatology. *Journal of Adolescence, 23*, 675–691.

Seiffge-Krenke, I., & Klesslinger, N. (2000). Long-term effects of avoidant coping on adolescents' depressive symptoms. *Journal of Youth and Adolescence, 29*, 617–630.

Seiffge-Krenke, I., Weidemann, S., Fentner, S., Aegenheister, N., & Poeblau, M. (2001). Coping with school-related stress and family stress in healthy and clinically referred adolescents. *European Psychologist, 6*, 123–132.

Sherbourne, C. D., & Stewart, A. L. (1991). The MOS social support survey. *Social Science & Medicine, 32*, 705–714.

Shevlin, M., Bunting, B., & Lewis, C. (1995). Confirmatory factor analysis of the Rosenberg Self-Esteem Scale. *Psychological Reports, 76*, 707–710.

Sjoberg, R. L., Nilsson, K. W., & Leppert, J. (2005). Obesity, shame, and depression in school-aged children: A population-based study. *Pediatrics, 116*, e389–e392.

Solomon, M. R. (2001). Eating as both coping and stressor in overweight control. *Journal of Advanced Nursing, 36*, 563–572.

Southall, D., & Roberts, J. E. (2002). Attributional style and self-esteem in vulnerability to adolescent depressive symptoms following life stress: A 14-week prospective study. *Cognitive Therapy and Research, 26*, 563–579.

State Crime Statistics. (2002). Retrieved August 11, 2008, from http://www.isp.state.il.us/crime/cii2002. cfm

Steiner, H., Erickson, S. J., Hernandez, N. L., & Pavelski, R. (2002). Coping styles as correlates of health in high school students. *Journal of Adolescent Health, 30*, 326–335.

Stockman, N. K., Schenkel, T. C., Brown, J. N., & Duncan, A. M. (2005). Comparison of energy and nutrient intakes among meals and snacks of adolescent males. *Preventive Medicine, 41*, 203–210.

Strauss, R. S. (2000). Childhood obesity and self-esteem. *Pediatrics, 105*, e15.

Taveras, E. M., Rifas-Shiman, S. L., Berkey, C. C., Rockett, H. R., Field, A. E., Frazier, A. L., et al. (2005). Family dinner and adolescent overweight. *Obesity Research, 13*, 900–906.

Thompson, B. (2000). Ten commandments for structural equation modeling. In: L. G. Grimm, & P. R. Yarnold (Eds.), *Reading and understanding more multivariate statistics* (pp. 261–284). Washington, DC: American Psychological Association.

U.S. Census Bureau. (2000). *Census 2000*. Retrieved April 19, 2006, from http://www.census.gov

Videon, T. M., & Manning, C. K. (2003). Influences on adolescent eating patterns: The importance of family meals. *Journal of Adolescent Health Behavior, 32*, 365–373.

Wadsworth, M. E., & Compas, B. E. (2002). Coping with family conflict and economic strain: The adolescent perspective. *Journal of Research on Adolescence, 12*, 243–274.

Wilburn, V. R., & Smith, D. E. (2005). Stress, self-esteem, suicidal ideation in late adolescents. *Adolescence, 40*, 33–45.

Yarcheski, A., & Mahon, N. E. (1999). The moderator-mediator role of social support in adolescents. *Western Journal of Nursing Research, 21*, 685–698.

APPENDIX A-3

Effects of a Supervised Exercise Intervention on Recovery From Treatment Regimens in Breast Cancer Survivors

City C. Hsieh, PhD; Lisa K. Sprod, MS; David S. Hydock, PhD; Susan D. Carter, MD; Reid Hayward, PhD; Carole M. Schneider, PhD

City C. Hsieh, PhD, is a professor in the Department of Physical Education at the National HsinChu University of Education in Taiwan; Lisa K. Sprod, MS, is a doctoral candidate and David S. Hydock, PhD, is a lecturer, both in the School of Sport and Exercise Science at the University of Northern Colorado in Greeley; Susan D. Carter, MD, is the medical director at the Rocky Mountain Cancer Rehabilitation Institute at the University of Northern Colorado and director of the Regional Breast Center of Northern Colorado in Greeley; Reid Hayward, PhD, is an associate professor in the School of Sport and Exercise Science and a director at the Rocky Mountain Cancer Rehabilitation Institute; and Carole M. Schneider, PhD, is a director at the Rocky Mountain Cancer Rehabilitation Institute and professor in the School of Sport and Exercise Science. No financial relationships to disclose. Mention of specific products and opinions related to those products do not indicate or imply endorsement by the *Oncology Nursing Forum or* the Oncology Nursing Society.

Purpose/Objectives: *To investigate the effects of supervised exercise training on cardiopulmonary function and fatigue in cancer survivors undergoing various clinical treatments.*

Design: *Pretest and post-test quasiexperimental.*

Setting: *Outpatient Oncology Rehabilitation Center.*

Sample: *96 breast cancer survivors undergoing various clinical treatments.*

Methods: *Subjects were divided into four groups based on the specific type of clinical treatment: surgery alone (n = 22); surgery and chemotherapy (n = 30); surgery and radiation (n = 17); and surgery, chemotherapy, and radiation (n = 27). Following a comprehensive screening and medical examination, cardiovascular endurance, pulmonary function, and fatigue were assessed, leading to the development of an individualized exercise prescription and a six-month exercise intervention. Repeated-measures analysis of variance and covariance were used to compare the effectiveness of the intervention and differences among treatment groups.*

Source: Oncology Nursing Forum, 2008, Vol. 35, No. 6, 909–915.

Main Research Variables: *Systolic and diastolic blood pressure, resting heart rate, forced vital capacity, forced expiratory volume, predicted oxygen consumption, time on treadmill, and fatigue.*

Findings: *Cardiopulmonary function (predicted maximal oxygen consumption and time on treadmill) significantly increased in all groups after exercise training. In addition, resting heart rate and forced vital capacity significantly improved in those receiving surgery, chemotherapy, and radiation. Psychologically, the exercise intervention resulted in significant reductions in behavioral, affective, sensory, cognitive and mood, and total fatigue scale scores in all three groups who received treatment with surgery. The breast cancer survivors in the surgery-alone group showed significant reductions in behavioral, affective, and total fatigue scale scores but not in sensory and cognitive and mood fatigue scale scores.*

Conclusions: *The results suggest that moderate intensity, individualized, prescriptive exercise maintains or improves cardiopulmonary function with concomitant reductions in fatigue regardless of treatment type. Moreover, cancer survivors receiving combination chemotherapy and radiotherapy following surgery appear to benefit to a greater extent as a result of an individualized exercise intervention.*

Implications for Nursing: *Clinicians need to be aware of adjuvant therapies such as moderate exercise that attenuate negative side effects of cancer treatments. Symptom management recommendations should be given to cancer survivors concerning the effectiveness of exercise throughout the cancer continuum and the importance of participating in a cancer rehabilitation exercise program.*

■ KEY POINTS

Cancer therapy not only impacts tumors and mutant cells but also can cause deleterious side effects on healthy tissue, resulting in acute and chronic physiologic and psychological negative symptoms.

Research indicates that the severity of cancer treatment–related symptoms may depend on the type of treatment.

Exercise training results in many positive physiologic and psychological benefits.

The American Cancer Society (ACS, 2008) estimated that 1,437,180 people will be diagnosed with new cases of cancer in 2008. Advances in technology and the effectiveness of cancer treatments have helped to significantly increase cancer survival rates. Cancer treatments include numerous therapeutic modalities such as surgery, chemotherapy, and radiotherapy. The type and technique of therapy used, alone or in combination with another treatment, are selected based on factors such as response rate, drug sensitivity, and side effects (Schneider, Dennehy, & Carter, 2003).

However, the impact of surgery, chemotherapy, or radiation is not limited to tumors or mutant cells; these treatments also cause deleterious effects on healthy tissues, resulting in acute and chronic physiologic and psychological negative symptoms in cancer survivors (Chabner & Longo, 2001; Gianni et al., 2001). Surgery has been correlated with fatigue in breast cancer survivors (Cimprich, 1993), whereas chemotherapy often leads to general fatigue (Byar, Berger, Bakken, & Cetak, 2006; de Jong, Kester, Schouten, Abu-Saad, & Courtens, 2006) and impaired exercise tolerance (Pihkala et al., 1995). Nail, Jones, Greene, Schipper, and Jensen (1991) reported that fatigue afflicts up to 96% of cancer survivors receiving chemotherapy. Radiation therapy has been implicated in the occurrence of interstitial myocardial fibrosis (Renzi, Straus, & Glatstein, 1992) and coronary and carotid artery arteriosclerosis (Rubin, Finkelstein, & Shapiro, 1992). Hickok, Morrow, McDonald, and Bellg (1996) demonstrated that radiotherapy resulted in fatigue in 78% of cancer survivors. Chemotherapy and radiation have been linked to impairments in left ventricular function, often manifested as altered ventricular morphology, abnormal pressure and volume relationships, and decreased left ventricular ejection fraction (d'Avella et al., 1998; Rubin et al., 1992). When used concomitantly, the effect of these therapies on the cardiovascular and muscular systems appears to be magnified (Bezwada et al., 1998). The magnitude and variability of these alterations suggest that cancer treatment–related fatigue is the result of a myriad of factors and specifically may be affected by the course of treatment.

Studies have shown that exercise training results in many positive physiologic and psychological benefits in cancer survivors (Coleman et al., 2003; Dimeo, Stieglitz, Novelli-Fischer, Fetscher, & Keul, 1999; Drouin et al., 2006; Mock et al., 1997, 2001; Mutrie et al., 2007; Pinto, Clark, Maruyama, & Feder, 2003; Schneider, Hsieh, Sprod, Carter, & Hayward, 2007; Schwartz, 1999, 2000; Segal et al., 2001; Turner, Hayes, & Reul-Hirche, 2004). Researchers have investigated the benefits of exercise training in breast cancer survivors receiving surgery, chemotherapy following surgery, radiotherapy following surgery, or chemotherapy and radiotherapy following surgery. For example, Gaskin, LoBuglio, Kelly, Doss, and Pizitz (1989) and Turner et al. (2004) investigated the effects of an exercise intervention on breast cancer survivors after surgery. Others (Dimeo et al., 1997, 1999; Schwartz, 1999, 2000; Segal et al., 2001) have reported the effects of exercise intervention on breast cancer survivors receiving chemotherapy following surgery. In addition, studies (Mock et al., 1997, 2005) have reported the effects of exercise on breast cancer survivors receiving radiotherapy following surgery. Moreover, the effects of exercise have been studied in breast cancer survivors who had completed surgery, chemotherapy, and/or radiation (Courneya et al., 2003; Mock et al., 2001; Mutrie et al., 2007; Pinto et al., 2003).

Initial research indicates that the severity of cancer treatment–related symptoms may be dependent on the type of treatment. For example, chemotherapeutic agents each impart unique side effects and long-term sequelae. In addition, chemotherapy and radiotherapy produce distinct detriments in cancer survivors that may be partially responsible for the variance in reported fatigue levels. Cancer survivors who had received a combination of chemotherapy and radiotherapy following surgery experienced higher levels of fatigue and scored lower during a functional capacity assessment than those survivors receiving chemotherapy or radiotherapy exclusively (Woo, Dibble, Piper, Keating, & Weiss, 1998). However, no investigation has specifically determined if the benefits of supervised exercise intervention are influenced by the type of treatment received by cancer survivors. Therefore, the purpose of the present study was to investigate the effects of supervised exercise training on cardiopulmonary function and fatigue in cancer survivors undergoing differing clinical treatments.

■ METHODS

Participants

Subjects were chosen from women who were referred by local oncologists to the Rocky Mountain Cancer Rehabilitation Institute (RMCRI) for rehabilitative exercise immediately following treatment for breast cancer. The university institutional review board approved all study procedures. Informed consent was obtained prior to participation in the study.

Assessment and Reassessment

Trained, certified cancer exercise specialists completed all assessments, exercise interventions, and reassessments. Cancer exercise specialists completed coursework, assessment observations, shadowing, and reliability testing before working with cancer survivors.

The cancer survivors received comprehensive screening followed by an initial medical examination prior to inclusion in the study. Cardiovascular endurance, pulmonary function, and fatigue were assessed leading to the development of individualized exercise prescriptions. Cardiovascular endurance (the ability of the heart, lungs, and circulatory system to supply oxygen to working muscles efficiently, therefore allowing for the production of energy for activities of daily living) was evaluated using the three-minute stage of the Bruce Treadmill Protocol, a multistage, variable speed, and elevation treadmill protocol. The Bruce protocol correlation coefficient is $r = 0.91$ with a standard error of estimate of 2.7 ml/kg per minute. Heart rate, blood pressure, oxygen consumption (predicted VO_{2max}), time on treadmill, and oxygen saturation were obtained from the Bruce protocol results. Participants continued to a predetermined heart rate or voluntary fatigue, dependent on the recommendation of the medical director of the institute.

Pulmonary function was assessed using a Flowmate™ spirometer, which measures forced vital capacity (FVC) and forced expiratory volume (FEV_1). Three tests were performed and were reproducible within 5% of each other. The participant's measured result was compared to predicted normative data tables for FVC and FEV_1 based on the participant's age, gender, height, and weight to obtain the percentage of predicted ($FVC\%_{pred}$ and $FEV_1\%_{pred}$). An $FVC\%_{pred}$ less than 75% suggests a restrictive disorder, and an $FVC\%_{pred}$ less than 60% suggests ventilatory disorder. Likewise, an $FEV_1\%_{pred}$ less than 75% suggests an obstructive disorder and less than 60% suggests a ventilatory disorder.

The revised Piper Fatigue Scale (Piper et al., 1998) was used to assess cancer-related fatigue. The behavioral fatigue subscale includes six questions and was used to assess the impact of fatigue on school and work, interacting with friends, and the overall interference with activities that are enjoyable. The affective fatigue subscale includes five questions and was used to assess the emotional meaning attributed to fatigue. The sensory fatigue subscale includes five questions and was used to assess the mental, physical, and emotional symptoms of fatigue. The cognitive and mood fatigue subscale includes six questions and was used to assess the impact of fatigue on concentration, memory, and the ability to think clearly. The average score on the 22 total questions from the subscales provided the total fatigue score (Piper et al., 1998). Patients are to circle the number that best describes the fatigue they are experiencing now. The Likert scale on the Piper Fatigue Scale ranges from 0 (none) to 10 (a great deal) of fatigue. The higher the score, the greater the patient fatigue. The revised Piper Fatigue Scale has a standardized Cronbach alpha of 0.97 with subscales reliability estimates ranging from 0.92–0.96. Reassessments were obtained following a six-month individually prescribed exercise intervention. The same physiologic and psychological parameters were assessed using identical protocols during the initial assessment and reassessment to obtain program effectiveness outcomes.

Exercise Prescription and Intervention

Certified cancer exercise specialists developed individualized exercise prescriptions and exercise interventions to meet the specific needs of each breast cancer survivor based on results from the medical and cancer history, the physical examination, and the initial physiologic and psychological assessments. Participants attended individually supervised exercise sessions two or three days per week for six months. Prior to each training session, the cancer exercise specialists asked each participant a series of questions that would clarify the need to alter the exercise intervention, if necessary. Questions focused on how participants felt after the last exercise session, if participants had any soreness or specific problems that would affect training, and if changes in medication or treatment had been implemented since the last exercise session. The exercise sessions lasted 60 minutes and were based on a "whole-body" approach (Schneider et al., 2003). Each exercise session was individualized for the cancer survivor but generally included a 10-minute warm-up, 40 minutes of aerobic exercise, resistance training and stretching, and concluded with a 10-minute cooldown. Exercise intensity was based on the cancer survivors' treadmill assessment results, and ranged from 40%–75% of heart rate reserve depending on the participants' health status. The Karvonen or percent heart rate reserve method was used to determine exercise heart rate intensity using the formula (exercise target heart rate = [(220 − age) − resting heart rate] × percent of exercise intensity + resting heart rate). The mode of aerobic exercise selected for each participant was based on the mode offering the greatest anticipated benefit. Options included outdoor or treadmill walking, stationary cycling, recumbent stepping, or walking on an AquaCiser® underwater treadmill. Resistance training and flexibility consisted of exercises emphasizing all of the major muscle groups. The exercise sessions concluded with an extremely low-intensity cooldown targeting all of the major muscle groups. Follow-up examinations revealed that participants' adherence to the exercise intervention was approximately 90%, which can be attributed to cancer exercise specialists who prescribed individualized cancer interventions that fit patients' circumstances.

Statistical Analyses

Participants' characteristics in the four groups were compared using one-way analysis of variance (ANOVA). The main effect of supervised exercise training was determined before and after the exercise intervention using repeated-measures ANOVA. Following main effects significance, Tukey honestly significant difference post-hoc tests were used to determine where significance occurred. The primary analyses compared changes from before and after the exercise intervention and between treatment groups using univariate analyses of covariance procedures in which the postvalue was the dependent variable, the prevalue of the same variable was the covariate, and treatment group was the grouping variable. Statistical analyses were performed using SPSS®. Significance was set at a probability of <0.05.

■ RESULTS

The study included 96 breast cancer survivors with a mean age of 57.9 ± 10.4 years. The convenience sample of participants was divided into four groups based on the type of clinical treatment they had received: surgery alone ($n = 22$); surgery and chemotherapy ($n = 30$); surgery and radiation ($n = 17$); and surgery, chemotherapy, and radiation ($n = 27$). All participants had surgery, with 53% having a mastectomy, 28% lumpectomy, and 16% bilateral mastectomy. Twelve percent of the women were on antidepressants. Skinfold body fat averaged $33.4 \pm 6.7\%$ before the exercise intervention and $33.4 \pm 5.8\%$ following the exercise intervention. The cancer survivors' initial characteristics are shown in Table A3.1. No significant differences were observed in age, height, and weight between groups. Table A3.2 shows cardiopulmonary function changes in all four groups before and after the exercise intervention. Following the six-month exercise intervention, predicted VO_{2max} and time on treadmill in all four treatment groups ($p < 0.05$) improved significantly. In addition, breast cancer survivors in the surgery, chemotherapy, and radiation group showed significant reductions in resting heart rate ($p < 0.05$) and concurrent increases on $FVC\%_{pred}$ after the supervised exercise intervention. Although the four treatment groups showed varying levels of improvement in cardiopulmonary function, no significant differences were noted between the four groups in regard to before exercise versus after exercise improvement.

Table A3.3 displays alterations on the four fatigue domains and total fatigue before and after the exercise intervention for all treatment groups. The exercise intervention resulted in significant reductions in behavioral fatigue, affective fatigue, sensory fatigue, cognitive and mood fatigue, and total fatigue in the surgery and chemotherapy; surgery and radiation therapy; and surgery, chemotherapy, and radiation therapy groups ($p < 0.05$). However, the breast cancer survivors in the surgery alone group showed significant reductions in

Table A3.1

Characteristics of the Breast Cancer Population

CHARACTERISTIC	SURGERY ALONE (N = 22)		SURGERY AND CHEMOTHERAPY (N = 30)		SURGERY AND RADIATION THERAPY (N = 17)		SURGERY, CHEMOTHERAPY, AND RADIATION THERAPY (N = 27)	
	$\bar{X}$	SD	$\bar{X}$	SD	$\bar{X}$	SD	$\bar{X}$	SD
Age (years)	155.6	11.3	155.6	11.0	157.2	19.4	163.1	19.8
Height (inches)	164.4	13.1	163.7	13.0	164.2	12.7	164.4	12.4
Weight (pounds)	167.4	31.0	164.2	38.1	164.9	42.0	173.5	40.4

Table A3.2

Cardiopulmonary Function Before and After the Exercise Intervention

VARIABLE	n	BEFORE EXERCISE $\bar{X}$	SD	AFTER EXERCISE $\bar{X}$	SD	% CHANGE
Systolic blood pressure (mm Hg)						
Surgery	22	132	17	127	12	−3.79
Surgery and chemotherapy	30	125	19	123	13	−1.60
Surgery and radiation therapy	17	126	17	121	14	−3.97
Surgery, chemotherapy, and radiation therapy	27	125	11	123	10	−1.60
Diastolic blood pressure (mm Hg)						
Surgery	22	80	7	76	8	−5.00
Surgery and chemotherapy	30	78	10	76	11	−2.56
Surgery and radiation therapy	17	78	10	76	8	−2.56
Surgery, chemotherapy, and radiation therapy	27	79	8	78	8	−1.27
Resting heart rate (bpm)						
Surgery	22	81	11	80	11	−1.23
Surgery and chemotherapy	30	86	13	83	13	−3.49
Surgery and radiation therapy	17	83	10	81	10	−2.41
Surgery, chemotherapy, and radiation therapy	27	86	13	81	11	−5.80*
FVC%$_{pred}$						
Surgery	22	98	18	102	19.4	3.36
Surgery and chemotherapy	30	96	20	100	20.6	4.81
Surgery and radiation therapy	17	96	18	95	21.0	−0.73
Surgery, chemotherapy, and radiation therapy	27	90	16	95	14.6	4.70*
FEV$_1$%$_{pred}$						
Surgery	22	92	24	99	21.1	6.95
Surgery and chemotherapy	30	91	22	99	19.3	9.17
Surgery and radiation therapy	17	90	19	88	22.7	−1.67
Surgery, chemotherapy, and radiation therapy	27	87	19	91	13.5	4.38
pVO$_{2max}$ (ml/kg/minute)						
Surgery	22	20	15	25	5.2	23.00*
Surgery and chemotherapy	30	21	6	24	5.4	15.17*
Surgery and radiation therapy	17	20	7	24	6.0	19.70*
Surgery, chemotherapy, and radiation therapy	27	21	7	25	5.2	18.93*
Treadmill time (minutes and seconds)						
Surgery	22	4:56	2:40	6:46	2:32	37.16*
Surgery and chemotherapy	30	5:33	2:06	7:03	2:02	27.03*
Surgery and radiation therapy	17	5:08	2:47	6:36	2:34	28.57*
Surgery, chemotherapy, and radiation therapy	27	5:28	2:33	7:18	2:31	33.54*

*$p < 0.05$.
bpm—beats per minute; FEV$_1$%$_{pred}$—forced expiratory volume percent of predicted; FVC%$_{pred}$—forced vital capacity percent of predicted; pVO$_{2max}$—predicted maximal oxygen consumption.

Table A3.3

Fatigue Before and After the Exercise Intervention

VARIABLE	n	BEFORE EXERCISE $\bar{X}$	SD	AFTER EXERCISE $\bar{X}$	SD	% CHANGE
Behavioral fatigue						
Surgery	22	49.60	2.79	2.39	1.62	−51.81*
Surgery and chemotherapy	30	14.40	2.69	2.82	2.29	−35.91*
Surgery and radiation therapy	17	14.29	2.36	2.10	2.22	−51.05*
Surgery, chemotherapy, and radiation therapy	27	15.21	2.64	3.08	2.49	−40.88*
Affective fatigue						
Surgery	22	15.29	2.52	3.96	2.27	−25.14*
Surgery and chemotherapy	30	15.52	2.52	3.85	2.98	−30.25*
Surgery and radiation therapy	17	15.39	2.49	3.43	2.28	−36.36*
Surgery, chemotherapy, and radiation therapy	27	15.90	1.92	3.99	2.04	−32.37*
Sensory fatigue						
Surgery	22	15.20	2.44	4.05	1.78	−22.12
Surgery and chemotherapy	30	15.53	2.36	4.18	2.29	−24.41*
Surgery and radiation therapy	17	15.54	2.16	2.99	2.07	−46.03*
Surgery, chemotherapy, and radiation therapy	27	15.80	1.71	3.71	1.64	−36.03*
Cognitive and mood fatigue						
Surgery	22	15.08	2.48	4.26	1.78	−16.14
Surgery and chemotherapy	30	14.77	1.97	3.93	1.95*	−17.61
Surgery and radiation therapy	17	14.64	2.08	3.42	1.99*	−26.29
Surgery, chemotherapy, and radiation therapy	27	15.25	1.99	3.29	1.25*	−37.33
Total fatigue						
Surgery	22	15.12	2.40	3.63	1.55*	−29.10
Surgery and chemotherapy	30	14.97	1.99	3.59	2.16*	−27.77
Surgery and radiation therapy	17	14.89	1.97	2.96	2.01*	−39.47
Surgery, chemotherapy, and radiation therapy	27	15.40	1.82	3.29	1.44*	−39.07

*$p < 0.05$.

fatigue on the behavioral and affective subscales and the total fatigue score ($p < 0.05$) but not on sensory and cognitive and mood subscales ($p > 0.05$) after exercise training. Moreover, no significant differences were observed between groups on any of the fatigue domains.

■ DISCUSSION

The present study is the first to compare the effects of an exercise intervention on cardiopulmonary function and fatigue in breast cancer survivors who received different types of clinical treatments. Cardiovascular toxicity, pulmonary toxicity, and extreme debilitating fatigue often are experienced by breast cancer survivors following surgery with adjuvant chemotherapy or radiotherapy. The study found that moderate intensity, individualized, prescriptive exercise could alleviate negative side effects of cancer treatment, as evidenced by an improvement in pVO_{2max} and the length of treadmill exercise time in all groups.

The side effects of cancer treatments can last days, months, and even years. Breast cancer survivors in the study were assessed within weeks following the end of treatment. The results showed that the breast cancer survivors did not experience prolonged decrements in physiologic or psychological parameters following treatment but were able to maintain their cardiovascular fitness (systolic blood pressure, diastolic blood pressure, resting heart rate) and pulmonary fitness (FVC and FEV_1) in the surgery alone, surgery with chemotherapy, and surgery with radiation groups as a result of the exercise intervention. Interestingly, breast cancer survivors in the group who had completed surgery plus adjuvant chemotherapy and radiotherapy showed significant improvements in resting heart rate (-5.8%) and FVC ($+4.7\%$) as a result of the exercise intervention, whereas systolic blood pressure, diastolic blood pressure, and FEV_1 maintained their initial levels.

The results are, to some extent, consistent with the findings of Courneya et al. (2003) who observed a beneficial effect of a structured training intervention on peak oxygen consumption ($+17.4\%$) compared with a control group in breast cancer survivors who started the intervention several months after surgical treatment and adjuvant chemotherapy. In addition, MacVicar, Winningham, and Nickel (1989) also showed improved pVO_{2max} following a 10-week interval-training cycle ergometer protocol compared with a stretching and flexibility exercise program in breast cancer survivors following chemotherapy. Similarly, an increase in pVO_{2max} between 15%–23% among all clinical treatment groups was observed. In addition, the significant improvements in resting heart rate and $FVC\%_{pred}$ in the surgery, chemotherapy, and radiation group imply that individualized exercise training can benefit cancer survivors independent of treatment type.

The pVO_{2max} of breast cancer survivors improved as result of exercise training in the study, regardless of the type of treatment. The mechanism by which exercise training increased pVO_{2max} and time on treadmill in breast cancer survivors following surgery and adjuvant chemotherapy and/or radiotherapy remains elusive. During exercise training, more than 80% of the consumed oxygen is used by working skeletal muscle. Maximum oxygen uptake is an integrative indicator of the maximum working capacity of the cardiopulmonary and muscular systems (lungs, heart, blood, working skeletal muscles) involved in the aerobic process from the delivery of atmospheric oxygen to the mitochondria of the muscle fibers. Therefore, any increase in maximum oxygen uptake brought about by exercise training involving large muscle mass is mostly attributable to an improvement of cardiopulmonary function but also of blood oxygen transport and muscle aerobic capacity (McArdle, Katch, & Katch, 2001). In addition, Chicco, Schneider, and Hayward (2006) and Hayward et al. (2004) found that exercise training preserved intrinsic cardiovascular function following treatment with various chemotherapeutic agents. These cardioprotective effects were associated with an exercise-induced increase in endothelial nitric oxide synthase, myocardial heat shock protein content, and attenuation in chemotherapy-induced myocardial lipid peroxidation. Therefore, several mechanisms may have contributed to the physiologic adaptations observed in this investigation.

Fatigue is a common effect of cancer treatment (Portenoy & Itri, 1999). Prevalence rates of fatigue as high as 96% have been reported following chemotherapy and radiotherapy. Fatigue may be described as lack of energy, muscle weakness, somnolence, dysphoric mood, or impaired cognition. Possible causes of fatigue include pain, sleep problems, infection, poor nutrition, side effects of medications, anemia, and deconditioning (Berger, 2003). Fatigue has been considered the most prevalent and distressing symptom of cancer therapies, as well as the most common unmanaged symptom. The presence of one or a combination of the symptoms has the potential to adversely affect quality of life and general well-being. For example, the presence of fatigue often leads to a decrease in daily activity level, which in turn lowers an individual's capacity to perform daily tasks in the future. As breast cancer survivors become too tired to participate fully in the roles and activities that make life meaningful, quality of life is adversely influenced.

Limitations

The convenience sample was a limitation of the study as well as the sample composition of women from one geographic area. In addition, the strength of the study could have been enhanced if a nonexercise group was included.

■ IMPLICATIONS FOR NURSING

The results of the study suggest that moderate intensity, individualized, prescriptive exercise maintains or improves cardiopulmonary function with concomitant reductions in fatigue regardless of treatment received for breast cancer. Nurses can help cancer survivors improve their quality of life by making appropriate referrals to initiate supportive therapies such as exercise interventions to help cancer survivors combat the side effects of cancer treatments whether surgery, chemotherapy, radiation, or combination therapy. The present study investigated moderate intensity exercise; future research must determine if higher intensity exercise also is safe for cancer survivors.

References

American Cancer Society. (2008). *Cancer facts and figures 2008.* Retrieved October 8, 2008, from http://www.cancer.org/downloads/STT/2008CAFFfinalsecured.pdf

Berger, A. (2003). Treating fatigue in cancer patients. *Oncologist, 8*(Suppl. 1), 10–14.

Bezwada, H. P., Granick, M. S., Long, C. D., Moore, J. H., Jr., Lackman, R. L., & Weiss, A. J. (1998). Soft-tissue complications of intra-arterial chemotherapy for extremity sarcomas. *Annals of Plastic Surgery, 40*(4), 382–387.

Byar, K. L., Berger, A. M., Bakken, S. L., & Cetak, M. A. (2006). Impact of adjuvant breast cancer chemotherapy on fatigue, other symptoms, and quality of life [Online exclusive]. *Oncology Nursing Forum, 33*(1), E18–E26. Retrieved September 24, 2008, from http://ons.metapress.com/content/um1281005428t806/fulltext.pdf

Chabner, B. A., & Longo, D. L. (2001). *Cancer chemotherapy and bio-therapy: Principles and practice* (3rd ed.). Philadelphia, PA: Lippincott Williams & Wilkins.

Chicco, A. J., Schneider, C. M., & Hayward, R. (2006). Exercise training attenuates acute doxorubicin-induced cardiac dysfunction. *Journal of Cardiovascular Pharmacology, 47*(2), 182–189.

Cimprich, B. (1993). Development of an intervention to restore attention in cancer patients. *Cancer Nursing, 16*(2), 83–92.

Coleman, E. A., Coon, S., Hall-Barrow, J., Richards, K., Gaylor, D., & Stewart, B. (2003). Feasibility of exercise during treatment for multiple myeloma. *Cancer Nursing, 26*(25), 410–419.

Courneya, K. S., Mackey, J. R., Bell, G. J., Jones, L. W., Field, C. J., & Fairey, A. S. (2003). Randomized controlled trial of exercise training in post-menopausal breast cancer survivors: Cardiopulmonary and quality of life outcomes. *Journal of Clinical Oncology, 21*(9), 1660–1668.

d'Avella, D., Cicciarello, R., Angileri, F. F., Lucerna, S., La Torre, D., & Tomasello, F. (1998). Radiation-induced blood-brain barrier changes: Pathophysiological mechanisms and clinical implications. *Acta Neurochirurgica, 71,* 282–284.

de Jong, N., Kester, A. D., Schouten, H. C., Abu-Saad, H. H., & Courtens, A. M. (2006). Course of fatigue between two cycles of adjuvant chemotherapy in breast cancer patients. *Cancer Nursing, 29*(6), 467–477.

Dimeo, F. C., Stieglitz, R. D., Novelli-Fischer, U., Fetscher, S., & Keul, J. (1999). Effects of physical activity on the fatigue and psychologic status of cancer patients during chemotherapy. *Cancer, 85*(10), 2273–2277.

Dimeo, F. C., Tilmann, M. H., Bertz, H., Kanz, L., Mertelsmann, R., & Keul, J. (1997). Aerobic exercise in the rehabilitation of cancer patients after high dose chemotherapy and autologous peripheral stem cell transplantation. *Cancer, 79*(9), 1717–1722.

Drouin, J. S., Young, T. J., Beeler, J., Byrne, K., Birk, T. J., Hryniuk, W. M., et al. (2006). Random control clinical trial on the effects of aerobic exercise training on erythrocyte levels during radiation treatment for breast cancer. *Cancer, 107*(10), 2490–2495.

Gaskin, T. A., LoBuglio, A., Kelly, P., Doss, M., & Pizitz, N. (1989). STRETCH: A rehabilitative program for patients with breast cancer. *Southern Medical Journal, 82*(4), 467–469.

Gianni, L., Dombernowsky, P., Sledge, G., Martin, M., Amadori, D., Arbuck, S. G., et al. (2001). Cardiac function following combination therapy with paclitaxel and doxorubicin: An analysis of 657 women with advanced breast cancer. *Annals of Oncology, 12*(8), 1067–1073.

Hayward, R., Ruangthai, R., Schneider, C. M., Hyslop, R. M., Strange, R., & Westerlind, K. C. (2004). Training enhances vascular relaxation after chemotherapy-induced vasoconstriction. *Medicine and Science in Sports Exercise, 36*(3), 428–434.

Hickok, J. T., Morrow, G. R., McDonald, S., & Bellg, A. J. (1996). Frequency and correlates of fatigue in lung cancer patients receiving radiation therapy: Implications for management. *Journal of Pain and Symptom Management, 11*(6), 370–377.

MacVicar, M. G., Winningham, M. L., & Nickel, J. L. (1989). Effects of aerobic interval training on cancer patients' functional capacity. *Nursing Research, 38*(6), 348–351.

McArdle, W. D., Katch, F. I., & Katch, V. L. (2001). *Exercise physiology. Energy, nutrition and performance* (5th ed.). Philadelphia, PA: Lippincott Williams & Wilkins.

Mock, V., Dow, K. H., Meares, C. J., Grimm, P. M., Dienemann, J. A., Haisfield-Wolfe, M. E., et al. (1997). Effects of exercise on fatigue, physical functioning, and emotional distress during radiation therapy for breast cancer. *Oncology Nursing Forum, 24*(6), 991–1000.

Mock, V., Frangakis, C., Davidson, N. E., Ropka, M. E., Pickett, M., Poniatowski, B., et al. (2005). Exercise manages fatigue during breast cancer treatment: A randomized controlled trial. *Psycho-Oncology, 14*(6), 464–477.

Mock, V., Pickett, M., Ropka, M. E., Lin, E., Stewart, K. J., Rhodes, V. A., et al. (2001). Fatigue and quality of life outcomes of exercise during cancer treatment. *Cancer Practice, 9*(3), 119–127.

Mutrie, N., Campbell, A. M., Whyte, F., McConnachie, A., Emslie, C., Lee, L., et al. (2007). Benefits of supervised group exercise programme for women being treated for early stage breast cancer: Pragmatic randomised controlled trial. *BMJ, 334*(7592), 517.

Nail, L. M., Jones, L. S., Greene, D., Schipper, D. L., & Jensen, R. (1991). Use and perceived efficacy of self-care activities in patients receiving chemotherapy. *Oncology Nursing Forum, 18*(5), 883–887.

Pihkala, J., Happonen, J. M., Virtanen, K., Sovijarvi, A., Siimes, M. A., Pesonen, E., et al. (1995). Cardiopulmonary evaluation of exercise tolerance after chest irradiation and anticancer chemotherapy in children and adolescents. *Pediatrics, 95*(5), 722–726.

Pinto, B. M., Clark, M. M., Maruyama, N. C., & Feder, S. I. (2003). Psychological and fitness changes associated with exercise participation among women with breast cancer. *Psycho-Oncology, 12*(2), 118–126.

Piper, B. F., Dibble, S. L., Dodd, M. J., Weiss, M. C., Slaughter, R. E., & Paul, S. M. (1998). The revised Piper Fatigue Scale: Psychometric evaluation in women with breast cancer. *Oncology Nursing Forum, 25*(4), 677–684.

Portenoy, R. K., & Itri, L. M. (1999). Cancer-related fatigue: Guidelines for evaluation and management. *Oncologist, 4*(1), 1–10.

Renzi, R. H., Straus, K. L., & Glatstein, E. (1992). Radiation-induced myocardial disease. In F. M. Muggia, M. D. Green, & J. L. Speyer (Eds.), *Cancer treatment and the heart* (pp. 289–295). Baltimore, MD: Johns Hopkins University Press.

Rubin, P., Finkelstein, J., & Shapiro, D. (1992). Molecular biology mechanisms in the radiation induction of pulmonary injury syndromes: Inter-relationship between the alveolar macrophage and the septal fibroblast. *International Journal of Radiation Oncology, Biology, Physics, 24*(1), 93–101.

Schneider, C. M., Dennehy, C. A., & Carter, S. D. (2003). *Exercise and cancer recovery.* Champaign, IL: Human Kinetics.

Schneider, C. S., Hsieh, C. C., Sprod, L. K., Carter, S. D. & Hayward, R. (2007). Effects of supervised exercise training on cardiopulmonary function and fatigue in breast cancer survivors during and after treatment. *Cancer, 110*(4), 918–925.

Schwartz, A. L. (1999). Fatigue mediates the effects of exercise on quality of life. *Quality of Life Research, 8*(6), 529–538.

Schwartz, A. L. (2000). Exercise and weight gain in breast cancer patients receiving chemotherapy. *Cancer Practice, 8*(5), 231–237.

Segal, R., Evans, W., Johnson, D., Smith, J., Colletta, S., Gayton, J., et al. (2001). Structured exercise improves physical functioning in women with stages I and II breast cancer: Results of a randomized controlled trial. *Journal of Clinical Oncology, 19*(3), 657–665.

Turner, J., Hayes, S., & Reul-Hirche, H. (2004). Improving the physical status and quality of life of women treated for breast cancer: A pilot study of a structured exercise intervention. *Journal of Surgical Oncology, 86*(3), 141–146.

Woo, B., Dibble, S. L., Piper, B. F., Keating, S. B., & Weiss, M. C. (1998). Differences in fatigue by treatment methods in women with breast cancer. *Oncology Nursing Forum, 25*(5), 915–920.

APPENDIX A-4

Predictors of Life Satisfaction in Stroke Survivors and Spousal Caregivers After Inpatient Rehabilitation

Sharon K. Ostwald, PhD, RN, FGSA; Kyler M. Godwin, MPH;
Stanley G. Cron, MSPH

A global measure of life satisfaction has become increasingly important as an adjunctive outcome of health care interventions for people with disabilities, including those caused by stroke. Life satisfaction of stroke survivors may affect caregiving spouses as well. The purpose of this study was to identify, among many physical and psychosocial variables, specific variables that were associated with life satisfaction at 12 months after discharge from inpatient rehabilitation, and variables that were predictive of life satisfaction 1 year later (at 24 months). Between 12 and 24 months, life satisfaction decreased for stroke survivors, while it increased for caregiving spouses. The relationship between the couple (mutuality) was the only variable that was a significant predictor of life satisfaction for both stroke survivors and their spouses.

Keywords: *caregiver, cardiovascular accident, life satisfaction, relationship, stroke, spouse, stroke survivor.*

Almost 6 million stroke survivors are alive today in the United States; most of them live at home with family (American Heart Association, 2008). Increases in survivorship often are accompanied by physical, psycho-social, affective, and cognitive disabilities that affect life satisfaction of people who have had a stroke and their family, especially their spouses. A 2006 National Stroke Association survey of long-term stroke survivors found that 87% of subjects had ongoing motor problems, 54% had difficulty walking, 52% had difficulty with hand movements, and 58% experienced spasticity (Jones, 2006). Continuing disabilities significantly decrease survivors' life satisfaction and the life satisfaction of their spouses.

As a result of new rehabilitation techniques and a change in our understanding of brain plasticity, nurses now care for stroke survivors who receive therapy not only immediately after their stroke, but also during subsequent hospitalizations for months and even years after the initial event. Consequently, a more complete understanding of the factors that influence a couple's life satisfaction after stroke is necessary. The purpose of this article is to report predictors of life satisfaction in stroke survivors and their spousal caregivers 12–24 months after discharge from inpatient rehabilitation.

■ LITERATURE REVIEW

Considerable literature exists on the meaning of terms such as life satisfaction, well-being, and quality of life (QOL). Ostwald provided an extended discussion of this literature (2008). There is general agreement that QOL is a complex, multidimensional concept

Source: Rehabilitation Nursing, July/August 2009, Vol. 34, No. 4, 160–174.

that includes both objective and subjective elements (Lau & McKenna, 2001; Low, Payne, & Roderick, 1999). In this article, life satisfaction is defined as a global measure of QOL that represents a general subjective appraisal of one's life and does not necessarily mean satisfaction with all aspects of life (Campbell, 1981; Diener, 1984; Musschenga, 1997). A person's subjective appraisal of life may be different from objective appraisals made by others (Veenhoven, 2000). Life satisfaction can only be understood from an individual perspective (Campbell, 1981). Although life satisfaction generally is considered to be stable (Schimmack, Diener, & Oishi, 2002), changes in health, relationships, and work have been shown to significantly decrease life satisfaction (Lucas, Clark, Georgellis, & Diener, 2003).

A recent narrative review found that most studies report lower life satisfaction in stroke survivors and their spousal caregivers than in the general population (Ostwald, 2008). However, variations in instruments, settings, and time in recovery have led to inconsistent conclusions. Only a few studies have followed stroke survivors for longer than 12 months, and even fewer have looked at life satisfaction in their caregiving spouses. In general, decreased life satisfaction in stroke survivors most often has been reported as related to motor impairments, limitations in daily activities, persistent aphasia (Bays, 2001), and poststroke depression (King, 1996). Viitanen, Fugl-Meyer, Bernspang, and Fugl-Meyer (1988) reported that 61% of stroke survivors were dissatisfied with their lives 4–6 years after their strokes. Long-term stroke survivors (longer than 5 years) report stagnation in recovery of function, which is associated with decreased life satisfaction (Teasdale & Engberg, 2005).

Depression and poor life satisfaction in stroke survivors have been shown to be positively related to depression and burden in caregivers (Anderson, Linto, & Stewart-Wynne, 1995). Decreased spousal life satisfaction has been shown to be associated with a stroke survivor's physical and cognitive impairments (Forsberg-Warleby, Moller, & Blomstrand, 2004) and a couple's lack of reintegration into normal patterns of living (White, Poissant, Cote-LeBlanc, & Wood-Dauphinee, 2006). Only 50% of spousal caregivers were satisfied with their lives "as a whole" 1 year after the stroke (Visser-Meily, Post, Schepers, & Lindeman, 2005). Spouses experienced more strain, worry, and disruption in their daily lives than adult children caregivers. For at least 1 year poststroke, spouses of stroke survivors are at greater risk for poorer health, restricted social contacts, and poorer life satisfaction (Franzen-Dahlin, Larson, Murray, Wredling, & Billing, 2007).

In the chronic disease literature, the relationship between caregiver and care recipients (Archbold, Stewart, Greenlick, & Harvath, 1990), the meaningfulness and manageability of caregiving (Haley, LaMonde, Han, Burton, & Schonwetter, 2003), and family functioning (Palmer & Glass, 2003) have been associated with life satisfaction. Spouses of stroke survivors who had cognitive and emotional impairments were the most likely to be dissatisfied with their relationship (Forsberg-Warleby et al., 2004). In a study of stroke survivors and spouses at 12 months poststroke, Carlsson, Forsberg-Warleby, Moller, and Blomstrand (2007) reported that satisfaction with life as a whole and the domains of leisure and sexual functioning were most affected for both stroke survivors and spouses after a stroke. Relationship with a partner was the only domain in which stroke survivors reported greater satisfaction than their spouses.

■ METHODS

Study Design and Sample Population

The sample for this study included 131 stroke survivors and their spousal caregivers who completed 12 months of the Committed to Assisting with Recovery after Stroke (CAReS) Study (NR005316). CAReS was a prospective longitudinal intervention study that randomized stroke survivors and their spousal caregivers into either a mild or intensive intervention upon discharge from inpatient rehabilitation. (For more information about the intervention, see Ostwald, Davis, Hersch, Kelley, & Godwin, 2008.)

CAReS participants had to be cohabitating, English-speaking couples with one member hospitalized with a diagnosis of stroke. The stroke survivor had to be at least 50 years of age, without global aphasia, with no additional major physical or psychiatric conditions (such as severe Parkinson's disease or dementia), and not on hospice. The sample was recruited between November 2001 and December 2005 from five hospitals within the Texas Medical Center, a large medical complex located in Houston. They were followed for 24 months. (For more information on recruitment and retention of the CAReS sample, see Schultz, Wasserman, & Ostwald, 2006.) CAReS was approved by the university institutional review board (IRB) and by the IRB committees of the hospitals from which patients were recruited.

■ DATA COLLECTION

A trained research nurse collected data from stroke survivors and spousal caregivers in their homes 12 months after discharge from inpatient rehabilitation. Caregivers completed the paper-and-pencil instruments while data were gathered from stroke survivors by interview. Data on life satisfaction were collected by telephone from stroke survivors and their spouses at 18 and 24 months postdischarge. All data were collected using standardized instruments that have proved valid and reliable. Sociodemographic data (age, gender, race/ethnicity, occupation, and educational level) were collected, and the four-factor Hollingshead scale was used to calculate socioeconomic status (SES) based on the couple's occupation and educational level (Hollingshead, 1979).

■ INSTRUMENTS

The variables shown in Table A4.1 have been demonstrated in previous studies to be related to life satisfaction in patients with chronic illnesses (Anderson et al., 1995; Archbold et al., 1990; Bays, 2001; Forsberg-Warleby et al., 2004; Haley et al., 2003; King, 1996). Only instruments measuring variables shown to be significant predictors of life satisfaction for stroke survivors or their spouses in the final models (Table A4.2 and Table A4.3) are discussed below.

The Satisfaction With Life Scale (SWLS) is a 5-item scale measuring global life satisfaction and has been shown to have high internal consistency and temporal reliability (Diener, Emmons, Larsen, & Griffen, 1985). Participants respond on a 7-point scale with

Table A4.1

Variables Assessed in Linear Mixed Models for Association With Life Satisfaction (SWLS)

MODEL	BLOCK	VARIABLES
Caregiver	12-month demographic and contextual variables	Age, gender, ethnicity, socioeconomic status, caregiver self-rated health, stroke survivor function, caregiver depression, caregiver-perceived stress, caregiver burden, caregiver mutuality
	12-month mediating variables	Coping strategies, social support, caregiver preparedness
Stroke survivor	12-month demographic and contextual variables	Age, gender, ethnicity, socieconomic status, stroke survivor self-rated health, stroke survivor function, stroke survivor depression, stroke survivor-perceived stress, stroke survivor mutuality
	12-month mediating variables	Overall perceived recovery, perceived physical ability, perceived emotional ability, perceived memory ability, perceived communication ability, perceived social participation

1 being *strongly disagree* and 7 being *strongly agree*. All items are summed to give a total score. Higher scores indicate greater satisfaction.

The Self-Rated Health Status is a single-question subjective measure of a person's perceived health status; it has been shown to be a valid health status indicator (Idler & Benyamini, 1997; Miilunpalo, Vuori, Oja, Pasanen, & Urponen, 1997). Participants respond to the question, "In general, would you say your health is …," on a 5-point scale (1 = *excellent* to 5 = *poor*). Lower scores indicate better perceived health status.

Table A4.2

Predictors of Stroke Survivor Satisfaction With Life Scores 12–24 Months After Discharge From Inpatient Rehabilitation

VARIABLE	ESTIMATE	*df*	*F*	*p* VALUE
Time (days)	−0.004	1, 89.9	4.43	.04
12-month age (years)	0.09	1, 117	4.98	.03
12-month geriatric depression scale	−0.52	1, 123	7.61	.01
12-month mutuality score	1.71	1, 114	8.22	.01
12-month stroke impact (emotion subscale)	0.11	1, 118	15.16	<.01

Table A4.3

Predictors of Caregiver Satisfaction With Life Scores 12–24 Months After Discharge From Inpatient Rehabilitation

VARIABLE	ESTIMATE	df	F	p VALUE
Time (days)	0.002	1, 98.6	1.74	0.19
12-month self-rated health status	−1.13	1, 117	9.27	<0.01
12-month perceived stress scale	−0.27	1, 115	20.46	<0.01
12-month mutuality score	2.49	1, 112	22.62	<0.01
12-month preparedness scale	1.23	1, 127	4.48	0.04
Time × 12-month perceived stress scale	0.0005	1, 97.9	6.24	0.01

Mutuality, a 15-item scale assessing the strength of the relationship between the caregiver and the care recipient, is measured on a 4-point scale (Archbold et al., 1990). Total mutuality scores range from 1 to 4 after averaging responses to the 15 items. High scores indicate the relationship between the caregiver and care recipient is characterized by love, shared pleasurable activities, common values, and reciprocity. High internal consistency has been reported with Cronbach's alpha ranging from .91 to .95 (Archbold et al., 1990; Carter et al., 1998).

The Perceived Stress Scale (PSS; Cohen & Wills, 1985) is a widely used instrument for measuring the degree to which participants perceive life to be stressful (in terms of being unpredictable, uncontrollable, and overloading) during the past month (Gallagher-Thompson, Brooks, Bliwise, Leader, & Yesavage, 1992; Gottlieb, Golander, Bar-Tal, & Gottlieb, 2001; Fredman & Daly, 1997; Keir et al., 2006; McCallum, Sorocco, & Fritsch, 2006). Participants make their ratings on a 5-point scale (0 = *never* to 4 = *very often*), with total scores ranging from 0 to 40. The scale has high internal consistency (.78) and has demonstrated moderate correlations with other measures of appraised stress.

The Geriatric Depression Scale (GDS-15) is a brief scale designed to assess depression in older adults (Sheikh & Yesavage, 1986). Items are summed for a total score; the scale has a cutoff of 4/5 for significant depressive symptomatology. The GDS-15 has a high level of internal consistency (Cronbach's alpha = 0.80), and all of the individual items are significantly associated ($p < .01$) with the total score (D'Ath, Katona, Mullan, Evans, & Katona, 1994).

The Stroke Impact Scale (SIS), Version 2, is a stroke-specific QOL instrument measuring the physical, mental, and emotional impact of stroke (Duncan et al., 1999). The SIS includes 59 questions in eight domains: strength, hand function, mobility, activities of daily living, emotion, memory, communication, and social participation. Higher scores indicate a higher QOL. The first four domains can be combined into the SIS physical domain score. The 1-week test-retest reliability correlation coefficients for the eight SIS domains ranged from .70 to .92, with the exception of the emotion domain, which was .57 (Duncan et al., 1999). Cronbach's alpha for the SIS emotion domain in the CAReS study was .81, however.

Caregiver Preparedness is an eight-item scale measuring general, physical, social, and emotional preparedness for caregiving. Participants answer questions on a 5-point Likert scale (0 = *not at all prepared* to 4 = *very well prepared*). The responses to the eight items are averaged with scores ranging from 1 to 4. Higher scores indicate greater caregiver preparedness (Archbold et al., 1990).

■ DATA ANALYSIS

Longitudinal analyses of SWLS scores between 12 and 24 months were conducted with linear mixed models (Brown & Prescott, 2006). Separate models were developed for stroke survivors and their spousal caregivers. A sequential method (Tabachnick & Fidell, 2001) was used to determine factors that are significant predictors of life satisfaction from the list of variables presented in Table A4.1. For the stroke survivor model, demographic and other 12-month contextual variables were entered as a block to comprise the initial model. A second model was constructed by adding 12-month instrument scores for the SIS. Significant variables resulting from this second model were tested for their interaction with time (in days) to determine if their association with life satisfaction changed between 12 and 24 months. A similar process was used for the caregiver model with demographic and other 12-month contextual variables entered as a block to create the initial model. A second model was constructed by adding 12-month instrument scores for coping, social support, and preparedness to variables that were found to be significant predictors ($p < .05$) of life satisfaction in the first model. The procedure for determining the final model for spousal caregiver life satisfaction was the same, except in the final model the 12-month PSS values were centered to their mean value (13.2). To improve interpretability of the caregiver models, the values for time were centered to the midpoint of follow-up (179.5 days). The final model included only those variables and interactions with $p < .05$. All statistical analyses were performed using SAS for Windows, Version 9.1 (SAS Institute, 2004).

■ RESULTS

Participant Profile

Among the stroke survivors in this sample, 77% were men. Considerable diversity existed in terms of age, ethnicity, and SES (Table A4.4). Although the average age of spouses was 63 (ages ranged from 41 to 86 years), minorities comprised 42% of the sample, with almost equal numbers being African American and Hispanic, which is representative of the Houston area. In addition, participants came from a wide range of socioeconomic backgrounds, with a range on the SES scale of 13–66 and a mean of 43.5.

■ KEY PRACTICE POINTS

1. Younger stroke survivors may experience more difficulty regarding social issues, including loss of work and child care, that may negatively affect their life satisfaction.
2. Preparing for the caregiving role is not a one-time event; as the needs of the stroke survivor change, spousal caregivers require ongoing information and support.

Table A4.4

Sociodemographic and Stroke-Related Characteristics of Stroke Survivors and Their Spousal Caregivers 12 Months After Discharge From Inpatient Rehabilitation ($N = 131$)

STROKE SURVIVORS			CAREGIVERS		
VARIABLE	n	%	VARIABLE	n	%
Male	101	77.1	Male	30	22.9
African-American	23	17.6	African-American	22	16.8
Asian	5	3.8	Asian	5	3.8
Hispanic	22	16.8	Hispanic	23	17.6
White, non-Hispanic	76	58.0	White, non-Hispanic	77	58.8
Other	5	3.8	Other	4	3.1

	X	SD	RANGE		X	SD	RANGE
Age	66.9	9.1	51.1–88.6	Age	63.0	10.6	41.1–87.1
Socioeconomic status	43.5	12.0	13–66	Socioeconomic status	43.5	12.0	13–66
Health status	2.61	0.89	1–5	Health status	2.9	1.0	1–5
Depression	3.2	2.7	0–15	Depression	2.88	2.86	0–14
Stress	10.5	7.3	0–30	Stress	13.2	7.2	0–35
Mutuality	3.3	0.7	1.3–4	Mutuality	3.0	0.8	0.5–4
SIS physical	69.1	23.1	6–100	Preparedness	2.9	0.7	0–4
SIS emotion	80.9	16.2	11–100				
SIS memory	85.0	16.2	11–100				
SIS communication	88.3	18.6	11–100				
SIS social participation	72.7	21.1	0–100				

Note. SIS, Stroke Impact Scale.

3. The quality of the relationship is the only predictor of life satisfaction for both stroke survivor and spousal caregiver.
4. Nurses must help couples surviving stroke assess their strengths and challenges in terms of marital relationship, family support, and lifestyle priorities.

Life Satisfaction Changes Over Time

Mean scores on the SWLS show changes in the opposite direction for stroke survivors and their spouses (Fig. A4.1). The life satisfaction scores of stroke survivors decreased from a mean of 23.79 ($SD = 6.62$) at 12 months to a mean of 22.42 ($SD = 6.73$) at 24 months, demonstrating a significant decrease over the 12-month follow-up. Life satisfaction scores for caregivers showed a trend in the opposite direction, however, with an increase in satisfaction from 24.25 ($SD = 6.73$) at 12 months to 25.16 ($SD = 5.94$) at 24 months. The difference in scores between spouses widened from being almost identical (0.46 points difference) at 12 months to being almost 3 points different (2.74 points) at 24 months.

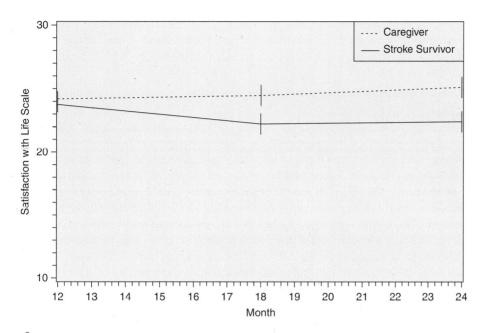

^aVertical bars represent the SEM of the mean for a group at a time point.

FIGURE A4.1   Mean Satisfaction With Life Scale (SWLS) scores over time for stroke survivors and spousal caregivers.

Predictors of Life Satisfaction in Stroke Survivors

Linear mixed model analysis of 12–24-month stroke survivor scores on the SWLS can be seen in Table A4.2. A significant decrease in life satisfaction occurred between 12 and 24 months ($p = .04$). The presence of depression at 12 months was a strong predictor of decreased life satisfaction. However, being older, having high scores on the mutuality scale and perceiving that they were recovering emotionally from the stroke (higher SIS emotion subscores) were all predictors of higher life satisfaction between 12 and 24 months after inpatient rehabilitation. None of these associations with stroke survivor life satisfaction were found to change significantly over time.

Predictors of Life Satisfaction in Spousal Caregivers

Linear mixed model analysis of 12-to-24-month caregiver SWLS scores showed an improvement in caregiver life satisfaction over time (slope estimate for time of .002 per day). This increase was not found to be statistically significant, however. Caregivers who perceived their health was poorer (higher scores on the Self-Rated Health Status Scale) and perceived greater stress (PSS score) at 12 months demonstrated decreased life satisfaction between 12 and 24 months. The negative association of PSS score with life satisfaction was found to change significantly over time ($p = .01$), with the estimate of the slope (.0005) indicating that this association became less negative over time. Increased caregiver life satisfaction was associated with increased 12-month Mutuality and Preparedness scores. Those who had a good relationship with their spouse and felt prepared for the caregiving role reported higher life satisfaction.

■ DISCUSSION

A global measure of QOL has become increasingly important as an adjunctive outcome of health care interventions. Satisfaction with health care and resultant satisfaction with living with a disability or chronic disease have become issues of interest to clinicians and researchers.

Scores on the SWLS in this sample of stroke survivors at 12 months were only slightly below the norms for older community-dwelling individuals (24.25; Pavot, Diener, Colvin, & Sandvik, 1991). Although some studies of long-term stroke survivors have found relatively high rates of life satisfaction (Lindmark & Hamrin, 1995), most studies have shown that life satisfaction norms are below those of the general population (Ostwald, 2008). The lack of large differences in this study is consistent with Campbell's (1981) assertion that most people seek to maximize their sense of well-being and perceive their life as positively as possible. Using a technique referred to as a "standard gamble," Hallan, Asberg, Indredavik, and Wideroe (1999) concluded that most stroke survivors did not view stroke as an overwhelming catastrophe.

This study, however, found that between 12 and 24 months after inpatient rehabilitation, life satisfaction scores declined in these stroke survivors. Poststroke depression at 12 months was a strong predictor of poor life satisfaction over the ensuing year. This is consistent with other studies that have found a strong relationship between poststroke depression and life satisfaction up to 3 years poststroke (Bays, 2001; Löfgren, Gustafson, & Nyberg, 1999). Physical function was not a significant predictor of life satisfaction in this study, as has been reported in other studies. However, these survivors may have experienced stagnation in their physical recovery, leading to depression and decreased life satisfaction, as reported by Teasdale and Engberg (2005) in their 5–15 year follow-up. Being older was associated with a higher level of life satisfaction. Others have reported that younger survivors may have additional social issues, including work and child care, that may negatively affect their life satisfaction (Teasell, McRae, & Finestone, 2000). Rehabilitation nurses need to be alert for signs of continuing poststroke depression and advocate for pharmacological, psychological, and social therapies that may help relieve depression and increase life satisfaction.

Spousal caregivers' mean on the SWLS was identical at 12 months (24.25) to the older community-dwelling population mean, and actually surpassed the population mean at 24 months. This is contrary to other studies that have reported significantly lower life satisfaction among caregivers at 12 months compared to the general population (Forsberg-Warleby et al., 2004). For caregivers, their own health, a perception of their preparedness for the caregiving role, and the stress associated with daily life were significantly related to life satisfaction. These findings suggest that preparation for the caregiving role is not a one-time event that occurs at the time of the stroke. Over time, the needs of stroke survivors change physically and emotionally, and the health status of caregivers may decline. Nurses encountering spousal caregivers need to continue to assess the caregiver's current knowledge, skills, and resources and provide appropriate learning opportunities and referrals. This education may focus on the caregiver's own health needs, needs of the stroke survivor, or stress-management techniques and community resources.

The only variable that was a significant predictor of life satisfaction for both stroke survivors and their spousal caregivers was their relationship. Couples who expressed a high degree of mutuality (e.g., love, enjoyment of each other) were most satisfied with their lives. This predictor did not change over time and was as strong at 24 months as it was at 12 months. Strokes occur within the context of an existing relationship, which may or may not be mutually rewarding. Although nurses cannot change a long-term marital relationship, they do need to be aware of the stresses that a stroke can place on any relationship. Research has demonstrated that physical and cognitive impairments, family dysfunction, lack of ability to communicate, and lack of ability to function socially or sexually may interfere with a couple's relationship, adjustment to the stroke, and life satisfaction (Clark & Smith, 1999; Eriksson, Tham, & Fugl-Meyer, 2005; Forsberg-Warleby et al., 2004; Korpelainen, Nieminen, & Myllyla, 1999).

Rehabilitation nurses need to help couples anticipate and cope with changes the stroke will cause in many areas of their lives. Although the rehabilitation team focuses on physical, cognitive, occupational, and speech therapy, nurses must also help couples access their strengths and challenges in terms of family support, their marital relationship, coping strategies, spiritual resources, lifestyle priorities, and financial and environmental challenges. Working with couples to increase long-term life satisfaction will require making realistic plans to meet short- and long-term challenges. Kautz (2007) provides excellent suggestions for ways in which rehabilitation nurses can intervene to effectively enhance intimacy among couples. Interventions to improve relationships often require an interdisciplinary effort that may include social workers, psychologists, clergy, and peer counselors, as well as referrals to community agencies and support groups.

■ LIMITATIONS

This study has two major limitations. First, the couples' satisfaction with life and the quality of their marital relationship were not known before the stroke, so it is not possible to know how much effect the stroke had on either life satisfaction or mutuality scores. Second, because life satisfaction was not measured until 12 months after discharge, it is not known whether life satisfaction changed in a positive or negative direction during the first 12 months after discharge. However, other studies that have looked at life satisfaction during the first 12 months have reported a negative impact of the stroke on life satisfaction of stroke survivors and their caregiving spouses.

■ IMPLICATIONS FOR REHABILITATION NURSES

This study has implications for rehabilitation nurses who are responsible for helping stroke survivors and their caregiving spouses experience long-term life satisfaction. Assessing stroke survivors for post-stroke depression during every encounter and providing continuing treatment may be an important strategy to increase life satisfaction. Stroke survivors who perceived that they were doing well emotionally at 12 months had higher levels of life satisfaction at 24 months, a further confirmation of the need to treat depression. Spousal caregivers who had good health felt confident about their caregiving ability, and those who reported less stress at 12 months had higher life satisfaction at 24 months. Nurses have an important role in teaching and supporting spouses in their caregiving roles and encouraging them to care for their own health. Finally, rehabilitation nurses need to be knowledgeable about stroke's effect on marital relationships and help couples identify challenges and develop realistic plans to minimize the negative effects of the stroke and strengthen their relationship as they face life after a stroke.

■ ACKNOWLEDGMENTS

This work was supported in part by the National Institutes of Health, National Institute for Nursing Research RO1 NR005316 (Sharon K. Ostwald, PI), and the Isla Carroll Turner Friendship Trust. The authors wish to thank Karen Janssen, MSN, RN, Celia Schulz, PhD, OTR, and Joan Wasserman, DrPH, RN, for their assistance with this project.

■ ABOUT THE AUTHORS

Sharon K. Ostwald, PhD, RN, FGSA, is a professor and Isla Carroll Turner Chair in Gerontological Nursing at University of Texas Health Science Center in Houston.

Kyler M. Godwin, MPH, is a research associate at the Center on Aging, School of Nursing, University of Texas in Houston.

Stanley G. Cron, MSPH, is a research instructor at the Center for Nursing Research at University of Texas Health Science Center in Houston.

References

American Heart Association. (2008). *Heart disease and stroke statistics.* Retrieved April 1, 2009, from www.americanheart.org/presenter.jhtml?identifier=1928

Anderson, C. S., Linto, J., & Stewart-Wynne, E. (1995). A population-based assessment of the impact and burden of care-giving for long-term stroke survivors. *Stroke, 26,* 843–849.

Archbold, P. G., Stewart, B. J., Greenlick, M. R., & Harvath, T. A. (1990). Mutuality and preparedness as predictors of care-giver role strain. *Research in Nursing & Health, 12,* 375–384.

Bays, C. L. (2001). Quality of life of stroke survivors: A research synthesis. *Journal of Neuroscience Nursing, 33*(6), 310–316.

Brown, H., & Prescott, R. (2006). *Applied mixed models in medicine* (2nd ed.). Hoboken, NJ: John Wiley & Sons.

Campbell, A. (1981). *The sense of well-being in America.* New York, NY: McGraw-Hill.

Carlsson, G. E., Forsberg-Warleby, G., Moller, A., & Blomstrand, C. (2007). Comparison of life satisfaction within couples one year after a partner's stroke. *Journal of Rehabilitation Medicine, 39*(3), 219–224.

Carter, J. H., Stewart, B. J., Archbold, P. G., Inoue, I., Jaglin, J., & Lannon, M., et al. (1998). Living with a person who has Parkinson's disease: The spouse's perspective by stage of disease. Parkinson's Study Group. *Movement Disorders, 13*(1), 20–28.

Clark, M. S., & Smith, D. S. (1999). Changes in family functioning for stroke rehabilitation patients and their families. *International Journal of Rehabilitation Research, 22*(3), 171–179.

Cohen, S., & Wills, T. A. (1985). Stress, social support, and the buffering hypothesis. *Psychological Bulletin, 98,* 310–357.

D'Ath, P., Katona, P., Mullan, E., Evans, S., & Katona, C. (1994). Screening, detection and management of depression in elderly primary care attenders. I: The acceptability and performance of the 15 item Geriatric Depression Scale (GDS15) and the development of short versions. *Family Practice, 11*(3), 260–266.

Diener, E. (1984). Subjective well-being. *Psychological Bulletin, 95*(3), 542–575.

Diener, E., Emmons, R., Larsen, R., & Griffen, S. (1985). The satisfaction with life scale. *Journal of Personality Assessment, 49*(1), 71–75.

Duncan, P. W., Wallace, D., Lai, S. M., Johnson, D., Embretson, S., & Laster, L. J. (1999). The stroke impact scale version 2.0. Evaluation of reliability, validity, and sensitivity to change. *Stroke, 30*(10), 2131–2140.

Eriksson, G. K., Tham, K., & Fugl-Meyer, A. R. (2005). Couples' happiness and its relationship to functioning in everyday life after brain injury. *Scandinavian Journal of Occupational Theapy, 12*(1), 40–48.

Forsberg-Warleby, G., Moller, A., & Blomstrand, C. (2004). Life satisfaction in spouses of patients with stroke during the first year after stroke. *Journal of Rehabilitation Medicine, 36*(1), 4–11.

Franzen-Dahlin, A., Larson, J., Murray, V., Wredling, R., & Billing, E. (2007). Predictors of psychological health in spouses of persons affected by stroke. *Journal of Clinical Nursing, 16,* 885–891.

Fredman, L., & Daly, M. P. (1997). Weight change: An indicator of caregiver stress. *Journal of Aging and Health, 9*(1), 43–69.

Gallagher-Thompson, D., Brooks, J. O., III, Bliwise, D., Leader, J., & Yesavage, J. A. (1992). The relations among caregiver stress, "sundowning" symptoms, and cognitive decline in Alzheimer's disease. *Journal of the American Geriatrics Society, 40*(8), 807–810.

Gottlieb, A., Golander, H., Bar-Tal, Y., & Gottlieb, D. (2001). The influence of social support and perceived control on handicap and quality of life after stroke. *Aging, 13*(1), 11–15.

Haley, W. E., LaMonde, L. A., Han, B., Burton, A. M., & Schonwetter, R. (2003). Predictors of depression and life satisfaction among spousal caregivers in hospice: Application of a stress process model. *Journal of Palliative Medicine, 6*(2), 215–224.

Hallan, S., Asberg, A., Indredavik, B., & Wideroe, T. E. (1999). Quality of life after cerebrovascular stroke: A systematic study of patients' preferences for different functional outcomes. *Journal of Internal Medicine, 246*(3), 309–316.

Hollingshead, A. (1979). *Four factor index of social status.* Unpublished manuscript.

Idler, E. L., & Benyamini, Y. (1997). Self-rated health and mortality: A review of twenty-seven community studies. *Journal of Health & Social Behavior, 38*(1), 21–37.

Jones, V. N. (2006). The forgotten survivor [Electronic version]. *Stroke Smart.* Retrieved April 1, 2009, from www.stroke.org/site/PageServer?pagename=SS_MAG_so2006_feature_forgot

Kautz, D. D. (2007). Hope for love: Practical advice for intimacy and sex after stroke. *Rehabilitation Nursing, 32*(3), 95–103.

Keir, S. T., Guill, A. B., Carter, K. E., Boole, L. C., Gonzales, L., & Friedman, H. S. (2006). Differential levels of stress in care-givers of brain tumor patients—Observations from a pilot study. *Supportive Care in Cancer, 14*(12), 1258–1261.

King, R. (1996). Quality of life after stroke. *Stroke, 27,* 1467–1472.

Korpelainen, J. T., Nieminen, P., & Myllyla, V. V. (1999). Sexual functioning among stroke patients and their spouses. *Stroke, 30,* 715–719.

Lau, A., & McKenna, K. (2001). Conceptualizing quality of life for elderly people with a stroke. *Disability & Rehabilitation, 23*(6), 227–238.

Lindmark, B., & Hamrin, E. (1995). A five-year follow-up of stroke survivors: Motor function and activities of daily living. *Clinical Rehabilitation, 9*(1), 1–9.

Löfgren, B., Gustafson, Y., & Nyberg, L. (1999). Psychological well-being 3 years after severe stroke. *Stroke, 30*, 567–572.

Low, J. T. S., Payne, S., & Roderick, P. (1999). The impact of stroke on informal carers: A literature review. *Social Science & Medicine, 49*, 711–725.

Lucas, R. E., Clark, A. E., Georgellis, Y., & Diener, E. (2003). Reexamining adaptation and the set point model of happiness: Reactions to changes in marital status. *Journal of Personality & Social Psychology, 84*(3), 527–539.

McCallum, T. J., Sorocco, K. H., & Fritsch, T. (2006). Mental health and diurnal salivary cortisol patterns among African American and European American femal dementia family caregivers. *American Journal of Geriatric Psychiatry, 14*(8), 684–693.

Miilunpalo, S., Vuori, I., Oja, P., Pasanen, M., & Urponen, H. (1997). Self-rated health status as a health measure: The predictive value of self-reported health status on the use of physician services and on mortality in the working-age population. *Journal of Clinical Epidemiology, 50*(5), 517–528.

Musschenga, A. W. (1997). The relation between concepts of quality-of-life, health and happiness. *Journal of Medicine & Philosophy, 22*(1), 11–28.

Ostwald, S. K. (2008). Predictors of life satisfaction among stroke survivors and spousal caregivers: A narrative review. *Aging Health, 4*(3), 241–252.

Ostwald, S. K., Davis, S. D., Hersch, G., Kelley, C., & Godwin, K. M. (2008). Evidence-based educational guidelines for stroke survivors following discharge home. *Journal of Neuroscience Nursing, 40*(3), 173–179, 191.

Palmer, S., & Glass, T. (2003). Family function and stroke recovery: A review. *Rehabilitation Psychology, 48*, 255–265.

Pavot, W., Diener, E., Colvin, R., & Sandvik, E. (1991). Further validation of the Satisfaction with Life Scale: Evidence for the cross-method convergence of well-being measures. *Journal of Personality Assessment, 57*(1), 149–161.

SAS Institute Inc. (2004). SAS Online Doc® 9.1.3. Retrieved May 6, 2009, from http://support.sas.com/documentation/onlinedoc/91pdf/index.html

Schimmack, U., Diener, E., & Oishi, S. (2002). Life-satisfaction is a momentary judgment and a stable personality characteristic: The use of chronically accessible and stable sources. *Journal of Personality, 70*(3), 345–384.

Schultz, C., Wasserman, J., & Ostwald, S. K. (2006). Recruitment and retention of stroke survivors: The CAReS experience. *Journal of Physical & Occupational Therapy in Geriatrics, 25*(2), 17–29.

Sheikh, J. I., & Yesavage, J. A. (1986). Geriatric Depression Scale: Recent evidence and development of a shorter version. *Clinical Gerontology, 5*, 165–173.

Tabachnick, B. G., & Fidell, L. S. (2001). *Using multivariate statistics* (4th ed.). Needham Heights, MA: Allyn & Bacon.

Teasdale, T. W., & Engberg, A. W. (2005). Psychological consequences of stroke: A long-term population-base follow-up. *Brain Injury, 19*(12), 1049–1058.

Teasell, R. W., McRae, M. P., & Finestone, H. M. (2000). Social issues in the rehabilitation of younger stroke patients. *Archives of Physical Medicine and Rehabilitation, 81*(2), 205–209.

Veenhoven, R. (2000). The four qualities of life. *Journal of Happiness Studies, 1*(1), 1–39.

Visser-Meily, A., Post, M., Schepers, V., & Lindeman, E. (2005). Spouses' quality of life 1 year after stroke: Prediction at the start of clinical rehabilitation. *Cerebrovascular Diseases, 20*(6), 443–448.

Viitanen, M., Fugl-Meyer, K. S., Bernspang, B., & Fugl-Meyer, A. R. (1988). Life satisfaction in long-term survivors after stroke. *Scandinavian Journal of Rehabilitative Medicine, 20*(1), 17–24.

White, C. L., Poissant, L., Cote-LeBlanc, G., & Wood-Dauphinee, S. (2006). Long-term caregiving after stroke: The impact on caregivers' quality of life. *Journal of Neuroscience Nursing, 38*(5), 354–360.

■ COMMENTARY

Cathy L. Bays, PhD, RN

Ostwald, Godwin, and Cron's research on predictors of life satisfaction in stroke survivors and their spousal caregivers is important because of its population and research design (see this issue's Continuing Education article on page 160). As the authors state, the majority of the approximate 6 million stroke survivors in the United States live at home with family. Moreover, strokes are the leading cause of serious, long-term disability in the United States (American Heart Association, 2009), affecting four out of five American families (National Stroke Association, 2009). This study's research design was important because few studies have followed stroke survivors for longer than 12 months, and even fewer have looked at life satisfaction in their caregiving spouses. Plus, this new study's 24-month longitudinal design included both survivors and their caregivers, which yielded a diverse sample and added to the existing body of knowledge on life satisfaction of stroke survivors and caregivers.

Ostwald, Godwin, and Cron's article identified feasible practice implications. Their suggestions for translating research into practice center around mutuality, survivor depression, caregiver preparation, and future research. Because mutuality was the one significant predictor of life satisfaction for both stroke survivors and caregivers, assessing the quality of relationships before stroke and designing interventions that strengthen relationships are essential practice and research areas of emphasis. The authors also advocate for early intervention with depressive symptoms. The strong correlation between life satisfaction and depression in stroke survivors warrants implementation of intensive primary preventative strategies to maintain and enhance the mental health of stroke survivors before depressive symptoms arise. Expanding on the authors' recommendation, specific intensive attention needs to be given to the initial preparation for and continual refinement of responsibilities in the dynamic caregiving role. Future research that can replicate and expand this study design to begin at stroke onset, continue for 3–5 years poststroke, and include stroke survivors with nonspousal caregivers will further enhance knowledge on life satisfaction in stroke survivors and their caregivers.

References

American Heart Association. (2009). *Stroke rehabilitation.* Retrieved May 7, 2009, from www.americanheart.org/presenter.jhtml?identifier=4713

National Stroke Association. (2009). *Caregivers and families.* Retrieved May 7, 2009, from www.stroke.org/site/PageServer?pagename=CARE

APPENDIX A-5

The Use of Narratives to Identify Characteristics Leading to a Productive Life Following Acquired Brain Injury

Michael R. Fraas, Margaret Calvert
University of New Hampshire, Durham

Purpose: *To determine the factors leading to successful recovery and productive lifestyles after acquired brain injury (ABI).*

Method: *Qualitative investigation examined semistructured interviews of 31 survivors of ABI. Thematic analysis followed a phenomenological approach and revealed 4 major themes and 28 subthemes in the interviews. Four participants stood out as exemplars of the themes embodied by all the participants in this investigation. Quotes from each are used to highlight the prevailing themes.*

Results: *The following 4 major themes emerged from the interviews: development of social support networks, grief and coping strategies, acceptance of the injury and redefinition of self, and empowerment.*

Conclusions: *The issues raised in these interviews may serve to inspire other survivors and provide them with hope and motivation as they progress through the recovery process. Suggestions on how clinicians can help to facilitate this process are discussed.*

Keywords: *acquired brain injury, narrative stories, identity, quality of life, community integration.*

Acquired brain injury (ABI) affects the lives of millions of Americans each year (Centers for Disease Control, 2006; Kissela et al., 2001; Langlois et al., 2003; Thurman, Alverson, Dunn, Guerrero, & Sniezek, 1999). ABI is the result of physical, functional, or metabolic change to the integrity of the brain not due to congenital, hereditary, or degenerative causes (Brain Injury Association of America, 2008). The causes of ABI can include trauma, vascular disruption, stroke, infectious disease, and tumor. The prevalence of ABI survivors continues to grow because of medical advances that have decreased the mortality rate for survivors (Sneed & Davis, 2002). In addition, people are living longer with their injuries, with life expectancies closing in on those of the uninjured population (Warren, Wrigley, & Yoels, 1996).

Many survivors of ABI face the challenge of a loss of identity, due to their many limitations, including physical, cognitive, and emotional function. This loss has a tremendous impact on the survivors' ability to integrate back into their communities and have a productive and meaningful quality of life. For many survivors, the struggle to integrate back into their communities is insurmountable. They have difficulties developing and maintaining relationships, they are no longer able to return to their previous occupations, and they report an increase in emotional dysfunction (Dawson & Chipman, 1995). However, many other survivors of ABI do go on to integrate into their communities and live productive and fulfilling

Source: American Journal of Speech-Language Pathology, November 2009, Vol. 18, 315–328.

lives. These individuals appear to redefine themselves, releasing the concepts of their former selves and developing new identities (Ellis-Hill & Horn, 2000; Tyerman & Humphrey, 1984). The sense of optimism, empowerment, and contentment in the face of continuing physical, cognitive, and emotional disability is inspiring.

What accounts for this ability to reestablish identity and overcome these persistent challenges? Ylvisaker and Feeney (1998) developed a comprehensive approach to meeting these needs that was based on a number of theoretical models. As the researchers incorporated the theoretical concepts into their clinical practices, they were able to determine a series of critical themes that lead to successful rehabilitation. Two themes in particular seem to relate strongly to the idea of establishing a new identity in order to achieve an enhanced quality of life. These include engagement in meaningful life activities and reconstruction of a satisfying sense of self (Ylvisaker & Feeney, 2000). The authors indicated that survivors are likely to be unsuccessful if they are not engaged in meaningful types of activities. In addition, abilities and activities of a survivor can be enhanced by restructuring their "schematic model of self." According to Ylvisaker and Feeney (2000), two theories help to explain these findings: the interacting cognitive subsystems approach (Teasdale & Barnard, 1993) and the self-as-metaphor hypothesis (Lakoff & Johnson, 1999).

The Teasdale and Barnard (1993) model illustrates two codes that encode for higher levels of meaning: the propositional and implicational codes. These two codes are responsible for storing explicit and implicit information, respectively. The propositional codes refer to semantic information and are tied to specific facts that can be verified (e.g., "I have a brain injury"). The implicational code is linked with emotions and affect, which can have an influence on the development of personal beliefs in oneself. The meanings developed by the implicational system are not the result of literal language but develop through the expression of linguistic styles such as metaphor, poetry, imagery, and narrative. Implicational codes can be expressed as either positive (e.g., "I am able") or negative beliefs (e.g., "I am disabled"), which can either motivate or stifle the survivor's progress (Teasdale, 1997). Implicational codes can not only motivate an individual but also lead to positive decision making and action (Ylvisaker & Feeney, 2000).

Another theory that helps to explain how individuals can reestablish their identities is the self-as-metaphor model developed by Lakoff and Johnson (1999). According to this model, all thinking about the self is metaphorical. This metaphorical manner of identity construction can be accomplished in a positive or negative fashion as well. As a survivor progresses through rehabilitation, his or her mental model of the self is ever evolving. Positive and negative emotions can lead to the development of positive and negative perceptions of the self, respectively. For the survivor to successfully reconstruct a positive and effective identity, the goals and the activities he or she pursues for attaining them must be consistent with his or her mental model of self.

In addition to the theoretical models posited above, a number of clinical studies have reported factors that also influence the ability of survivors of ABI to reestablish their identities and begin living a productive and meaningful quality of life. Addressing the interplay between cognitive processes such as memory and executive function and emotional concerns such as anxiety and depression has been linked to improved identity (Dewar & Gracey, 2007), as well as the individual's ability to integrate into the community, display a positive affect, and establish social support networks (Kalpakjian, Lam, Toussaint, & Merbitz, 2004). Meanwhile, negative sense of self, reduced social activity, and psychological morbidity lead to an inability to successfully reconstruct identity and live meaningful lives (Ellis-Hill & Horn, 2000). Steadman-Pare and colleagues reported the need for ongoing support for survivors of ABI many years after onset of injury to help integrate them into their communities, provide them with emotional support, and give them opportunities for work and leisure (Steadman-Pare, Colantonio, Ratcliff, Chase, & Vernich, 2001).

Clinical investigations such as these have provided us with significant evidence outlining the issues associated with successful reconstruction of identity and recovery from ABI; however, they fall short of providing us with a holistic perspective of the struggles that these individuals face in trying to live a productive and satisfying life. Narratives can provide the reader with a glimpse into the physical, psychological, social, and economic impact of an injury and how that injury affects the individual, the family, and the community (Greenhalgh & Collard, 2003).

Narratives can be used to effectively shape our own identities and to share with others the critical characteristics of ourselves (Thorne & McLean, 2003). The evolutionary psychologist Steven Pinker has argued that stories (i.e., narratives) are an important tool for learning and developing relationships with others in one's own social group (Pinker, 2007). Narratives are stories that allow us to conceptualize our lives and our identities and share them with others. In the clinical setting, our interactions with our clients become incorporated into their identities, becoming part of their life story. Difficult to define moments in the clinical process can be explored using a narrative approach (Hinckley, 2008). The stories that emerge from these encounters can be used as effective tools for educating colleagues, students, and other clients.

Hinckley examined published narratives to answer the question "What does it take to live successfully with stroke and aphasia?" (Hinckley, 2006). Four major themes emerged from Hinckley's analysis: the need for social support, adaptation of perception of self, lifelong goal setting, and taking charge of communication improvement. She concluded that the stories that emerged from these narratives can provide clinician, client, and community member alike with an enhanced sense of understanding the rehabilitation process.

Case study illustrations can also be used as an effective means of educating individuals about the rehabilitation process. Ylvisaker and Feeney (1996) used this approach to highlight the effectiveness of a community-based remediation of executive dysfunction following traumatic brain injury (TBI). The authors identified seven themes that emerged from these illustrations that defend their proposal for "supported cognition" to remediate executive dysfunction (Ylvisaker & Feeney, 1996).

The purpose of this investigation is to establish and report the shared characteristics of survivors who have demonstrated successful recovery from ABI and who indicate that they live productive lives. Interviews were conducted with members of a community-based, postrehabilitation day program for adults with ABI. Several themes emerged from these narratives that were reported as necessary for living a productive and successful life. Individual case study accounts will serve as exemplars of the qualities exhibited by study participants. It is felt that this research will lend significant insight into the challenges and the triumphs faced by survivors of ABI. In addition, it is hoped that the findings from this investigation can facilitate a means of education among clinicians, students, clients, and the general public about the journey through the brain injury recovery process.

■ METHOD

Participants

The participants in this investigation formed a convenience sample. They included members of a community-based, postrehabilitation program for adults with ABI. The program provides members with an opportunity to address their long-term physical, cognitive, social, emotional, and vocational needs. The 31 members who participated are survivors of ABI. Twenty-one (68%) are male, and 10 (32%) female. Their ages ranged from 21 to 66, with an average age of 43.52 (SD = 13.53) years. Their diagnoses comprised cerebral vascular accident (CVA; $n = 11$, 35.5%), TBI ($n = 16$, 51.6%), and other ($n = 4$, 12.9%; includes seizure disorder and tumor).

The participants had an average time after injury onset of 124.89 (SD = 101.93) months (range = 22–432 months). They were members of the program for an average of 37.81 (SD = 23.17) months (range = 8 72 months). The majority of participants had a high school education ($n = 14$, 45.2%), 1 participant had less than 8 years of school (1.5%), 3 reported 8–11 years of school (9.7%), 5 had a postsecondary degree (16.1%), 5 had a college degree (16.1%), and 3 participants reported an advanced degree (9.7%). Demographic information is displayed in Table A5.1.

The Neurobehavioral Functioning Inventory (NFI; Kreutzer, Seel, & Marwitz, 1999) was administered to each participant to provide an indication of level of functioning. Six domains are included: depression, somatic, attention/memory, communication, aggression, and motor abilities. The NFI was selected because it allows the researcher to collect information on a wide spectrum of behaviors and symptoms commonly associated with ABI. It is a useful measure for evaluating health-related quality of life. The measure consists of

Table A5.1

Participants' Demographic Information

GENDER	AGE	TIME AFTER INJURY (MONTHS)	PROGRAM DURATION (MONTHS)	EDUCATION (YEARS)	DIAGNOSIS		
					TBI	CVA	OTHER
Male ($n = 21$)	43.10	109.36	35.76	12.95	11	8	2
SD	12.25	101.85	23.18	3.01			
Female ($n = 10$)	44.40	157.50	42.10	13.80	5	3	2
SD	16.61	99.19	23.78	2.39			

Note. Program duration is time (in months) that participants were involved in a community-based program. TBI, traumatic brain injury; CVA, cerebral vascular accident; OTHER, tumor or seizure disorder.

Table A5.2

Mean *t* Scores and Standard Deviations for Participants in Neurobehavioral Functioning Inventory (NFI) Domains, and Percentage of Participants Scoring Within Normed Data Ranges

SCORE	NFI DOMAIN					
	D	S	A/M	C	A	M
Normed *t*-score range	47.16	48.32	48.42	51.61	50.61	50.67
SD > or < M	9.07	8.71	9.27	11.11	8.20	10.50
Very high ≥ 65 (>1.5 SDs > M)	0%	0%	0%	3%	3%	0%
High = 57–65 (>2/3 SDs > M)	19%	16%	23%	26%	23%	51%
Average = 44–56 (2/3 SDs > or < M)	49%	65%	58%	45%	51%	23%
Low = 35–43 (>2/3 SDs < M)	19%	13%	3%	16%	23%	16%
Very low ≤ 35 (>1.5 SDs < M)	13%	6%	16%	10%	0%	10%

Note. Normed *t*-score range is from NFI (Kreutzer et al., 1999). D, depression; S, somatic; A/M, attention/memory; C, communication; A, aggression; M, motor abilities.

76 items that measure the frequency of behaviors on a 5-point Likert scale including never, rarely, sometimes, often, and always. Cronbach's alpha analysis of the NFI indicates high internal reliability for all scales ranging from .86 to .95. Administration of the NFI takes approximately 30 min.

Group *t*-score means and standard deviations for each NFI domain are provided in Table A5.2. In addition, normed *t*-score ranges (with standard deviations above or below the mean) are provided for comparison (Kreutzer et al., 1999). The percentage of participants in this investigation who fell into each of those normed ranges is provided. For example, participants in this investigation had an average t score of 51.61 (SD = 11.11) on the NFI communication domain. Compared with other patients of similar age and injury severity, a "very high" score on this domain would be a *t* score greater than or equal to 66, or >1.5 SDs above the normed *t*-score mean. Only 3% of the participants in this investigation demonstrated *t* scores on the communication domain that were in this range. Similarly, 26% of our participants scored in the high range between 57 and 65 (>2/3 SDs above the mean), 45% scored in the average range, 16% in the low range, and 10% in the very low range (>1.5 SDs below the normed *t*-score mean).

Interviews

The data used for this qualitative investigation consisted of narrative life stories collected as part of the ABI program's Oral History Project. Participants volunteered to be a part of the project, which was developed as a way for members to share their stories with each other and to educate the community about ABI. At the time of this investigation, 31 of approximately 160 registered members had been interviewed. The 31 participants represent a core group of members who attend the program on a regular basis (i.e., weekly). No members were excluded from participating. Members who had not participated by the time of this investigation either declined to participate or were unable to be interviewed due to scheduling constraints.

Although not a perfect means for ensuring external validity, it is felt that the heterogeneity of these 31 participants provides an accurate reflection of not only the membership at large (the 160 total members) but also the greater brain injury community in general. One caveat to this would be their membership in the community-based day program for adults with ABI. This issue will be addressed below.

Thirty of the 31 participants provided answers to interview questions independently. One participant, who displayed severe memory impairment secondary to tumor resection, was assisted by his father in answering some of the questions. Two members, whose speech was unintelligible secondary to dysarthria following TBI, used augmentative and alternative communication devices to assist them in providing their answers. All participants provided informed consent to allow their responses to be used for research purposes.

Each oral history was conducted as a semistructured interview between two members of the program. The interviews were facilitated by one of the researchers (the second author), who provided technical assistance (e.g., help with recording equipment) and facilitated the cognitive-linguistic needs of members when required (e.g., help with word finding). Following informed consent, interview participants were provided a list of the interview questions. Any questions or concerns that they had were addressed at this time.

The interviews were conducted by members of the program as well. Therefore, members interviewed members. Six members interviewed between 2 and 10 members each, making up the total 31 interviews evaluated for this study. Each interviewer provided his or her oral history (i.e., interview) before conducting an interview. This served to decrease the risk that responses from a previous interview influenced future responses by a participant (i.e., interviewee). The interviewers offered to serve in this capacity; they were not selected for any particular reason. Scheduling dictated, more than anything, who interviewed whom. No one was denied an opportunity to interview if he or she inquired.

Interviewers were provided with a list of eight questions that served as a framework for the interview. This provided an element of structure; however, the interviewers were free to explore other issues in further detail as they arose. Interviewers were provided with guidelines for conducting the interviews. They were instructed to follow the framework of the interview questions but were encouraged to provide follow-up questions at any time. The interview facilitator did not direct the interviewer or interviewee but was present to ensure that the conversation did not diverge too far off topic. If the conversation did diverge too far from the eight-question interview framework, the facilitator asked the interviewer to provide the next question on the list.

The eight-question framework (see Appendix A5.A) was developed by the researchers as a means of capturing a picture of the interviewees' lives before and after their injuries. In addition, the questions were designed to explore how long-term deficits affect other areas of functioning and recovery. These deficits (e.g., communication, physical, and emotional) have been found many years after injury onset (Corrigan, Whiteneck, & Mellick, 2004; Kaitaro, Koskinen, & Kaipio, 1995; O'Connor, Colantonio, & Polatajko, 2005). The questions also probed for information regarding the member's life prior to the injury, what happened to him or her (i.e., the accident), the recovery process, challenges he or she continued to face, and current goals. All eight questions were responded to by each interviewee. Interviews lasted between 7 and 45 min, depending on expressive abilities and content shared.

Interviews were recorded digitally on a Sony Hi-MD Walkman Digital Music Player MZ-RH910 using Microphone Madness MM-BSM-7 Binaural Stereo microphones.

The interviews were then edited to eliminate personally identifying information and/or offensive language.

Data Analysis

This qualitative investigation examined semistructured interviews of members of a community-based, postrehabilitation program for adults with ABI. Qualitative analysis was used because of its effectiveness in providing subjective interpretations of successful quality of life reported by survivors of ABI (Glover, 2003; Koskinen, 1998). The interviews were transcribed by a graduate student who was instructed on transcription methods. The interviews were analyzed following Seidman's phenomenological approach to interviewing as qualitative research (Seidman, 1998).

The authors began with a random sample of nine interviews. Each transcribed interview was analyzed, and extensive field notes were taken. This approach was chosen because the case study has been considered a "transparadigmatic and transdisciplinary heuristic that involves the careful delineation of the phenomena for which evidence is being collected" (VanWynsberghe & Khan, 2007). In other words, the case study is a universally accepted paradigm that allows the researcher to circumscribe the unit of analysis.

Thematic analysis was completed using manual techniques associated with theme coding and theme grouping (Seidman, 1998). First, interesting ideas were identified from these initial interviews. The winnowing process continued by grouping the ideas into categories. As the categories began to emerge from this analysis, names for these categories (i.e., themes) began to arise. We independently identified the list of categories from each of the nine interviews as they emerged, and we avoided using past experience or knowledge of the literature to identify categories. This approach lends itself to this process because it prohibits the researcher from stating the unit of analysis at the outset of the research. The unit of analysis must come into focus as the research progresses (VanWynsberghe & Khan, 2007).

The authors compared their findings with each other and, subsequently, were able to extract 28 subthemes from the raw data. Successive analysis by the authors hierarchically coded the subthemes into major themes. Four major themes emerged, and definitions were applied to each. For example, statements were coded into "social support networks" if they included any of the subthemes initially identified. A mutual agreement was reached between authors on the identification and naming of themes.

Four main themes emerged from the data analysis. The first is the need for strong social support networks composed of family and the community. Second, participants indicated that the ability to cope with their situation and control their emotions was an important factor in their success after their injury. Third, acceptance of the "new self" was important to

Table A5.3

Major Themes Leading to Successful Recovery From Acquired Brain Injury and Subsequent Productive Lives as Reported by Study Participants		
	PARTICIPANTS	
THEME	N	%
1. Social support networks	27	87
2. Grief and coping	30	98
3. Acceptance of injury and redefinition of self	26	84
4. Empowerment	18	58

a successful and productive life postinjury. Finally, participants indicated that they engaged in activities that brought them a sense of empowerment.

The authors subsequently used the four themes as a checklist, which they applied to each of the 31 transcribed interviews. If the theme was identified in the participant's interview, a check was placed in the column for that theme. Reliability analysis to determine whether an interviewee reported a particular theme was conducted by the authors, who independently reviewed each interview. The authors came to a 97% agreement in identifying which themes were acknowledged in each interview ($M = 120$, SD $= 0.033$, range $= 118–122$). The percentage of members who reported that theme was calculated for each. See Table A5.3 for a list of themes and the percentage of members who reported it in their interviews.

Case Studies

From the initial sample of 31 interviews, 4 case studies were chosen that gave defined examples of each of these themes in very different individuals with highly contrasting situations. These 4 individuals were selected from the pool of 31 interviews because they stood out as exemplars of the themes embodied by all the participants in this investigation. Based on personal experience with each of these participants, the researchers agreed that the 4 could best speak to the issues raised by the 31 participants. In addition, these 4 reported each of the four themes in their interviews, and they were leading what they reported as successful and productive lives. The stories from these individuals serve as expert accounts of life following ABI and the struggle to make a successful recovery and live a productive life.

The 4 participants highlighted in this investigation were contacted either in person or by telephone to supply follow-up information. Participants were asked to clarify statements made in their interviews and to provide demographic and medical history information. The participants provided informed consent to have their stories recounted in this article.

Case Study Participants

Participant 1.   Participant 1 was 55 years old when he suffered a left hemisphere CVA. Prior to his accident, he was married, employed as a certified public accountant, and actively involved in his local town political system. Participant 1 was in a coma for 3 weeks and hospitalized for 6 months, where he received speech, occupational, and physical therapy. He continued to receive speech therapy for 4 years after his accident, about which he said, "There must have been a screwup with insurance for me to receive so much therapy." However, he credited his current level of expressive language to his extended access to speech therapy. Participant 1 continues to exhibit expressive language problems and hemiparesis of the right side of his body; however, he is effective with oral communication, and he walks with the use of a cane.

Participant 1 has been a member of the ABI program since its inception in 2000. He leads the weekly aphasia support group at the ABI program and also facilitates a monthly aphasia support group within the greater community. Participant 1 has been honored by the National Aphasia Association for his work in advocating for individuals with aphasia. He remains married. He recently received a grant allowing him to develop an advocacy video to educate law enforcement and emergency medical personnel on the characteristics of aphasia.

Participant 2. Participant 2 was 25 years old when she suffered a cerebellar stroke on the day after Christmas. She had been married for 1 year and had recently completed a master's degree in social work. She reported, "I was in the best shape of my life at the time and was playing professional women's football." She was taken to a hospital for what her family thought was dehydration. A nurse in the emergency room refused to give her a wheelchair because she suspected that Participant 2 was "having a drug overdose." A doctor finally diagnosed the onset of a stroke, and an emergency craniotomy was ordered. Participant 2 reported that she was not in a coma, but she was hospitalized and received extensive rehabilitation services for 6 months.

Participant 2 became involved in the ABI program after a friend of the family made the recommendation. She has been involved for 4 years and helps facilitate several mental health groups offered to members during the programming week. She remains married. She marked the fifth anniversary of her stroke by completing the Honolulu, HI, marathon sponsored by the American Heart Association, an organization with which she has begun work as a stroke spokeswoman.

Participant 3. Participant 3 was 26 years old when an aneurysm ruptured as the result of an arterial venous malformation (AVM). Participant 3 was bilingual (French and English) and worked as a cook and caterer for a local restaurant. He had recently begun a business selling gourmet salad dressings, which was beginning to gain him some regional attention. The day of his AVM, Participant 3 had planned to quit his job at the restaurant and focus all his energies on his business.

Following his accident, Participant 3 went through multiple surgeries to repair his AVM. He was in a coma for 4 weeks. When he emerged from coma, he received several months of intensive rehabilitation before being sent home. His doctors and therapists informed Participant 3 that he would "never walk or talk again." Four years later, he found a speech pathologist willing to address his language deficits. In the 12 years since his AVM, Participant 3 has made significant recovery. He continues to demonstrate mild right-sided hemiparesis (upper and lower extremities) and to display expressive language difficulties when speaking English, although he ambulates independently and uses oral language to communicate. He has never regained the ability to speak French, his first language.

Participant 3 became involved in a local brain injury support group that was the foundation for the ABI program, and he has been a member since 2000. He was able to go back to school and subsequently gained a degree as a master gardener. He works part-time landscaping gardens for family and friends, although he reports that he is unable to work full-time because "I will lose my [federally funded] disability compensation." Participant 3 facilitates several functional skill training groups at the ABI program, including gardening and cooking.

Participant 4. Participant 4 was 21 years old when he sustained a TBI in a motor vehicle accident. The driver of the car in which he was riding fell asleep at the wheel. Participant 4 was thrown from the car and sustained multiple injuries and remained in a coma for several weeks. After emerging from his coma, he received speech, occupational, and physical therapy for "6 months, five times a week." Participant 4 continues to exhibit short-term memory impairment and word-finding problems, and reports difficulty "remembering names and faces."

Prior to his accident, Participant 4 fathered a son at the age of 15 years. He indicated that he did not have a good relationship with his family and was often in trouble. "I was a bad person, I was an unhappy person," he reported. Since his accident, Participant 4 now feels that he is a better father and is more involved as a family member. "I'm a much better person now; I have a better relationship with my family." Participant 4 has been involved with the ABI program for 2 years. He has recently gained competitive employment and moved into his own apartment.

■ RESULTS

Numerous subthemes ($N = 28$) were identified from analysis of the transcribed interviews. These subthemes were then organized into four main themes: development of social support networks, grief and coping, acceptance of injury and redefinition of self, and empowerment. Themes and subthemes are defined in Appendix A5.B. Included is the percentage of participants who reported each theme and subtheme. Introductions to each theme, and supporting quotes from the 4 exemplar case studies, are provided below. Several subthemes were expressed with more frequency among the participants. These prominent subthemes will be specifically addressed under their corresponding main theme. Additionally, there were a few subthemes that overlapped with some of the more prominent subthemes; they too will be discussed briefly.

Social Support Networks

Social support networks were an important variable reported by participants in redeveloping a productive life following ABI. However, during the initial recovery period, participants were not always able to maintain strong social support networks, particularly with friends. The majority of the 31 participants (71%) indicated that social support networks began to deteriorate following recovery from their injuries.

> I used to have a huge cluster of friends, and now I do have a handful of friends and everybody else is an acquaintance, [be]cause I now understand I don't know how many

people thought they would come and support me in rehab and how many didn't, not very much. (Participant 3)

I've lost friends because they can't deal with this. But, but that's what goes on. (Participant 1)

Sometimes this deterioration of social supports was the result of emotional distress felt by the survivors that was associated with changes in cognitive, linguistic, or physical functioning following their accident. Participant 4 expressed how his aphasia hastened fear and anxiety that limited his ability to maintain friendships with former peers:

Other friends I don't like to talk to. Most people don't understand aphasia. I'm always scared that people think I'm dumb. But I'm not. They just don't understand about the aphasia. So I would rather not to talk with other people. It really upsets me. Sometimes with strangers it doesn't really bother me because I'm never going to see them again. Who cares?

In addition, dating was an act identified by several participants (19%) that brought them a tremendous amount of anxiety following their injuries. Participant 4 indicated that one of his primary goals was to develop the confidence to date again:

I would love to find a girlfriend. That would be the absolute best thing. It has been 2 years, 22 years since my accident. That is one thing that I can't do is go over and ask a girl to go out. I have to be strong with myself, but it's hard. When I would go ask someone it would make me very worried.

Role of Family in Recovery.   Despite the initial challenges of maintaining social support networks faced by the participants in this analysis, they reported strong bonds with immediate family and friends. In fact, 87% of the participants in this investigation reported that strong support (e.g., family and friends) was a key to their successful recovery. In all of the interviews, a deep sense of gratitude toward friends and family was seen. Survivors knew the extent of sacrifice that their loved ones made and also what they continued to do to make their life easier. Each exhibited a deep sense of understanding that it was because of this sacrifice that they were able to be where they were.

And that was the strength of my family to be that way so after they did my operations they had to do rehabs. Well, I went from Boston to Concord. They did their best. We are a strong-willed family. (Participant 3)

I'm a better person because I realize that my family are the most important people. Not my old friends, not people who I thought were cool. It was my family that cared about me, that did things for me. I am different, and I try to be as nice to my family as I can. (Participant 4)

I don't understand how we were able to make this. I give this [credit] to my wife, she the biggest [best]. Yesterday I was down, crying. She got me and she said you know, listen, it's okay; think how you were last year or 2 years ago. You're doing fine, you know. She had to keep reminding me of everything. (Participant 1)

Marriage.   Marriage survival was an issue that, for some, was instrumental to the recovery process (16%). Participants 1 and 2 were both married at the time of their injuries. They continued to be married at the time of the interviews.

I'm grateful that we made it, and you ask me how it's going now, and it's wonderful. We're in love. (Participant 1) [My husband] was the source of my strength throughout the recovery process. I know that the divorce rate for many survivors is quite high, which makes our ability to stay together that much more special. (Participant 2)

Importance of Supports for Family. Finally, participants felt that the ability of their families to provide support was directly affected by the extent to which the family members themselves had access to caregiver supports and resources (61%).

I think the caregivers have a tougher job than the patients. At least in my case because they have to deal with "Yes, your loved one has a problem, and she, he may not live, but you have to keep going," and she had to take on the burden. (Participant 1)

Grief and Coping Following ABI

Nincty-eight percent of the interviewees reported that grief was a prominent issue in their recovery process and that modification of coping strategies (e.g., religious beliefs or spirituality) was a necessary requirement for their success. As Participant 3 said, "When I first came to [the ABI program], I had so much anger and frustration and I couldn't speak much; it was really hard."

Grief. The participants in this study reported a progression though several stages of grieving before they were able to accept their postinjury self. This progression was necessary for the survivor to understand the emotional procession of accepting the changes in his or her life. The stages of grief reported by the participants included denial (87%), anger (84%), and depression (84%).

I thought for at least a year that I, um, everybody else, they were either faking or they were, um, it wasn't me and it was a dream, or something is wrong with them. (Participant 1)
Well it took me almost 3 years to fully embrace and understand that this is my life now. (Participant 2)
And it took me a long time to realize that wait a minute, it's been a long time now, maybe I am, maybe something is wrong. Then I got a lot of depression. (Participant 1)
The participants also reported a period of withdrawal from social situations.
After my accident, I didn't want friends because I have aphasia and I don't know how to say words. It was very difficult, and I felt dumb being with other friends. So I didn't want to spend time with other people. (Participant 4)

Coping. The participants in this investigation indicated that adaptations in their coping styles had to be made before they achieved success following their injuries (35%). Participant 3 reflected on his ability to instill a positive attitude following his injury: "I've been to the bottom of the pit and to the top of the pit. I just try my best and think positive, and if it doesn't [work] there is a reason I can't, so I can stop and try something totally different."

Participant 4 indicated the importance of changing from a negative coping strategy to one that was more positive and effective: "I used to drink too much. I was not happy so I would drink. Now I do not at all. I don't want it because I don't want to be who I used to [be]."

Belief System (Spirituality). The idea of a belief system serving as a coping mechanism surfaced in a significant number of the interviews (39%). Many described a newfound belief, while some described a renewed belief. Participant 4 reported about his newfound belief in God:

> He has saved my life. He is someone I can talk with. I can't talk about my problems with other people. But when I'm with my God, it doesn't matter, He understands. I didn't go to church before the accident but I go to church everyday now. He loves me and I love Him, and that is all I need to know.

Participant 3 indicated that he redeveloped his spiritual belief system. In doing so, he felt that it provided him with a sense of balance in his life:

> Well, I was born Catholic, Roman Catholic. But the way that I am, I am not, I can't be in the Roman Catholic like my whole family. I now believe from the Unitarian is to help one another. I'm a person likes to help one another. So I've been going to the Unitarian, and it's a good one cause you don't have to be there every Sunday, it helps me be more level.

Acceptance of Injury and Redefinition of Self

Another common theme identified by 84% of the participants in this investigation was the concept of injury acceptance and redefinition of the self. Many survivors reported that the emotional and psychological changes necessary to finally accept their injuries took a long period of time to fully emerge (68%). Participant 1 indicated that he suffered a long emotional battle before coming to accept his situation:

> Well it's been 1, 2, 3, 4, 5, 6, 62 years that it's been since I had my stroke. And it is getting better, sometimes I can see different things, but it's not and I don't think it's ever going to be perfect, you know. But that you know. But the other thing is I finally realized that that's okay, you know, I have to do, I have to, I can't just sit here and um and um on a log.

The individuals in this investigation sought new meaning by developing aspects of their lives that they neglected for one reason or another before their injury (65%). For example, Participant 4 talked about how he had become a nicer person and a better son as well as father to his own son. He highly valued his role within the family. He also realized that this role had changed as a result of his injury (e.g., reduced ability/desire to participate in activities that took him away from his family role before the injury).

> When I'm at [the ABI program], I'm a nicer person. But I'm just a normal person with them. We all have our problems, from an accident or a stroke. But when we are all there together everyone completely understands. (Participant 4)
> I am 180% another person. I'm much more calm; I don't have anger anymore; I don't have fits. For a while, I just wanted to get back to my old self [and] my little life, and just be normal again. Well, I will never be normal; I don't want to be normal. I like the person who I am. (Participant 3) Everything has done an about-face. And part of my changing has been accepting the fact that I do have a disability and what that means in my life. (Participant 2)

In addition, the participants were able to accept themselves for who they had become (81%). Furthermore, they had come to accept that they were not who they used to be.

When it came to everyone else I was fine. I didn't have any prejudices. But me being disabled is a whole different ball of wax. Looking at what I had previously and dealing with being disabled was all negative. All of my thought processes were, oh, if I'm disabled that means this whole slew of things. That means being "weak"; that means being "lazy." And understanding changing my perception and of what that means for me, that has been a tremendous feat for me. I'm still going through it. (Participant 2)

These participants acknowledged that they had new roles to play and new goals to achieve (68%), and their sense of self differed greatly from who they were before. In reaching this stage, they had found a way to fit their new selves into their lives.

I will never go back to the old [me]. That [person] died when they did the operation. I'm a whole new person, I'm more able and more stronger than I never thought I would get. (Participant 3)

. . . but I present pretty well and I think that that can fool myself and other people, definitely myself. I don't think it has probably been until the last month or so that I have really embraced the difficulties I still have, and that has been a really, well it took me almost 3 years to fully embrace and understand this is my life now. (Participant 2)

Empowerment

The participants in this investigation have achieved a number of accomplishments that have empowered them to become independent, resourceful, and eager to give back to their communities. In addition to living independent lives and being able to drive, the participants indicated that their lives were productive and fulfilling. This sense seemed to stem from their advocacy of brain injury awareness and their desire to help others who have gone through similar experiences. Fifty-eight percent of the interviewees reported some element of empowerment that they contributed to their ability to live a productive life.

Developing a Sense of Independence.   Many of the participants in this investigation reported living independent lives (32%). They demonstrated the ability to reintegrate into their communities, drive themselves, and set their own goals for achievement. However, they reported that the early stages of the recovery process were challenging, as decisions were often made by family members, schedules were determined by therapy routines, and choices were often limited based on their functionality.

Yes, I'm living alone. My mom and dad wanted me to live back with [them]. I love my mom and dad, but I can be such an opinionated person I said I wanted to live alone. So I can get this way if I have my family, and my mom will say and do anything my mom will do this for me, so what am I going to say, "Mom will do it, mom will do it," so I can just sit and relax so everyone can give me pity? No I'm not like that. (Participant 3)

Many of the interviewees reported that they took the opportunity to explore activities and set their own goals, and then with support, integrate themselves into the community (42%). For Participant 2, being able to tap into her social work background was a key component to her empowerment. From there she was able to begin working as a spokesperson for the American Heart Association.

> I have actually been trying to maneuver into being a spokesperson for stroke. So far I have probably done 15 different speaking engagements through [the ABI program] and through the American Heart Association and through Train to End Stroke, kind of a little bit of everything. (Participant 2)

Procuring Employment.   The ability to procure employment was not always attainable for many of the participants in this investigation. Many of them indicated how difficult it was to go from being actively employed to suddenly finding themselves unable to work.

> Well, it was very busy. I was a um a planner [financial planner] … at night, I was the counsel, head of the counsel of Newmarket. I was very busy almost 1, 2, 3, 4, 5, 6, 7 days a week. I was very involved with the mills. They were going to close; they did close, so it was like what are we going to do with these mills? So I was in 1, 2, 3, 4, 5, 6, 7, 8, 9 years I was involved with the mills and the um the um closure. And so I was very involved so I didn't have, and I also built my house, so I was really I was very busy and then all of a sudden nothing. (Participant 1)

The majority of the participants (92%) in this investigation were employed to some capacity premorbidly (e.g., full-time, part-time, or student). However, only a fraction (19%) remained employed in a part-time capacity following their injuries. Extending the definition of employment to include volunteer work and return to the classroom increases the percentage substantially (42%). Nevertheless, of the 4 exemplar cases, only 1 currently maintained gainful employment (Participant 4). None of the 4 participants had returned to his or her preinjury profession. Regardless, this did not preclude them from living productive and fulfilling lives.

> I will never, quote, work. It's too hard for me because I get tired in the afternoon so I tried to work and um I wanted to be independent and I'm really hard. I like to do hard work and stuff, but I now know my ability that I can do, not disability. But there is no job out there for me to have a "normalish" job. (Participant 3)
>
> The most difficult thing before my stroke, I would say that 100% my belief had always been a career woman and that was kind of my ideal. That is why I went from high school to college to grad school all right in a row because I was always going to work and then when it became time my husband was going to stay home with our children. Whereas before, a couple months ago, I never said I'm not working. I just said I'm not working right now, you know I'm volunteering, I'm busy doing all this stuff, and that is true, but I don't see working in my future. (Participant 2)

Driving.   Driving was mentioned as either one of the biggest contributors to empowerment or one of the main goals for regaining their sense of independence by the participants in this study (55%).

> For a year I didn't drive. That was horrible. I just really, I have always been a driver. As people know now that I have my license, I was never a passenger. I never liked other people driving. I get car sick pretty easily and over that year I had to ask for other people to drive and wow that was just really hard, accepting other people's, I'm not very good at asking for help either. I had no choice, I had to ask for help and not only that but asking for help but in the same breath being frustrated. (Participant 2)

When asked what his biggest goal was for the future, Participant 4 reported, "I would love to be able to drive. I had a seizure about 2 months ago so now I'm not allowed to drive." (At the time of this writing, Participant 4 was seizure-free and had regained his driver's license.)

ABI Advocacy and a Need to Give Back.   The individuals in this investigation have had to find a way to meet past vocational pursuits within postinjury abilities. This has taken different forms, all of which have included getting highly involved in providing support for other survivors. This has not only empowered the participants but also given them the opportunity to support the ABI community. The interviewees reported that the ABI program in which they participated has given them the opportunity to support the ABI community in ways that were empowering to both the individual and the group as a whole. Participant 1 did this by facilitating several aphasia support and strategy groups, Participant 2 facilitated several emotional support groups, Participant 3 facilitated gardening and cooking groups, and Participant 4 has been active in music groups.

Participant 1 discussed his desire to give back to the aphasia community:

I says I gotta do something. I mean I didn't expect that. I mean, I says what can we do? Look at the people, the people that came that just had a stroke and have aphasia. I want to start a foundation, so when we came to home we said let's do it. So we um, I got people that had aphasia, I had a therapist, pathologist, I have doctors that will help.

Participant 1 now runs the Aphasia Advocacy Foundation both within the ABI program infrastructure and as an independent organization that provides support and education at the community and state levels.

The desire to contribute, advocate (48%), and give back (52%) has empowered many of the participants in this investigation. It has given them a sense of purpose and a sense of belonging. Participant 3 concluded his interview by offering to extend the same support to others that was provided to him by the ABI program: "[The ABI program] has helped me so much. I'm so grateful to be here and would gladly be here to support anyone else who needs support."

■ DISCUSSION

The participants in this study represented a sample of individuals who have made remarkable progress during their recovery from ABI. Analysis of the interviews conducted with these survivors identified several themes congruent with each that were influential to postinjury successes. The four primary themes identified in this investigation were social support networks, grief and coping following ABI, acceptance of the injury and redefinition of self, and empowerment.

The themes reported in this investigation were similar to those identified by Hinckley (2006). First, the need for strong social support networks was identified in both studies. Second, the ability to make adjustments and adaptations to the new self was evident in both analyses. Thirdly, empowerment (defined as becoming independent and/or giving back to their communities) was an important factor to productivity and quality of life. Hinckley's description of looking to the future and setting new goals had similar parallels to the empowerment theme reported in this investigation. In addition, Hinckley identified "taking charge of one's own continued communication improvement" as a separate theme.

This could easily be grouped under the empowerment theme in this investigation. Although communication was mentioned often by the participants in this investigation, it was often being referred to as a deficit and a source of anxiety or frustration that limited social support networks and led to feelings of grief. In addition, not all participants in this investigation demonstrated communicative impairments; therefore, the theme did not emerge as strongly as in the Hinckley study, where all participants were reported to exhibit aphasia (Hinckley, 2006).

There were also strong similarities between the identified themes in this investigation and those highlighted by Ylvisaker and Feeney (2000). These researchers suggest that two themes in particular have a significant influence in successful rehabilitation of individuals with ABI. The first is the ability of the individual to reconstruct a satisfying sense of self. The theme "acceptance of injury and redefinition of self" in the current investigation mirrors Ylvisaker and Feeney's findings. The participants in our investigation were able to accept and redefine themselves through vocational adjustment (61%), overcome emotional barriers (68%), address neglected aspects of themselves (81%), and identify new roles and goals for themselves (68%).

The second of Ylvisaker and Feeney's major themes associated with successful recovery involves the survivor's ability to engage in meaningful activities. The ability of the participants in the current investigation to develop meaningful activities led to our fourth goal of "empowerment." Examination of the four exemplars in this investigation reveals that they all not only reconstructed a satisfying sense of self but were able to participate in activities that established their independence (42%) and subsequently motivated them to advocate for themselves and others with ABI (48%) and give back to their communities (52%).

Taken together, the accounts of Hinckley (2006) and Ylvisaker and Feeney (2000) arguably support all four themes identified in this investigation. First is the development of social support networks. Hinckley demonstrated that successful recovery from stroke is often facilitated through participation in strong social support networks. It has also been demonstrated that in order for survivors of ABI to reestablish their identities, integrate back into their communities, and have a meaningful quality of life, they must establish strong support networks (Kalpakjian et al., 2004). However, survivors of ABI often find that their social support networks begin to weaken or disappear following their injury. This was reported by the majority of the participants in this investigation (71%). A lack of resources to address the long-term needs of survivors and the existence of misconceptions held by family and friends can cause a great deal of strain on these personal relationships (Knight, Devereux, & Godfrey, 1998). Clinicians can support the patient and family by educating them about the recovery process and informing them of support networks in the community.

Next is the issue of grief and coping. After brain injury, a variety of personal adjustments must be made. These adjustments often require the survivor to accept that some parts of his or her life will never go back to the way they were before the accident. This realization can produce a variety of emotional responses, such as anger, anxiety, and depression, which were prevalent in the participants of this investigation. Emotional sequelae, which have been previously reported by survivors of ABI, affect not only quality of life but also goal setting, motivation, and long-term recovery (Curran, Ponsford, & Crowe, 2000).

While neither Hinckley nor Ylvisaker and Feeney directly identified grief and coping as major themes in their investigations, it can be argued that the process of grieving and the development of functional coping mechanisms allow survivors to accept their injury, redefine themselves, and develop a sense of empowerment. Ylvisaker and Feeney (2000) demonstrated that under the interacting cognitive subsystems model outlined by Teasdale (1997), maladaptive emotions (e.g., anger or denial) could be avoided if the survivor were taught to construct alternative models of the self, which could be automatically triggered in the advent of a negative emotional response. In essence, the survivor is developing an internal coping strategy to address issues of grief. Clinicians can help their patients to cope effectively by helping them to develop methods that address actual issues and stay clear of avoidant methods, such as substance abuse, that can lead to further emotional decline. Research strongly indicates that providing patients with psychoeducational information early in the recovery process can have a dramatic effect on their ability to cope with ABI (Mittenberg, Tremont, Zielinski, Fichera, & Rayls, 1996; Ponsford et al., 2002). Teaching patients how to detect problems or stressors before they occur and instructing them on coping strategies to regulate their lifestyle and environment can lead to an increased quality of life.

Successful recovery from ABI is also affected by survivors' ability to accept their injuries and redefine who they are. Reports from Hinckley (2006) and Ylvisaker and Feeney (2000) both support our findings of the need for the survivor to accept his or her injury and redefine the self in order to successfully recover from ABI. Hinckley's analysis of aphasia narratives found that change in self-concept was a critical factor to readjustment and personal development for people with aphasia.

Similarly, Ylvisaker and Feeney (2000) observed great success in the rehabilitation of their participant Jason following "identity reconstruction." Through identity reconstruction, Jason began to see himself metaphorically as "Jason-as-Clint-Eastwood"; Jason associated Clint Eastwood with power, success, control, and independence, which were characteristics that Jason valued. In doing so, Jason was able to succeed by developing positive emotions and scripts for common situations, and using support personnel effectively. In a similar manner, the participants in this investigation were also able to effectively reconstruct their own identities by developing a sense of purpose, making emotional connections, and developing new goals for themselves.

The motto of the postrehabilitation, community-based day program that the participants in this investigation belong to is "You are not who you were; be who you are." This sentiment is lived by each of these participants. They have accepted their injuries (81%), developed new goals for themselves (68%), overcome emotional barriers (68%), and forged lasting and supportive social networks (87%). When clinicians provide a focus on goal setting, emotional adjustment, and social integration early on in therapy, survivors can be better equipped to make the necessary adjustments to meet the long-term challenges associated with ABI.

Finally, the issue of empowerment is evident in each of these investigations. In the last 10 years, the mental health literature has explored what aspects of life lead to feelings of empowerment. Three major categories emerge that define empowerment: self-esteem/self-efficacy (e.g., developing independence), actual power (e.g., being assertive and learning new skills), and community activism (e.g., giving back to the community and ABI advocacy;

Chamberlin, 1997; Rogers, Chamberlin, Ellison, & Crean, 1997). Hinckley (2006) identified from her narrative analyses that living successfully following stroke required participation in lifelong goal setting by the survivor. Similarly, our participants also reported that developing and following through with new goals was an empowering endeavor (68%). Ylvisaker and Feeney (2000) emphasized that in order to be successful the survivor must engage in activities that are meaningful. The participants in our investigation reported that the activities that empowered them such as ABI advocacy (48%) and the need to give back to their communities (52%) were also highly meaningful.

Implications of Narratives for the Clinician

Narratives, such as the ones described in this investigation, can help to enlighten clinicians about the recovery process by providing them with a holistic look at the needs of their patients. It has been demonstrated that the attitudes and beliefs about ABI recovery held by practicing speech-language pathologists were significantly different after listening to interviews of ABI survivors (Fraas & Calvert, 2007). In particular, the researchers found that the speech-language pathologists' attitudes and beliefs about the recovery process significantly improved with regard to the psycho-social and vocational challenges of the survivors following their exposure to survivor narratives. Furthermore, poor attitudes and beliefs held by clinicians about patients' ability to recover have been linked to poor outcomes (Fischer, Trexler, & Gauggel, 2004; Tervo, Palmer, & Redinius, 2004).

In addition, clinicians may find the use of survivor narratives an effective treatment tool for several reasons. Narratives such as these can be used to educate patients and their families about the recovery process. The interviews in this investigation contain many examples of the stages of recovery experienced by survivors. Furthermore, a number of coping mechanisms were discussed that clinicians could implement with their patients. Narratives can be used to instill hope and provide a source of motivation to their patients. The survivors highlighted in this investigation all made tremendous strides to reach the level that they are at today. To do so, they had to redefine themselves and set new goals for their future. Clinicians can share these stories with their patients as a means to inspire them throughout the therapy process.

Clinicians should be assiduous in sharing such stories of recovery with their patients. They can help survivors and their families to identify useful suggestions offered in these narratives and apply modifications that will enable their greater success. By inspiring and empowering survivors and their families through increased education and improving the attitudes and beliefs about ABI held by health professionals, survivors of ABI will improve their rehabilitation process and experience a higher quality of life.

The Impact of Community-Based Programming

Although the purpose of this investigation was not to examine the effectiveness of community-based programming for adults with ABI, it should be mentioned that involvement in this type of programming may have affected the findings of this investigation. The participants in this investigation all belong to a community-based, postrehabilitation day program designed to address the long-term needs of its members. Group activities offered in the program provide members with ways to increase socialization and decrease emotional instability. In addition, the program emphasizes a health and wellness approach to empowering members toward occupation or meaning after injury. Future research should be conducted to examine the impact that these types of programs have on improving quality of life for their members.

Limitations

There are two limitations to this investigation that preclude definitive generalizations from being made. First is that the participants consisted of a convenience sample of members of a community-based program for adults with ABI. While the group as a whole is quite heterogeneous, they are from a small region of the United States and may not adequately represent survivors of ABI across the country.

In addition, the program that the participants are involved with addresses many of their long-term needs associated with their ABI. Few such programs exist nationally relative to the numbers of survivors with unmet long-term needs. It may be that membership in this program was responsible for shaping their interview responses. The ability of other community-based programs to meet the persistent needs of survivors of ABI has been documented (Hashimoto, Okamoto, Watanabe, & Ohashi, 2006; Jacobs, 1997; Jacobs & Demello, 1996; Malec, 2001; Powell, Heslin, & Greenwood, 2002). Whether participation in these types of programs leads to perceptions of living a productive life is an area that needs further investigation.

Conclusion

This investigation highlights the major themes shared by survivors of ABI. The themes appear to have had an impact on their successful postinjury accomplishments. Many survivors of ABI are not as fortunate as the participants highlighted in this investigation. However, stories of inspiration such as these may serve to provide hope and motivation to others as they progress through the recovery process.

■ ACKNOWLEDGMENTS

This project was funded in part by a generous grant from The Beaumont Foundation of America. The authors would like to thank The Krempels Brain Injury Foundation and its members for their participation in and support of this research.

References

Brain Injury Association of America. (2008). *Types of brain injury*. Retrieved May 27, 2008, from www.biausa.org/Pages/types_of_brain_injury.html#aquired

Centers for Disease Control and Prevention. (2006). *Stroke facts and statistics*. Retrieved December 13, 2006, from www.cdc.gov/stroke/stroke_facts.htm

Chamberlin, J. (1997). A working definition of empowerment. *Psychiatric Rehabilitation Journal, 20*, 23–26.

Corrigan, J. D., Whiteneck, G., & Mellick, D. (2004). Perceived needs following traumatic brain injury. *Journal of Head Trauma Rehabilitation, 19*, 205–216.

Curran, C. A., Ponsford, J. L., & Crowe, S. (2000). Coping strategies and emotional outcome following traumatic brain injury: A comparison with orthopedic patients. *Journal of Head Trauma Rehabilitation, 15*, 1256–1274.

Dawson, D. R., & Chipman, M. (1995). The disablement experienced by traumatically brain-injured adults living in the community. *Brain Injury, 9*, 339–353.

Dewar, B. K., & Gracey, F. (2007). "Am not was": Cognitive–behavioural therapy for adjustment and identity change following herpes simplex encephalitis. *Neuropsychological Rehabilitation, 17*, 602–620.

Ellis-Hill, C. S., & Horn, S. (2000). Change in identity and self-concept: A new theoretical approach to recovery following a stroke. *Clinical Rehabilitation, 14*, 279–287.

Fischer, S., Trexler, L. E., & Gauggel, S. (2004). Awareness of activity limitations and prediction of performance in patients with brain injuries and orthopedic disorders. *Journal of the International Neuropsychological Society, 10*(2), 190–199.

Fraas, M., & Calvert, M. (2007). Oral histories: Bridging misconceptions and reality in brain injury recovery. *Disability and Rehabilitation, 29*, 1449–1455.

Glover, A. (2003). An exploration of the extent to which attending Headway enhances quality of life after traumatic brain injury. *Disability and Rehabilitation, 25*, 750–760.

Greenhalgh, T., & Collard, A. (2003). *Narrative based health care: Sharing stories. A multi-professional workbook.* London: BMJ.

Hashimoto, K., Okamoto, T., Watanabe, S., & Ohashi, M. (2006). Effectiveness of a comprehensive day treatment program for rehabilitation of patients with acquired brain injury in Japan. *Journal of Rehabilitation Medicine, 38*(1), 20–25.

Hinckley, J. J. (2006). Findingmessages in bottles: Living successfully with stroke and aphasia. *Top Stroke Rehabilitation, 13*(1), 25–36.

Hinckley, J. J. (2008). *Narrative-based practice in speech-language pathology: Stories of a clinical life.* San Diego, CA: Plural.

Jacobs, H. E. (1997). The clubhouse: Addressing work-related behavioral challenges through a supportive social community. *Journal of Head Trauma Rehabilitation, 12*, 14–27.

Jacobs, H. E., & Demello, C. (1996). The clubhouse model and employment following brain injury. *Journal of Vocational Rehabilitation, 7*, 169–179.

Kaitaro, T., Koskinen, S., & Kaipio, M. L. (1995). Neuropsychological problems in everyday life: A 5-year follow-up study of young severely closed-head-injured patients. *Brain Injury, 9*, 713–727.

Kalpakjian, C. Z., Lam, C. S., Toussaint, L. L., & Merbitz, N. K. (2004). Describing quality of life and psychosocial outcomes after traumatic brain injury. *American Journal of Physical Medicine and Rehabilitation, 83*(4), 255–265.

Kissela, B., Broderick, J., Woo, D., Kothari, R., Miller, R., Khoury, J., et al. (2001). Greater Cincinnati/Northern Kentucky Stroke Study: Volume of first-ever ischemic stroke among blacks in a population-based study. *Stroke, 32*, 1285–1290.

Knight, R. G., Devereux, R., & Godfrey, H. P. (1998). Caring for a family member with a traumatic brain injury. *Brain Injury, 12*, 467–481.

Koskinen, S. (1998). Quality of life 10 years after a very severe traumatic brain injury (TBI): The perspective of the injured and the closest relative. *Brain Injury, 12*, 631–648.

Kreutzer, J. S., Seel, R., & Marwitz, J. H. (1999). *Neurobehavioral functioning inventory.* San Antonio, TX: The Psychological Corporation.

Lakoff, G., & Johnson, M. (1999). *Philosophy in the flesh: The embodied mind and its challenge to western thought.* New York, NY: Basic Books.

Langlois, J. A., Kegler, S. R., Butler, J. A., Gotsch, K. E., Johnson, R. L., Reichard, A. A., et al. (2003). Traumatic brain injury-related hospital discharges: Results from a 14-state surveillance system, 1997. *MMWR Surveillance Summary, 52*(4), 1–20.

Malec, J. F. (2001). Impact of comprehensive day treatment on societal participation for persons with acquired brain injury. *Archives of Physical Medicine and Rehabilitation, 82,* 885–895.

Mittenberg, W., Tremont, G., Zielinski, R. E., Fichera, S., & Rayls, K. R. (1996). Cognitive-behavioral prevention of post-concussion syndrome. *Archives of Clinical Neuropsychology, 11*(2), 139–145.

O'Connor, C., Colantonio, A., & Polatajko, H. (2005). Long term symptoms and limitations of activity of people with traumatic brain injury: A ten-year follow-up. *Psychological Reports, 97*(1), 169–179.

Pinker, S. (2007). Toward a consilient study of literature. *Philosophy and Literature, 31*(1), 162–178.

Ponsford, J., Willmott, C., Rothwell, A., Cameron, P., Kelly, A. M., Nelms, R., et al. (2002). Impact of early intervention on outcome following mild head injury in adults. *Journal of Neurology, Neurosurgery, and Psychiatry, 73*(3), 330–332.

Powell, J., Heslin, J., & Greenwood, R. (2002). Community based rehabilitation after severe traumatic brain injury: A randomised controlled trial. *Journal of Neurology, Neurosurgery, and Psychiatry, 72*(2), 193–202.

Rogers, E. S., Chamberlin, J., Ellison, M. L., & Crean, T. (1997). A consumer-constructed scale to measure empowerment among users of mental health services. *Psychiatric Services, 48,* 1042–1047.

Seidman, I. (1998). *Interviewing as qualitative research* (2nd ed.). New York, NY: Teachers College Press.

Sneed, S. L., & Davis, J. (2002). Attitudes of individuals with acquired brain injury towards disability. *Brain Injury, 16,* 947–953.

Steadman-Pare, D., Colantonio, A., Ratcliff, G., Chase, S., & Vernich, L. (2001). Factors associated with perceived quality of life many years after traumatic brain injury. *Journal of Head Trauma Rehabilitation, 16,* 330–342.

Teasdale, J. D. (1997). The transformation of meaning: The interacting cognitive subsystems approach. In M. Power & C. R. Brewin (Eds.), *The transformation of meaning in psychological therapies* (pp. 125–140). New York, NY: Wiley.

Teasdale, J. D., & Barnard, P. J. (1993). *Affect, cognition, and change: Re-modelling depressive thought.* Hillsdale, NJ: Erlbaum.

Tervo, R. C., Palmer, G., & Redinius, P. (2004). Health professional student attitudes towards people with disability. *Clinical Rehabilitation, 18,* 908–915.

Thorne, A., & McLean, K. C. (2003). Telling traumatic events in adolescence: A study of master narrative positioning. In R. Fivush & C. A. Haden (Eds.), *Connecting culture and memory: The development of an autobiographical self* (pp. 169–186). Mahwah, NJ: Erlbaum.

Thurman, D. J., Alverson, C., Dunn, K. A., Guerrero, J., & Sniezek, J. E. (1999). Traumatic brain injury in the United States: A public health perspective. *Journal of Head Trauma Rehabilitation, 14,* 602–615.

Tyerman, A., & Humphrey, M. (1984). Changes in self-concept following severe head injury. *International Journal of Rehabilitation Research, 7*(1), 11–23.

VanWynsberghe, R., & Khan, S. (2007). Redefining case study. *International Journal of Qualitative Methods, 6*(2), 1–10.

Warren, L., Wrigley, J. M., & Yoels, W. C. (1996). Factors associated with life satisfaction among a sample of persons with neurotrauma. *Journal of Rehabilitation Research and Development, 33,* 404–408.

Ylvisaker, M., & Feeney, T. J. (1996). Executive functions after traumatic brain injury: Supported cognition and self-advocacy. *Seminars in Speech and Language, 17*(3), 217–232.

Ylvisaker, M., & Feeney, T. (1998). *Collaborative brain injury intervention: Positive everyday routines.* San Diego, CA: Singular.

Ylvisaker, M., & Feeney, T. (2000). Reconstruction of identity after brain injury. *Brain Impairment, 1*(1), 12–28.

■ APPENDIX A5.A ORAL HISTORY QUESTIONS

1. Could you tell me about your life before your injury?
   Additional Probes:
   employment
   family
   goals
   education
   friends
   social life
   religion
2. Describe your injury.
   Additional Probes:
   How long ago did it happen?
   Where did it happen?
   What happened to you?
3. What was your rehab experience like?
   Additional Probes:
   What types of therapy did you have?
   Where did you have therapy?
   What was beneficial/nonbeneficial during therapy?
4. What changes have occurred since your injury?
   Additional Probes:
   Physical
   Emotional
   Communication
5. How has life been since your injury?
   Additional Probes:
   Social
   Family
   Vocation
   Financially
   Religion
6. How has your communication been affected since your injury?
7. What goals are you currently working toward? Or what would you like to achieve in your life now?
8. How has [the ABI program] played a part in your life?

■ APPENDIX A5.B DEFINITION OF THEMES AND SUBTHEMES AND PERCENTAGE OF OCCURRENCE

THEMES AND SUBTHEMES	DEFINITION	%
Social support networks	**Influence of friendships and family in the recovery process, including various forms of relationships (e.g., marriage and dating)**	87
Support of friends/family	Survivor's family and friends were supportive	87
Initial loss of friends	Friends of survivor stopped coming to visit during the recovery phase	71
Supports for family members	Survivor's family received support	61
Misconceptions/ misunderstandings	Some aspect of survivor's injury was misunderstood (e.g., aphasia)	52
Relationships	Survivor's ability to develop new relationships	45
Marriage	Survival of marriage was influential in recovery	16
Dating	Ability to begin dating	19
Grief and coping	**Includes various stages of grieving; forms of coping (both positive and negative) with ABI**	98
Denial	Survivor progressed through denial stage	87
Frustration, anger	Survivor progressed through periods of anger and frustration	84
Depression	Survivor overcame depression	84
Withdrawal	Survivor withdrew from social settings as a coping mechanism	42
Religion, spirituality	Survivor developed or rediscovered sense of spirituality or religion	39
Coping adaptations	Survivor learned to adapt coping styles to deal with limitations (e.g., communication, emotions)	35
Alcohol/drugs	Ability to find alternatives to alcohol/drugs in order to cope	19
Acceptance of injury and redefinition of self	**Includes issues pertaining to acceptance and redefinition of self; changing roles and goals**	84
Redefining self	Seeking new attributes to characterize themselves	84
Vocational adjustment	Survivor accepts that he or she is unable to conduct responsibilities of previous job	61
Reexplore neglected aspects of former self	Nurture issues neglected before accident (e.g., family, enjoyed activities)	65
Productivity	Become productive with his or her life instead of "sitting around"	77
Overcome barriers	Survivor is able to get past emotional and psychological barriers to recovery	68
Acceptance (negative and positive aspects) of self	Survivor embraces all attributes of self	81
New roles/new goals	Survivor defines a new role for himself or herself and sets goals to achieve it	68
Empowerment	**Issues related to new achievements; need to give back to others and to provide education to members of the community**	58
Motivation	Survivor reports that he or she became motivated	23
Make own decisions, set goals	Shift decision/goal setting from caregiver or clinician to survivor (i.e., independence)	32
Independence vs. dependency	Survivor identifies areas of dependency and determines ways to become more independent	42
Employment	Survivor identifies new means for gainful employment (e.g., volunteer)	42
Driving	Survivor able to regain driving status	55
Promote awareness, advocate	Survivor advocates for self and educates public about brain injury	48
The need to give back	Survivor is compelled to provide support for others with similar experiences	52

Note. Themes are indicated in boldface type.

APPENDIX A-6

Transition to Home Care: Quality of Mental Health, Pharmacy, and Medical History Information[*][†]

Ellen L. Brown, EdD, MS, RN
Stein Gerontological Institute
Patrick J. Raue, PhD
Amy E. Mlodzianowski, MS
Barnett S. Meyers, MD
Rebecca L. Greenberg, MS
Martha L. Bruce, PhD, MPH
Weill Medical College of Cornell University

Abstract

Objective: *To assess the completeness and accuracy of clinical information provided by referral sources to visiting nurses for patients admitted to receive home health care.*

Methods: *Clinical referral information for a representative sample of 243 older adults admitted to receive skilled home-health nursing was compared to medical record information from home-health charts and in-home research interviews to determine their concordance. Measures used included referral information, home-care chart documentation, in-home nurse review of medications, medication allergies, caregiver contact information, cognitive status, depression status, and follow-up plan.*

Results: *There were medication discrepancies between in-home nurse review and admission information in 215 cases (88.4%). Clinical information on medication allergies was lacking from referrers in 85 cases (34.9%). No information was provided by the referrers about cognitive status in 38 (73%) cases classified as cognitively impaired and in only 2 of 35 cases with major depression identified with the Structured Clinical Interview for Axis I Diagnostic and Statistical Manual of Mental Disorders, Fourth Edition (SCID), was depression related information provided by referrers.*

Conclusions: *The primary finding of this study is that during a transfer of an older adult to the home care service sector, essential clinical information is often missing, and there are significant discrepancies between medication regimens. These findings support*

Source: International Journal of Psychiatry in Medicine, Vol. 36, No. 3, 2006. 339–349. Copyright by Baywood Publishing Co., Inc., 2006.

---

[*]A version of this article was presented at the Annual Meeting of the American Geriatrics Society, held in May 11–15, 2005, Orlando.
[†]This study was supported by NIMH Grants R01 MH56482, K01 MH066942, and R24 MH64608. Dr. Bruce received research support from NIH. Consulting services were supported by NIH-funded grants to Washington University, University of Iowa, Rochester University, and MediSpin Company, and by a CDC funded grant to the University of Washington. Dr. Meyers received research support through Speaker's Bureau, Forest Laboratories.

the need for both educational initiatives and technology to address the complex care needs of older adults across settings to reduce the risk for medication errors and poor outcomes.

Keywords: *care transitions, home care, medical errors, geriatrics.*

■ INTRODUCTION

Inadequate communication of patient information between health care providers, when a patient is transferred or admitted to a new health care setting, puts older adults with complex care needs at increased risk for medication errors, potential harm, and poor medical outcomes (Agency for Healthcare Research and Quality, 2003; Coleman & Boult, 2003). Medically ill older adults are at risk for adverse outcomes related to transitioning between levels of service when relevant referral information is either incomplete or inaccurate. Home care agencies caring for mostly older adult medical patients may be at increased risk for receiving faulty or missing patient information. Home care nurses providing skilled care and physicians ordering and supervising home care service delivery need to be concerned about poor communication of patient information for persons entering the home care service sector.

A home care agency can receive referrals from many different hospitals, nursing homes, rehabilitative facilities, and physicians, making the establishment of routine clinical communication difficult. Presently, Medicare does not require specific patient information for a home care admission. However, the minimum clinical information that is needed for effective care transition from one service sector to another has been identified (Coleman, 2003).

In 2006, the Joint Commission on Accreditation of Healthcare Organizations (JCAHO) required home care agencies to establish a process for reconciling and monitoring patient medications across settings (Home Care National Patient Safety, 2006). Without integrated pharmaceutical information, system health care providers must communicate with providers across settings to verify what are many times complicated medication regimens. This "hand-off" of patients and information can be complicated by medication changes during a hospitalization, inability of providers across settings and disciplines to connect and communicate, and no established process designating the clinician responsible for medication reconciliation.

To our knowledge, this is the first study to examine the clinical information provided by referral sources to visiting nurses for older adult patients admitted to home health care. Examining the clinical information from many "referral sources" is important because it represents how care is usually delivered. A prior study, investigating medication reconciliation, reported that 14% of older adults, post hospitalization, experienced one or more medication discrepancies (Coleman, Smith, Raha, & Min, 2005). The study design utilized a health care delivery system with only one hospital, which limits its generalizability. In addition, the patients were primarily discharged to home, which indicates less medical burden than is found in the home health care population. Therefore, we believe the finding of this study underestimates the problem of medication reconciliation.

In the present study, we evaluated medication reconciliation and several other factors identified as essential for safe and effective care transition including medication allergies, caregiver contact information, follow-up plan, and cognitive status (Coleman, 2003). Additionally, depression assessment information provided by referral sources was evaluated for those home care recipients determined to be depressed. This study explored whether completeness and accuracy of the above information was related to a variety of system and patient variables, including referral site, complexity of patient medical status (e.g., medical comorbidity, number of medications), presence of major depression, and presence of cognitive impairment. These data support expert review of this problem and build on data collected from a systematically studied sample of home health care recipients (Bruce et al., 2002; Coleman & Boult, 2003).

■ METHODS

This study underwent full review and received approval from the Institutional Review Board of Weill Medical College of Cornell University. The setting for this study was the Visiting Nurse Services in Westchester (VNSW), a nonprofit, Medicare-certified, voluntary home care agency serving Westchester County, New York, a diverse region consisting of urban, suburban, and semi-rural areas.

Design

This study investigated the completeness and accuracy of clinical information provided by referrers for home care service admission. Published standards (Coleman, 2003), home health charts, and in-home patient research interviews were used to evaluate clinical information provided by referral sources. Referral documentation was assessed for the presence or absence of medication allergies, caregiver contact information, follow-up plan, cognitive status, and depressive status. Additionally, medication discrepancies were evaluated between referral documentation and in-home nurse review as documented in the plan of care (485 Form—described below).

Eligible Patient Subjects

As described in detail elsewhere (Bruce et al., 2002), the study obtained a random sample of newly admitted, elderly (age 65 and older) medical-surgical home care patients on a weekly basis between December 1997 and December 1999. Of the 889 eligible patients invited to participate in the study, 539 (60.6%) signed consent and were interviewed in their home. The analyses presented here are based on the sub-sample of 243 patients from the parent study who were admitted to home care between January 1999 and December 1999, the 2nd year of the study. Subjects were assessed in their homes on average within 23 ± 6.8 days of admission.

Measures

Study data came from patient medical records (CMS-485 Form [485 Form], referral documentation [RefD]), and in-home patient interviews. The plan of care (485 Form) is established by home care agency staff after the first home visit. It includes patient demographics (age, gender), primary admission diagnosis (International Classification of Diseases, 1980), patient assessment measures, and a list of medications, including dose and instructions.

Federal regulations require home care agencies to obtain a physician-signed 485 Form as soon as practical after the initiation of the plan of care and prior to submitting for reimbursement. The 485 Form provides written orders that detail the needed home care services.

The RefD is typical of the information received by home care agencies. RefD is provided using the format selected by the referral source (e.g., clinical note from a physician or a hospital discharge note) and does not require all referrers to use the same format or provide the same information. Examining the accuracy and completeness of the RefD clinical and functional patient information is the primary objective of this study. As discussed previously, the authors (EB, PR, AM) examined the RefD for medication allergies, caregiver contact information, follow-up plan, medications, including dose and instructions, cognitive status, and depressive status. A caregiver "contact" person is a family member or a close friend who carries responsibilities like a family member. A "follow-up plan" was coded "present" if there was a planned healthcare provider visit or medical test.

Using the medication list from the 485 Form as the "gold standard," a medication discrepancy was defined as discordance between the 485 Form and the RefD in medication agent, dose, or instruction. "Missing agent" was coded if a medicine appeared on the 485 Form but not the RefD. "Missing dose" (i.e., dose not present) and "missing instructions" (e.g., qd, bid, tid) were also coded, except in cases where a "missing agent" was documented. An "inconsistent agent" was coded if an agent appeared on the RefD but not on the 485 Form. "Inconsistent dose" (e.g., 20 mg dose on the RefD vs. 40 mg dose on the 485 Form) and "inconsistent instructions" (e.g., medication to be taken bid on the RefD vs. tid on the 485 Form) were also coded, except in cases where an "inconsistent agent" was documented. This method was applied to avoid assigning multiple errors (e.g., agent and dose) for a single prescribed agent.

Presence of depression-related information was examined on the RefD for those with a diagnosis of major depression assigned by research interviewers. Research assistants administered the Structures Clinical Interview for Axis I DSM-IV Disorders (SCID) (Spitzer, Gibbon, & Williams, 1995) in patients' homes to assess depressive symptoms and disorders. According to SCID criteria, a symptom was rated present if the patient reported that the symptom occurred most of the day nearly every day for any 2-week period in the past month. As described elsewhere (Bruce et al., 2002), due to the complexities of diagnosing major depression in elderly medically ill patients, diagnoses were assigned based on review of interview and medical record information by the study team.

To determine whether referral information included depression-related data, the RefD was reviewed for mention of mood (e.g., sad, hopeless, depressed, stable mood, euthymic), anhedonia (e.g., diminished interest in activities, lack of motivation or pleasure), and suicide ideation (e.g., thoughts of death, thoughts of suicide). If any of these symptoms were documented on the RefD, the reviewers considered depression-related information to be present.

Presence of clinical information about cognitive status was examined on the RefD for those with MMSE scores below 24. Research assistants administered the Mini Mental State Exam (MMSE) (Folstein, Folstein, & McHugh, 1975) to assess cognitive function. To determine whether referral information included clinical information about cognitive functioning, the RefD was reviewed for any mention of level of consciousness (e.g., alert, stuporous, lethargic), orientation (e.g., oriented, disoriented), and memory (e.g., forgetful, confused).

If any of the presence or absence of any of these symptoms was documented on the RefD, the reviewers considered an assessment of overall cognitive functional status to be present.

Overall functional disability, Activities of Daily Living (ADL) (Katz, Downs, & Cash, 1970), and Instrumental Activities of Daily Living (IADL) (Lawton, Moss, Falconer, & Kleban, 1982) was measured by a self-report count of activities in each domain that he or she was able to do without assistance. Sociodemographic data such as ethnicity and living arrangements were also obtained via in-home interviews. A Charlson Comorbidity Index (CCI) score (Charlson, Pompei, Ales, & MacKenzie, 1987) was determined by study physician review of patient-reported medical conditions and medical record.

Interrater Reliability

Interrater reliability among raters based on joint ratings of 20 charts was adequate to excellent for each category. Kappas of 0.89 were obtained for presence or absence of allergy information, 0.79 for caregiver contact information, 0.90 for plan of care, 0.66 for depression status, and 0.63 for cognitive status (Shoukri, 2004). A kappa of 0.83 was obtained for presence or absence of any medication discrepancy, and the Intraclass Correlation Coefficient (Shrout & Fleiss, 1979) was 0.93 for total number of medication discrepancies.

As described elsewhere (Bruce et al., 2002), interrater reliability in the assessment of SCID symptoms was excellent for the number of symptoms present (intraclass $r = 0.91$). Interviewer ratings were monitored throughout the study by the study psychologist (PR).

Statistical Analyses

Analyses were conducted using SAS, version 8.02 (SAS Institute, Inc., Cary, NC) and SPSS, version 13.0 (SPSS, Inc., Chicago, IL) statistical packages. Demographic, clinical, and functional characteristics were reported using descriptive statistics. Chi-square tests were performed to compare proportion of patients by each referral source (hospitals, nursing homes, physicians) on the presence of medication allergies, caregiver contact information, follow-up plan, and medication reconciliation. The sample size for depression and cognitive status was too small to compare proportion of patients by each referral source. Correlations were performed to identify associations between patient clinical and demographic factors (gender, age, race, number of IADL and ADL limitations, CCI, major depression, MMSE < 24, number of medications, referral source) and medication reconciliation.

Patient Sample

Demographic and clinical characteristics of the patient sample appear in Table A6.1. The most common ($n = 74$; 30.6%) primary admission diagnoses were diseases of the circulatory system (ICD-9: 401–459). Patients suffered substantial medical comorbidity (mean CCI was 2.5 ± 2; mean medications prescribed 6.3 ± 3.3), and functional disability (mean IADL limitations was 3.5 (range 0–6); mean ADL limitations was 1.2 ± 1.4 (range 0–6). Thirty-five subjects (14.4%) met criteria for a major depressive episode.

Most patients ($n = 151$; 72%) were referred for home care services following a hospitalization, $n = 38$ (15.6%) referred from a nursing home stay, $n = 30$ (12.3%) directly by

Table A6.1

Sociodemographic and Clinical Characteristics of Sample ($n = 243$)

DESCRIPTOR	VALUE[a]
Continuous Variables	
Age	78.6 (7.6)
Mini Mental State Examination	25.8 (3.2)
Charlson Comorbidity Index (CCI) Score	2.5 (2)
# Medications prescribed	6.3 (3.3)
Categorical Variables	
Gender	
Female	151 (62.1%)
Male	92 (37.9%)
Marital status	
Married	83 (34.1%)
Not married	160 (65.9%)
Living situation	
Alone	94 (38.6%)
Not alone	149 (61.4%)
MMSE < 24	52 (21%)

[a]Data are presented as mean (*SD*) for the continuous variables and as number (percentage) for the categorical variables.

a physician, $n = 12$ (5%) from a rehabilitative program, and $n = 12$ (5%) were self or family referred or other. Physician referrals are referrals made directly by the physician from their office (i.e., no hospital, nursing home, or rehabilitation center stay). Patients were referred from 37 hospitals, 17 nursing homes, 28 physicians, and 3 rehabilitation centers. Referral source information was unavailable for one subject.

■ RESULTS

Table A6.2 describes the clinical information that was assessed for presence or absence and reports the proportion of subjects with absent information in each category assessed. Referral documentation (RefD) provided by physicians was significantly less likely than RefD from nursing homes or hospitals to include a medication allergy list (physicians 23% vs. nursing homes 76% vs. hospitals 71%; Chi-Square $= 27.41$, $df = 2$, $p < .001$). RefD caregiver contact information or follow-up plan did not vary significantly by referral source. In subjects with MMSE scores < 24, no information was provided by the referral source about the patient's cognitive status in 38 cases (73%). In cases where a SCID diagnosis of DSM-IV major depression was identified by the research interview, depression status information was provided in only 2 of 35 cases.

In 215 cases (88.4%), there was a medication inconsistency between the referral documentation (RefD) and the in-home nurse review (485 Form). On average, the mean

Table A6.2

Data Absent on Admission to Home Care	
DATA	N (%)
Medication allergy list	85/243 (34.9)
Caregiver contact information	114/243 (46.9)
Follow-up plan (planned physician visit or medical test)	173/243 (71.1)
Cognitive functional status[a]	38/52 (73.1)
Depression status[b]	33/35 (94.3)

[a]In cases with MMSE < 24 ($n = 52$), MMSE range 0–30.
[b]In cases where a research diagnosis of major depression was established ($n = 35$).

number of medication inconsistencies was 3.2 ± 2.4 (range $= 1$–12). The most common medication inconsistencies were for a missing agent ($n = 167$; 77.7%) or an inconsistent agent ($n = 89$; 41.4%). There were no significant differences in presence of medication inconsistencies between referring hospitals, nursing homes, and physician offices. The only demographic or clinical characteristic associated with the presence of a medication inconsistency was greater number of medications prescribed ($r = 0.23$, $p < .01$).

■ DISCUSSION

The primary finding of this study is that home care admission information received by home care agencies for older adults is incomplete and inaccurate. These findings are disturbing and clearly improving the quality of care for older adults with complex care needs across health care settings is indicated. In particular, older adults entering the home care service sector are at increased risk for medication errors. This study found that greater than one-third of admissions did not include information about medication allergies, and that most medication regimens lacked reconciliation between information received upon admission and the medications being taken at home.

Recently, JCAHO has added to the "requirements and recommendations" regarding medication reconciliation, recognizing that many patients may be too ill or disabled to participate in the medication reconciliation process (Addendum to Sentinel Event Alert #35, 2006). This Alert addendum recommends that if a patient has requested assistance from another person(s) (e.g., family member, significant other, surrogate decision maker) and the patient is unable to actively or fully participate in the medication reconciliation process, this other authorized person should be involved in the process. The need to improve the medication reconciliation process is supported by the findings of this study. However, the effectiveness of involving a patient authorized "other" in the medication reconciliation process is unknown. Additionally, many older home care patients live alone and do not have or may not want to include others in their medical affairs. In this study, a significant minority of the patient referrals did not include contact information for a family or other person, possibly indicating that including another person in the medication reconciliation process may not be feasible in many cases.

Researchers have reported on the development of models for improving medication use and safety for home care recipients. These models require the addition of a pharmacist to the home care interdisciplinary team to identify and resolve medication-related problems (Meredith et al., 2003; Triller, Clause, Briceland, & Hamilton, 2003). However, the focus of these interventions was on improved medication use and management, not on resolving medication discrepancies.

Nonetheless, establishing a process where local pharmacists provide consultation for medication reconciliation is promising and delivery models should be developed and evaluated.

We were particularly surprised by the lack of cognitive status and emotional assessment information conveyed for those adults determined to be cognitively impaired or depressed. In the case of depression, there is evidence that late-life depression often goes unrecognized in home care (Brown et al., 2004; Brown, McAvay, Raue, Moses, & Bruce, 2003). These findings support the need for education in transitional care for clinicians and administrative support staff involved in transfer of patients.

There are four study limitations that should be considered in interpreting these findings. First, this study only evaluated data from one home care agency. However, patient characteristics, primary admission diagnoses, and living arrangements were similar to elderly home health care recipients nationally (Munson, 1990). As important, these data document inconsistencies in transmission or omission of information sent to this agency from 85 unique sources, strengthens the generalizability of these findings. Second, the study utilized liberal criteria for evaluating clinical referral information received by the home care agency concerning depression and cognitive functioning. Thus, the provision of depression and cognitive assessment information by referring hospitals, nursing homes, and physicians may be less adequate than revealed. Third, the small number of depressed and cognitively impaired did not permit analysis of this information by referral source. And fourth, the data presented was collected 7 to 9 years ago. However, there is no indication that the capitation of home health services (Prospective Payment) or other fiscal or regulatory changes have affected referral information. Specifically, referral sources have not been required to change or modify the information provided to a home care agency. However, future research is needed to determine if recent Joint Commission mandates and professional organizational initiatives have improved the quality of home care referral information.

These findings suggest that older adult home care patients are at increased risk for poor outcomes from inadequate transitional care procedures and support the need for required standardized national home care admission data. In the future, a universal electronic medical record should help improve the quality of transitional care, but at the present time clinicians and the organizations in which they work that "send" or "receive" patients should consider dedicating more time to this process. Policy makers should address the need for clinician communication and collaboration across sites in providing safe and effective transitional care and adequate reimbursement incentives for the time involved in medically complex discharges.

■ ACKNOWLEDGMENTS

The authors would like to thank the staff and patients of the Visiting Nurse Services in Westchester without which this study would not have been possible.

References

Addendum to Sentinel Event Alert #35. (2006). *Using medication reconciliation to prevent errors.* Joint Commission on Accreditation of Healthcare Organizations [online, updated February 9, 2006]. Retrieved June 8, 2006, from http://www.jointcommission.org/SentinelEvents/ SentinelEventAlert/sea_35.htm

Agency for Healthcare Research and Quality. (2003). *Patient safety initiative building foundations, reducing risk.* AHRQ Publication No. 04-RG005, 2003.

Brown, E. L., Bruce, M. L., McAvay, G. J., Raue, P. J., Lachs, M. S., & Nassisi, P. (2004). Recognition of late-life depression in home care: Accuracy of the outcome and assessment information set. *Journal of the American Geriatrics Society, 52,* 995–999.

Brown, E. L., McAvay, G. J., Raue, P. J., Moses, S., & Bruce, M. L. (2003). Recognition of depression in the elderly receiving homecare services. *Psychiatric Services, 54,* 208–213.

Bruce, M. L., McAvay, G. J., Raue, P. J., Brown, E. L., Meyers, B. S., Keohane, D. J., et al. (2002). Major depression in elderly home health care patients. *American Journal of Psychiatry, 159,* 1367–1374.

Charlson, M. E., Pompei, P., Ales, K. L., & MacKenzie, C. R. (1987). A new method of classifying prognostic comorbidity in longitudinal studies: Development and validation. *Journal of Chronic Diseases, 40,* 373–383.

Coleman, E. A. (2003). Falling through the cracks: Challenges and opportunities for improving transitional care for persons with continuous complex care needs. *Journal of the American Geriatrics Society, 51,* 549–555.

Coleman, E. A., & Boult, C. (2003). The American Geriatrics Society Health Care Systems Committee: Improving the quality of transitional care for persons with complex care needs. *Journal of the American Geriatrics Society, 51,* 556–557.

Coleman, E. A., Smith, J. D., Raha, D., & Min, S. J. (2005). Posthospital medication discrepancies: Prevalence and contributing factors. *Archives of Internal Medicine, 165*(16), 1842–1847.

Folstein, M. S., Folstein, S. E., & McHugh, P. R. (1975). Mini mental state: A practical method for grading the cognitive state of patients for the clinician. *Journal of Psychiatric Research, 12,* 189–198.

Home Care National Patient Safety. (2006). Goals 2006, #8. Joint Commission on Accreditation of Healthcare Organizations [online]. Retrieved June 8, 2006, from http://www.jointcommission.org/PatientSafety/NationalPatientSafetyGoals/06_npsg _ome.htm

International Classification of Diseases, 9th Revision. (1980). *Clinical Modification* (ICD-9-CM), volume 1: *Diseases Tabular List,* 2nd ed. DHHS Publication PHS 80-1260. Washington, DC: US Government Printing Office.

Katz, S., Downs, T. D., & Cash, H. R. (1970). Progress in the development of an index of ADL. *Gerontologist, 10,* 10–20.

Lawton, M. P., Moss, M., Falconer, M., & Kleban, M. H. (1982). A research and service oriented multilevel assessment instrument. *Journal of Gerontology, 37,* 91–99.

Meredith, S., Feldman, P., Frey, D., Giammarco, L., Hall, K., Arnold, K., et al. (2003). Improving medication use in newly admitted home healthcare patients: A randomized controlled trial. *Journal of the American Geriatrics Society, 50,* 1484–1491.

Munson, M. L. (1999). *Characteristics of elderly home health care users: Data from the 1996 National Home and Hospice Care Survey. Advance data from vital and health statistics; No. 309.* Hyattsville, MD: National Center for Health Statistics.

Shoukri, M. M. (2004). *Measures of interobserver agreement.* New York, NY: Chapman & Hall.

Shrout, P. E., & Fleiss, J. L. (1979). Intraclass correlations: Uses in assessing rater reliability. *Psychological Bulletin, 86*, 420–428.

Spitzer, R. L., Gibbon, M., & Williams, J.B. (Eds.). (1995). *Structured clinical interview for axis I DSM-IV disorders.* Washington, DC: American Psychiatric Association Press, Inc.

Triller, D. M., Clause, S. L., Briceland, L. L., & Hamilton, R. A. (2003). Resolution of drug-related problems in home care patients through a pharmacy referral service. *American Journal of Health Systems Pharmacists, 60*(9), 905–910.

APPENDIX A-7

Psychological Consequences Associated With Intensive Care Treatment

James Carr

Intensive Care Unit (ICU) treatment involves a range of physical and psychological stressors including serious illness, invasive medical procedures, and prolonged incapacity. In addition to physical health problems, those that survive ICU often experience long term psychological difficulties such as cognitive impairment, depression, anxiety, and post-traumatic stress disorder. This review will first consider the types of psychological problems that can occur both during ICU treatment and following discharge and some of the factors involved in their development. Second, consideration is given to medical and psychological intervention strategies that can be provided both during treatment and in follow-up.

Keywords: *intensive care, post-traumatic stress disorder, cognitive impairment, delirium, psychological difficulties.*

■ INTRODUCTION

Traditionally, research into intensive care unit (ICU) outcomes has focussed on physical health, length of hospital stay, and mortality rates. More recently the issue of quality of life has become of greater interest. This review considers an aspect of quality of life following ICU treatment; psychological outcomes. The review also considers psychological difficulties during ICU stay.

■ PSYCHOLOGICAL DISTRESS DURING ICU TREATMENT

The majority of ICU patients will have been unaware of their admission or the circumstances leading to it, which will often have been traumatic. It may not be until late into their admission that they become aware of where they are and how they arrived there. This, coupled with the stressful nature of the ICU environment may lead to a relatively high level of psychological distress. A number of studies have examined which specific aspects of ICU treatment are stressful for patients. The findings from these studies have been reasonably consistent in identifying the main stressors, which can be roughly categorized into physiological and psychological stressors. The main physiological stressors identified include; having tubes in the nose and mouth, pain, sleep disturbance, thirst, and the noise of buzzers and alarms (Biancofiore et al., 2005; Hweidi, 2007; Novaes, Aronovich, Ferraz, & Knobel, 1997; Rotondi et al., 2002). Psychological stressors include; not being in control of the situation, not being in control of ones own body, inability to communicate, missing family and friends, and not being given sufficient information (Biancofiore et al., 2005; Novaes et al., 1997, 1999; Van de Leur et al., 2004). Overall, patients tend to rate physiological stressors as more stressful than psychological stressors (Hweidi, 2007). A number of studies have

Source: Trauma 2007, Vol. 9, 95–102

compared staff perceptions of stressors with those of patients. Findings have tended to indicate a reasonable consistency between what staff and patients perceive to be stressful. However they also indicate that staff tend to rate the level of distress caused by particular stressors as being greater than patients do (Biancofiore et al., 2005; Novaes et al., 1999).

Psychological distress is relatively common during ICU treatment and includes anxiety, stress, withdrawal, denial, regression, anger, depression, and hallucinations and delusions (Mohta, Sethi, Tyagi, & Mohta, 2003). Those who have experienced traumatic injury will often, in the short term, experience periods of anxiety or worry and a number will also experience dissociative episodes which can involve disruption of memory and perception as well as feelings of unreality or detachment. Over the following weeks symptoms of PTSD can occur (Schnyder & Malt, 1998). Schnyder et al. (2000) assessed psychological reactions in accident victims shortly following the trauma. They found that 4.1% experienced post-traumatic stress disorder (PTSD) while 19.9% met criteria for sub-syndromal PTSD. The main symptoms of PTSD include the re-experiencing of a traumatic event via for example images, perceptions or dreams; avoidance of stimuli associated with the event and increased arousal. The term sub-syndromal PTSD is essentially applied to those that experience the core symptoms of PTSD but do not meet full diagnostic criteria. The incidence was higher in women, those with higher levels of stress in the two years prior to the accident, those with psychosocial risk factors such as prior sexual abuse and those lacking psychosocial protective factors such as having a good relationship with parental figures or carers. Objective measures of injury severity did not relate to PTSD incidence but the patients subjective appraisal did. Malt and Olafsen (1992) also found that subjective appraisal of accident severity not objective ratings predicted PTSD. Cognitive impairment has also been noted in ICU patients. Jones, Griffiths, Slater, Benjamin, and Wilson (2006) found that all non-delirious patients assessed while on the ICU exhibited cognitive impairment with regard to strategic thinking and problem-solving, of whom 67% also experienced memory impairment. Impairment was associated with longer ICU stay and older age.

Delirium is a common occurrence during ICU treatment with between 22 and 83% of ICU patients experiencing delirium with typically higher rates for those receiving mechanical ventilation (Bergeron, Skrobik, & Dubois, 2002; Lin et al., 2004). Delirium is defined in the American Psychiatric Associations Diagnostic and Statistical Manual IV (DSM-IV) as a disturbance of consciousness with reduced ability to focus, sustain or shift attention, a change in cognition, such as memory or language disturbance or a perceptual disturbance. Delirium develops over a short period of time (usually hours or days) and is of temporary duration (American Psychiatric Association, 2000). A number of factors have been identified as predictive of delirium in the ICU. Dubois, Bergeron, Dumont, Dial, and Skrobik (2001) identified hypertension, smoking history, abnormal bilirubin level, epidural use, and morphine as being predictive of delirium. McGuire, Basten, Ryan, and Gallgher (2000) report that common medical predictors include; metabolic disturbance, electrolyte imbalance, withdrawal symptoms, acute infections, seizures, head trauma, vascular disorders, and intracranial space occupying lesions. They also report that a range of medications are associated with delirium. The only pre-morbid factors identified include older age and lower cognitive functioning. No environmental or psychological characteristics were predictive of delirium leading to the conclusion that delirium has a physiological cause. Delirium has been associated with a range of negative outcomes such as increased mortality and longer admission (Ely et al., 2004; McGuire et al., 2000; Thomason et al., 2005) although this may reflect the effects of an underlying causal factor rather than a consequence of delirium itself (McGuire et al., 2000).

■ PSYCHOLOGICAL OUTCOMES FROM ICU

Psychological difficulties can persist long after discharge from ICU. Jones, Humphris, and Griffiths (1998) identified a range of psychological outcomes following ICU treatment such as recurrent nightmares, agoraphobia, panic attacks, anger, fear of dying, depression, and anxiety. Scragg, Jones, and Fauvel (2001) found that of patients recently treated in an ICU 30% reported clinically significant depression, 43% reported significant anxiety and 38% reported significant symptoms of PTSD of whom 15% would meet diagnostic criteria. Schelling et al. (1998) found that 27.5% of ICU survivors reported PTSD. Kapfhammer, Rothenhauslern, Krauseneck, Stoll, and Schelling (2004) examined prevalence rates of PTSD in ICU survivors. At discharge 43.5% reported PTSD and 8.7% reported sub-syndromal PTSD. At long-term follow-up (median 8 years) 23.9% reported PTSD and 17.4% sub-PTSD. Only length of ICU stay was predictive of this with demographic and illness factors being unrelated.

While rates of psychological distress vary between studies and may be affected by response rate, it is clear that levels of psychological distress are significantly higher in those leaving ICU than they are in the general population. For example, the lifetime prevalence rate of PTSD in the general population is estimated at between 1% and 9.2% (Breslau, Davis, Andreski, & Peterson, 1991; Helzer, Robins, & McEvoy, 1987). Rates following ICU treatment are significantly higher than this and are similar to those found in people having been exposed to major trauma (Curran et al., 1990; Kilpatrick & Resnik, 1993; Morgan, Scourfield, Williams, Jasper, & Lewis, 2003). Depression rates are also higher than those found in the general population where lifetime prevalence is estimated at between 4.4% and 19.5% (Roth & Fonagy, 2005). A number of factors have been examined to explain the high levels of psychological distress observed in ICU survivors. Scragg et al. (2001) found that being younger and having a longer ICU stay were predictive of higher rates of PTSD but not of anxiety or depression. Rattray, Johnston, and Wildsmith (2005) also found that younger age predicted anxiety and that female gender predicted higher levels of anxiety and depression. Objective measures of ICU treatment such as illness severity were not predictive of psychological outcome with the exception of length of stay. Kapfhammer et al. (2004) found that with the exception of duration of stay, no clinical or demographic factor distinguished between those who developed PTSD and those who did not. Deja et al. (2006) found an association between perceived levels of social support and PTSD following ICU treatment. Higher levels of social support were associated with lower levels of PTSD.

Patients frequently experience amnesia with regard to their time in ICU and events leading up to their admission. Rotondi et al. (2002) found that one third of participants had no recollection of their time in ICU, while Jones, Griffiths, and Humphris (2000) reported a rate of up to 40%. These patients were found to be on average more severely ill and to have spent longer on mechanical ventilation. They also found that patients were more likely to recall stressful experiences than non-stressful ones. Amnesia may be the result of a number of factors such as traumatic brain injury, delirium, sedation, and drug withdrawal (Jones, 2002). Due to poor recall of the events leading to ICU treatment and of their time in ICU, many patients do not realise how ill they have actually been or how long recovery is likely to take. This may lead to a discrepancy between expected and actual outcome. As a result, patients may develop feelings of frustration, hopelessness, and depression as the expected return to function does not occur (Jones, 2002; Jones & Griffiths, 2002).

Patients frequently report delusional and hallucinatory experiences during their time in ICU with reported rates varying from 26% to 82% (Bergbor-Engberg & Haljamae, 1988; Skirrow, 2002). Delusional experiences vary but several commonly occurring themes have been identified. These include benign hallucinatory experiences, hallucinations with a negative or delusional theme and pure delusions. Benign hallucinatory experiences are identical to other experiences except that the patient has no negative emotional reaction to them. Hallucinations with a negative delusional theme are hallucinations where the patients experience negative emotions and they may have themes such as having been kidnapped. Pure delusions are beliefs without hallucinations and may relate to reality. For example the patient may be aware that they are in hospital but believe that staff are trying to kill them (Skirrow, 2002). Capuzzo et al. (2004) found that memories of delusional experiences were more frequent in those who had no clear memory of the period in ICU and in those who had developed an infection. These patients tended to have been admitted more urgently and were more likely to have been mechanically ventilated. They also found that delusional memories persisted for longer than factual memories of ICU.

Delusional experiences are important in terms of psychological outcome. Jones, Griffiths, Humphris, and Skirrow (2001) found that those who had delusional recall of ICU had higher levels of PTSD symptoms particularly where they had not factual recall of their time in ICU. They propose that factual recall of ICU may be protective against later psychological difficulties. Jones et al. (2003) also found that higher rates of delusional memory were associated with higher levels of anxiety as well as higher levels of PTS symptoms. Granja et al. (2005) found that 51% of ICU patients reported dreams and nightmare during ICU and 14% were still disturbed by these 6 months following discharge. Those that had experienced dreams and nightmares scored significantly lower on measures of health related quality of life, including anxiety and depression.

■ COGNITIVE IMPAIRMENT

Cognitive impairments, such as memory executive difficulties can have profound effects on a person, affecting their ability to work, form and maintain relationships and may lead to long term care. Cognitive impairment has been identified in ICU patients in a number of studies. The levels and type of impairment have varied between studies and with type of illness. Jackson et al. (2007) found that 57% of trauma ICU survivors exhibited cognitive impairment at 1–2 years follow-up. Impairment was more frequent in those who had sustained skull fracture. Jackson et al. (2003) examined patients who had been in a medical ICU. They found that at six months 32% of patients exhibited cognitive impairment. Impairment was found in a range of different areas but was primarily found in working and visual memory, visual construction and processing speed. These patients were also found to have a higher incidence of depressive symptoms. Sukantarat, Burgess, Williamson, and Brett (2005) examined survivors of critical illness. They found that at three months post-discharge 55% scored below the 5th percentile on at least one cognitive assessment i.e. within the bottom 5% of the general population and 35% on two or more. However, at 9 months only 27% scored below the 5th percentile on one test and 4% on two or more. This suggests that while levels of cognitive impairment are relatively high following ICU treatment, there may be improvement over time in at least some patients. Rosene, Copass, Kastner, Nolan, and Eschenbach (1982) found that in women at 2–12 months following recovery from toxic shock syndrome, 50% exhibited symptoms such as difficulty concentrating, memory lapses, and other cognitive difficulties and also had associated neurological abnormalities. Two thirds showed electroencephalographic abnormalities. Hopkins et al. (1999) examined survivors of severe acute respiratory distress syndrome (ARDS). They found that all participants exhibited generalised cognitive impairment at discharge. At one year 30% continued to show general cognitive impairment and 78% showed impairment in at least one area of cognition.

Cognitive impairment is an obvious consequence of head trauma. However a number of other factors have been identified following ICU treatment such as hypoxaemia and sepsis (Rothenhausler, Ehrentraut, Stoll, Schelling, & Kapfhammer, 2001). In sepsis as many as 70% suffer from encephalopathy (Eidelman, Putterman, Putterman, & Sprung, 1996; Papadopoulos, Davies, Moss, Tighe, & Bennett, 2000). Wilson (1996) examined the impact of hypoxia on cognitive functioning in patients referred for neuropsychological assessment (i.e. those already identified or suspected of cognitive impairment). She found a wide range of impairment including amnesic syndrome, memory difficulties, executive dysfunction, visuo-spatial and visuo-perceptual deficits, and general intellectual impairment. Suave, Doolittle, Walker, Paul, and Scheinman (1996) examined the neuropsychological outcomes from cardiac arrest survivors. They found that while in hospital, 84% had deficits in one or more areas. Six months following discharge 50% remained impaired. The most frequent type of impairment was in delayed recall. It has been established that psychological difficulties such as depression and anxiety occur at a relatively high frequency following ICU treatment. There is a well recognised association between psychological problems such as depression and PTSD and cognitive impairment such as memory, attention, and information processing difficulties (Cohen, Lohr, Paul, & Boland, 2001; Jelinek et al., 2006; Paelecke-Habermann, Pohl, & Leplow, 2005; Samuelson et al., 2006; Yehuda et al., 2006). There may therefore be an association between the high rates of psychological difficulty and cognitive impairment identified following ICU treatment.

Cognitive impairment can influence other types of outcome following ICU treatment. For example cognitive impairment has been identified as a factor influencing work status following major trauma with those suffering cognitive impairment being less likely to return to work (Holstag, van Beeck, Lindeman, & Leenen, 2007; Jackson et al., 2007; Vles et al., 2005). Jackson et al. also found that those with cognitive impairment experienced greater difficulties in activities of daily living. Rothenhausler et al. (2001) found that at an average of six years post discharge, 24% of ARDS survivors showed cognitive impairments all of whom were classified as disabled compared to 23% of those without cognitive impairment.

■ INTERVENTION AND PREVENTION OF PSYCHOLOGICAL DIFFICULTIES

There is a paucity of literature specifically considering interventions for patients suffering from psychological problems during and following ICU treatment and clearly further research is required. Self help approaches have been found to provide some benefit. Jones et al. (2003) provided ICU patients with a self-help manual that detailed both exercise methods as well as advice around psychological and psychosocial issues. A normalising approach was emphasised throughout where it was emphasised that the experiences that the patients were having were normal for ICU survivors. They found that patients who had used the manual showed a trend towards less depression, but that there was no impact of anxiety or PTSD rates. Backmän (2002) recommends that a simple diary should be kept for each patient, detailing their stay in the ICU and including pictures. This is in order to facilitate patient understanding of what actually happened during their stay. Patients receiving the diaries reported that they were indeed helpful in facilitating understanding, although no objective outcome measures were used.

While these approaches appear beneficial, more serious psychological problems may require further treatment. The current recommended medical treatment of anxiety disorders includes the use of selective serotonin reuptake inhibitors (SSRI) or where this is not possible imipramine or clomipramine. Benzodiazapines are associated with poorer outcomes. For PTSD medication is not recommended as a front-line treatment, but trauma focused psychological therapy is. Psychological intervention studies indicate that cognitive behavioural therapy (CBT) probably has the best empirical support for both anxiety disorders generally and PTSD specifically. However other interventions such as behavioral therapy and in the case of PTSD, eye movement desensitisation reprocessing (EMDR), have also been shown to be effective (National Institute for Clinical Excellence, 2005, 2007a; Roth & Fonagy, 2005).

For mild depression guided self-help is recommended as the first line of treatment. For more severe cases, the recommended medications are SSRI's which can be combined with individual psychological therapy. There is some debate as to whether a combination of medication and psychological therapy is superior to either alone. CBT is the best supported and most recommended form of psychological therapy although there is also evidence supporting the use of Interpersonal Psychotherapy (National Institute for Clinical Excellence, 2007b; Roth & Fonagy, 2005).

For delirium, Poldemen and Smit (2005) recommend regular assessment of the patient to enable early identification (e.g. the Confusion Assessment Method for the ICU; Ely et al., 2001) and proactive management strategies. They also recommend preventative strategies such as preventing dehydration, sleep disturbance, electrolyte disorders and hypoxaemia and providing cognitive stimulation, visual and hearing aids, and early mobilisation. Delirium can be managed medically in the ICU. Lipowski (1989) recommends that this should address both the underlying cause of the delirium and its symptoms. Behavioral management may also be employed such as using clear communication with the patient and regular reality orientation, for example, letting them know where they are, what is happening, and who the therapist is (McGuire et al., 2000).

■ CONCLUSION

Psychological problems are common both during and following ICU treatment. These include organically based difficulties such as delirium and cognitive impairment and those of a more psychological nature such as stress, depression, anxiety, and PTSD. Psychological difficulties seem to be associated with a number of factors including mechanical ventilation, longer ICU stay, female gender, and pre-illness psychosocial factors such as social support. The presence of hallucinations and delusions during ICU treatment also seems to be an important factor in predicting psychological difficulties while factual recall may be protective. There is no evidence of an association between illness severity and psychological difficulties; rather it is perceived severity that is important. Cognitive impairment is common particularly in those who have received mechanical ventilation and suffered head trauma or sepsis. The effects of this can be long term, but there is evidence of improvement at least in some patients over time. Evidence for the efficacy of intervention strategies is relatively small but there is evidence that both medical and psychological strategies are likely to be effective in managing, preventing, and treating psychological difficulties.

References

American Psychiatric Association. (2000). *Diagnostic and statistical manual of mental disorders* (4th ed. Text Revision). Washington, DC: American Psychiatric Association.

Backmän, C. (2002). Patient diaries in ICU. In R. D. Griffiths & C. Jones (Eds.), *Intensive care aftercare* (pp. 125–130). Oxford: Butterworth-Heinemann.

Bergbor-Engberg, I., & Haljamae, H. (1988). A retrospective study of patients' recall of respirator treatment: Nursing care factors and feelings of security/insecurity. *Intensive Care Nursing, 4*, 95–101.

Bergeron, N., Skrobik, Y., & Dubois, M. (2002). Delirium in critically ill patients. *Critical Care, 6*, 181–182.

Biancofiore, G., Bindi, M. L., Romanelli, A. M., Urbani, L., Mosca, F., & Filipponi, F. (2005). Stress inducing factors in ICUs: What liver transplant recipients experience and what care givers perceive. *Liver Transplantation, 11*, 967–972.

Breslau, N., Davis, C., Andreski, P., Peterson, E. (1991). Traumatic events and PTSD in an urban population of young adults. *Archives of General Psychiatry, 40*, 216–222.

Capuzzo, M., Valpondi, V., Cingolani, E., De Luca, S., Gianstefani, G., Grassi, L., et al. (2004). Application of the Italian version of the intensive care unit memory tool in the clinical setting. *Critical Care, 8*, 48–55.

Cohen, R., Lohr, I., Paul, R., & Boland, R. (2001). Impairments of attention and effort among patients with major affective disorders. *The Journal of Neuropsychiatry and Clinical Neurosciences, 13*, 385–395.

Curran, P. S., Bell, P., Murray, G., Loughrey, G., Roddy, R., & Rocke, L. G. (1990). Psychological consequences of the Enniskillen bombing. *The British Journal of Psychiatry, 156*, 478–482.

Deja, M., Denker, C., Weber Carstens, S., Schröder, J., Pille, C. E., Hokema, F., et al. (2006). Social support during intensive care unit stay might improve mental impairment and consequently health related quality of life in survivors of severe acute respiratory distress syndrome. *Critical Care, 10*, 147–158.

Dubois, M. J., Bergeron, N., Dumont, M., Dial, S., & Skrobik, Y. (2001). Delirium in an intensive care unit: A study of risk factors. *Journal of Intensive Care Medicine, 27*, 1297–1304.

Eidelman, L. A., Putterman, D., Putterman, C., & Sprung, C. L. (1996). The spectrum of septic encephalopathy: Definitions, etiologies and mortalities. *The Journal of American Medical Association, 275*, 470–473.

Ely, E. W., Inouye, S. K., Bernard, G. R., Gordon, S., Francis, J., May, L., et al. (2001). Delirium in mechanically ventilated patients: Validity and reliability of the confusion assessment method for the intensive care unit (CAM-ICU). *The Journal of American Medical Association, 286*, 2703–2710.

Ely, E. W., Shintani, A., Truman, B., Speroff, T., Gordon, S. M., Harrell, F. E., Jr., et al. (2004). Delirium as a predictor of mortality in mechanically ventilated patients in the intensive care unit. *The Journal of American Medical Association, 291*, 1753–1762.

Granja, C., Lopes, A., Moriera, S., Dias, C., Costa-Pereira, A., & Carneiro, A.; JMIP Study Group. (2005). Patients recollections of experiences in the intensive care unit may affect their quality of life. *Critical Care, 9*, 96–109.

Helzer, J. E., Robins, L., & McEvoy, L. (1987). Post-traumatic stress disorder in the general population: Findings of the epidemiological catchment area survey. *The New England Journal of Medicine, 317*, 1630–1634.

Holstag, H. R., van Beeck, E. F., Lindeman, E., & Leenen, L. P. H. (2007). Determinants of long term functional consequences after major trauma. *The Journal of Trauma, 62*, 919–927.

Hopkins, R. O., Weaver, L. K., Pope, D., Orme, J. F., Bigler, E. D., & Larson-Lohr, V. (1999). Neuropsychological sequelae and impaired health status in survivors of severe acute respiratory distress syndrome. *American Journal of Respiratory Critical Care Mededicine, 160*, 50–56.

Hweidi, I. M. (2007). Jordanian patients' perception of stressors in critical care units: A questionnaire survey. *International Journal of Nursing Studies, 44*, 227–235.

Jackson, J. C., Hart, R. P., Gordon, S. M., Shintani, A., Truman, B., May, L., et al. (2003). Six month neuropsychological outcome of medical intensive care unit patients. *Critical Care Medicine, 31*, 1226–1234.

Jackson, J. C., Obremsky, W., Bauer, R., Greevy, R., Cotton, B. A., Anderson, V., et al. (2007). Long term cognitive, emotional and functional outcomes in trauma intensive care unit survivors without intracranial hemmorrrhage. *The Journal of Trauma, 62*, 80–88.

Jelinek, L., Jacobsen, D., Kellner, M., Larbig, F., Biesold, K. H., Barre, K., et al. (2006). Verbal and non-verbal memory functioning in posttraumatic stress disorder (PTSD). *Journal of Clinical Experimental Neuropsychology, 28*, 940–948.

Jones, C. (2002). Acute psychological problems. In R. D. Griffiths & C. Jones (Eds.), *Intensive care aftercare* (pp. 19–26). Oxford: Butterworth-Heinemann.

Jones, C., & Griffiths, R. D. (2002). Physical and psychological recovery. In R. D. Griffiths & C. Jones (Eds.), *Intensive care aftercare* (pp. 125–130). Oxford: Butterworth-Heinemann.

Jones, C., Griffiths, R. D., & Humphris, G. (2000). Disturbed memory and amnaesia related to intensive care. *Memory, 8*, 79–94.

Jones, C., Griffiths, R. D., Humphris, G. H., & Skirrow, P. (2001). Memory delusions and the development of acute post-traumatic stress disorder related symptoms after intensive care. *Critical Care Medicine, 29*, 573–577.

Jones, C., Griffiths, R. D., Slater, T., Benjamin, K. S., & Wilson, S. (2006). Significant cognitive dysfunction in non-delirious patients identified during and persisting following critical illness. *Intensive Care Medicine, 32*, 923–926.

Jones, C., Humphris, G. M., & Griffiths, R. D. (1998). Psychological morbidity following critical illness — The rationale for care after intensive care. *Clinical Intensive Care, 9*, 199–205.

Jones, C., Skirrow, P., Griffiths, R. D., Humphris, G. H., Ingleby, S., Eddleston, J., et al. (2003). Rehabilitation after critical illness: A randomised controlled trial. *Critical Care Medicine, 31*, 2456–2461.

Kapfhammer, H. P., Rothenhauslern, H. B., Krauseneck, T., Stoll, C., & Schelling, G. (2004). Post traumatic stress disorder and health related quality of life in long term survivors of acute respiratory distress syndrome. *The American Journal of Psychiatry, 161*, 45–52.

Kilpatrick, D. G., & Resnik, H. S. (1993). PTSD associated with exposure to criminal victimisation in clinical and community populations. In J. R. T. Davidson & E. B. Foa (Eds.), *PTSD in review: DSM-IV and beyond*. Washington, DC: American Psychiatric Association Press.

Lipowski, Z. J. (1989). Delirium in the elderly patient. *The New England Journal of Medicine, 320*, 578–582.

Lin, S. M., Liu, C. Y., Wang, C. H., Lin, H. C., Huang, C. D., Huang, P. Y., et al. (2004). The impact of delirium on the survival of mechanically ventilated patients. *Critical Care Medicine, 32*, 2352–2354.

Malt, U. F., & Olafsen, O. M. (1992). Psychological appraisal and emotional response to physical injury: a clinical phenomenological study of 109 adults. *Psychiatric Medicine, 10*, 117–134.

McGuire, B. E., Basten, C. J., Ryan, C. J., & Gallgher, J. (2000). Intensive care syndrome: A dangerous misnomer. *Archives of Internal Medicine, 160*, 906–909.

Mohta, M., Sethi, A. K., Tyagi, A., & Mohta, A. (2003). Psychological care in trauma patients. *Injury, 34*, 17–25.

Morgan, L., Scourfield, J., Williams, D., Jasper, A., & Lewis, G. (2003). The Aberfan disaster; 33 year follow-up of survivors. *The British Journal of Psychiatry, 182*, 532–536.

National Institute for Clinical Excellence. (2005). Post-traumatic stress disorder (PTSD). The management of PTSD in adults and children in primary and secondary care. National Institute for Clinical Excellence.

National Institute for Clinical Excellence. (2007a). Anxiety (amended): Management of anxiety (panic disorder with or without agoraphobia, and generalised anxiety disorder) in adults in primary, secondary and community care. National Institute for Clinical Excellence.

National Institute for Clinical Excellence. (2007b). Depression (amended): Management of depression in primary and secondary care. National Institute for Clinical Excellence.

Novaes, M. A., Aronovich, A., Ferraz, M. B., & Knobel, E. (1997). Stressors in the ICU: Patients evaluation. *Journal of Intensive Care Medicine, 23*, 1282–1285.

Novaes, M. A., Knobel, E., Bork, A. M., Pavão, O. F., Nogueira-Martins, L. A., & Ferraz, M. B. (1999). Stressors in the ICU: Perception of the patient, relatives and health care team. *Journal of Intensive Care Medicine, 25*, 1421–1426.

Paelecke-Habermann, Y., Pohl, J., & Leplow, B. (2005). Attention and executive functions in remitted major depression patients. *Journal Affective Disorder, 89*, 125–135.

Papadopoulos, M. C., Davies, D. C., Moss, R. F., Tighe, D., & Bennett, E. D. (2000). Pathophysiology of septic encephalopathy: A review. *Critical Care Medicine, 28*, 3019–3024.

Poldemen, K. H., & Smit, E. (2005). Dealing with the delirium dilemma. *Critical Care, 9*, 335–336.

Rattray, J. E., Johnston, M., & Wildsmith, J. A. W. (2005). Predictors of emotional outcomes of intensive care. *Anaesthesia, 60*, 1085–1092.

Rosene, K. A., Copass, M. K., Kastner, L. S., Nolan, C. M., & Eschenbach, D. A. (1982). Persistent neuropsychological sequelae of toxic shock. *Annals of Internal Medicine, 96*, 865–870.

Roth, A., & Fonagy, P. (2005). *What works for whom? A critical review of psychotherapy research* (2nd ed.). New York: Guilford Press.

Rothenhausler, H. B., Ehrentraut, S., Stoll, C., Schelling, G., & Kapfhammer, H. P. (2001). The relationship between cognitive performance and employment and health status in long term survivors of the acute respiratory distress syndrome: results of an exploratory study. *General Hospital Psychiatry, 23*, 90–96.

Rotondi, A. J., Celluri, L., Sirio, C., Mendelsohn, A., Schulz, R., Belle, S., et al. (2002). Patients recollections of stressful experiences while receiving prolonged mechanical ventilation in an intensive care unit. *Critical Care Medicine, 30*, 746–752.

Samuelson, K. W., Neylan, T. C., Metzler, T. J., Lenoci, M., Rothlind, J., Henn-Haase, C., et al. (2006). Neuropsychological functioning in posttraumatic stress disorder and alcohol abuse. *Neuropsychology, 20*, 716–726.

Schelling, G., Stoll, C., Haller, M., Briegel, J., Manert, W., Hummel, T., et al. (1998). Health related quality of life and post-traumatic stress disorder in survivors of the acute respiratory distress syndrome. *Critical Care Medicine, 26*, 651–659.

Schnyder, U., & Malt, U. F. (1998). Acute stress response patterns to accidental injuries. *Journal of Psychosomatic Research, 45*, 419–424.

Schnyder, U., Morgeli, H., Nigg, C., Klaghofer, R., Renner, N., Trentz, O., et al. (2000). Early psychological reactions to life threatening injuries. *Critical Care Medicine, 28*, 86–91.

Scragg, P., Jones, A., & Fauvel, N. (2001). Psychological problems following ICU treatment. *Anaesthesia, 56*, 9–14.

Skirrow, P. (2002). Delusional memories of ICU. In R. D. Griffiths & C. Jones (Eds.), *Intensive care aftercare*. Oxford: Butterworth-Heinemann.

Suave, M. J., Doolittle, N., Walker, J. A., Paul, S. M., & Scheinman, M. M. (1996). Factors associated with cognitive recovery after cardiopulmonary resuscitation. *American Journal of Critical Care, 5*, 127–139.

Sukantarat, K. T., Burgess, P. W., Williamson, R. C. N., & Brett, S. J. (2005). Prolonged cognitive dysfunction in survivors of critical illness. *Anaesthesia, 60*, 847–853.

Thomason, J. W., Shintani, A., Peterson, J. F., Pun, B. T., Jackson, J. C., & Ely, E. W. (2005). Intensive care delirium an independent predictor of longer hospital stay: a prospective analysis of 261 non-ventilated patients. *Critical Care, 9*, 375–381.

Van de Leur, J. P., Van der Schans, C. P., Loef, B. G., Deelman, B. G., Geertzen, J. H., & Zwaveling, J. H. (2004). Discomfort and factual recollection in intensive care unit patients. *Critical Care, 8*, 467–473.

Vles, W. J., Steverburg, E. W., Essink-Bot, M. L., van Beeck, E. F., Meeuwis, J. D., & Leenen, L. P. (2005). Prevalence and determinants of disabilities and return to work after major trauma. *The Journal of Trauma, 58*, 126–135.

Wilson, B. A. (1996). Cognitive functioning of adult survivors of cerebral hypoxia. *Brain Injury, 10*, 863–874.

Yehuda, R., Tischler, L., Golier, J. A., Grossman, R., Brand, S. R., Kaufman, S., et al. (2006). Longitudinal assessment of cognitive performance in holocaust survivors with and without PTSD. *Biological Psychiatry, 60*, 714–721.

APPENDIX A-8

Mixed Methods in Intervention Research: Theory to Adaptation

Bonnie K. Nastasi
Walden University, Minneapolis, Minnesota
John Hitchcock
Caliber, an ICF International Company, Fairfax, VA Walden University, Minneapolis, Minnesota
Sreeroopa Sarkar Gary Burkholder
Walden University, Minneapolis, Minnesota
Kristen Varjas
Georgia State University, Atlanta
Asoka Jayasena
Peradeniya University, Sri Lanka

The purpose of this article is to demonstrate the application of mixed methods research designs to multiyear programmatic research and development projects whose goals include integration of cultural specificity when generating or translating evidence-based practices. The authors propose a set of five mixed methods designs related to different phases of program development research: (a) formative research, Qual →/+ Quan; (b) theory development or modification and testing, Qual → Quan →/+ Qual → Quan . . . Qual → Quan; (c) instrument development and validation, Qual → Quan; (d) program development and evaluation, Qual →/+ Quan →/+ Qual →/+ Quan . . . Qual →/+ Quan, or Qual →←← Quan; and (e) evaluation research, Qual + Quan. We illustrate the application of these designs to creating and validating ethnographically informed psychological assessment measures and developing and evaluating culturally specific intervention programs within a multiyear research program conducted in the country of Sri Lanka.

Keywords: mixed methods, intervention research, evaluation research, culture specificity.

Given the current emphasis on both evidence-based practice and culturally competent practice, it is critical for researchers and interventionists to identify models for developing culturally appropriate evidence-based practice (e.g., Ingraham & Oka, 2006; Nastasi & Schensul, 2005). Mixed methods designs applicable to intervention research can take a number of forms depending on the specific purpose or stage of the project (for an in-depth discussion of mixed methods designs, see Tashakkori & Teddlie, 2003). Most mixed methods discussions (e.g., Creswell, 2003; Tashakkori & Teddlie, 2003) do not cover multiphase evaluation projects in detail, nor do they address the potential role of mixed methods designs for developing culturally appropriate practices in applied fields such as education and psychology. Morse (2003) discussed the application of mixed methods designs across

Source: Journal of Mixed Methods Research 2007, Vol. 1, No. 2, 164

individual studies within a program of research but did not present an integrative multi-phase model for conducting programmatic research. Furthermore, although qualitative research designs (e.g., ethnography) are well suited for understanding culture and context, the integration of qualitative and quantitative methods to facilitate development of culture-specific instruments (e.g., psychological assessment tools) and interventions has received minimal attention (see Hitchcock et al., 2005).

We propose that the process of program development research is best characterized by a recurring sequence of qualitative and quantitative data collection culminating in a recursive qualitative-quantitative process depicted as Qual → Quan → Qual → Quan . . . (Qual →← Quan). Qualitative methods (Qual) are used to generate formative data to guide program development, followed by quantitative evaluation (Quan) to test program effectiveness. Application in another setting can be facilitated by subsequent qualitative data collection (Qual) leading to program design adapted to the new context and participants, which is then followed by quantitative data collection (Quan) to test program outcomes. This sequence can occur across multiple settings and participant groups. Following initial adaptations to local context, program implementation and evaluation can be characterized by a recursive process (Qual →← Quan) in which collection of both qualitative and quantitative data inform ongoing modifications as well as implications for future program development and application.

The purpose of this article is to demonstrate the application of mixed methods research designs to multiyear programmatic research and development projects, whose goals include the integration of cultural specificity into development of an evidence base for practice. In particular, we illustrate the application of mixed methods designs to the development and validation of ethnographically informed psychological assessment measures, and the development and evaluation of culturally specific intervention programs.

■ A HEURISTIC MODEL: THEORY TO ADAPTATION

We propose a general heuristic for depicting multiyear research and development projects as an iterative research intervention process (see Fig. A8.1), based on the Participatory Culture-Specific Intervention Model (PCSIM; Nastasi, Moore, & Varjas, 2004). The research process begins with formative data collection to test the proposed conceptual model based on existing theory and research. At this stage, qualitative research methods are used to identify and define the constructs/variables specific to a particular culture or context (e.g., individual and environmental factors that explain/predict mental health, violent behavior, or academic achievement in a specific cultural group). Findings from the qualitative research are used to construct a modified model and develop assessment and intervention tools to test the model. Quantitative research methods are then used to test the model, for example, using instrument validation techniques and/or experimental or quasi-experimental designs. Evaluation research involves the triangulation of qualitative and quantitative methods to examine

Authors' Note: The initial phases of this work were funded by grants to the first author from the Society for the Study of School Psychology and the State University of New York at Albany. An earlier version of this article was presented at the annual meeting of the American Educational Research Association, San Francisco, April 2006.

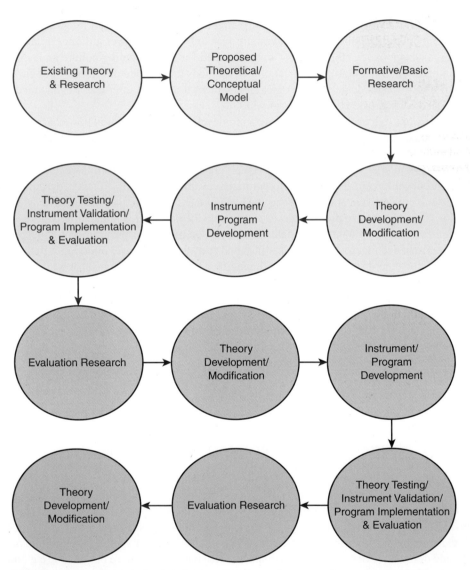

FIGURE A8.1 Mixed methods in intervention research process: theory to adaptation.

acceptability, integrity, and effectiveness of intervention methods as both a formative and summative process. The application of research as an ongoing formative evaluation process can assist in systematic modification of the intervention model and program design to meet context-specific needs (e.g., application of intervention to particular school or community). Summative research provides evidence of program effectiveness and informs application and translation to other settings. As interventions are applied to multiple populations and settings, the iterative use of mixed methods can help to inform adaptations and development of a general intervention model.

■ APPLYING MIXED METHODS DESIGNS TO MULTIYEAR RESEARCH AND DEVELOPMENT PROJECTS: AN ILLUSTRATION

As depicted in Figure A8.1, the multiple purposes for research within any given multiyear project (e.g., formative research, instrument development, evaluation research) necessitate the use of mixed methods designs. Drawing on the general model (Fig. A8.1), we propose a set of five designs applicable across various phases of the theory → adaptation process (see Table A8.1). The remainder of this article is focused on description and illustration of these five designs, based on our own intervention research experiences across an ongoing multiyear project, the Sri Lanka Mental Health Promotion Project (SLMHPP). (Although Figure A8.1 provides the heuristic for depicting the theory to adaptation process of program development, the remainder of this article is focused on representing the five designs depicted in Table A8.1. (For other examples of the application of mixed methods to multiyear research and development projects, see Nastasi et al., 1998–1999; Nastasi, Schensul, Balkcom, & Cintrón-Moscoso, 2004; Schensul, Mekki-Berrada, Nastasi, & Saggurti, in press; Schensul, Nastasi, & Verma, 2006; Schensul, Verma, & Nastasi, 2004.)

In the SLMHPP, conducted in the Central Province of Sri Lanka, we applied various mixed methods designs to (a) conduct formative research, (b) develop and test culture-specific theory, (c) develop and validate culture-specific instruments, and (d) develop and evaluate a culture-specific intervention program. Attempts to further test and modify culture-specific theory and mental health programming in India and other Sri Lankan contexts are ongoing. Although we attempt to represent the use of mixed methods for specific purposes or phases in the theory → adaptation process, the distinctions across phases are artificial (as reflected in Fig. A8.1). Thus, for example, formative research and theory development phases overlap as do theory testing and instrument development. Furthermore, the phases are not always sequential but may occur concurrently or recursively. (As noted throughout, some of the findings from various phases of the project have been published or presented elsewhere. This article, however, reflects an integration of the work within a multiphase mixed methods framework.)

■ FORMATIVE/BASIC RESEARCH PHASE: QUAL →/+ QUAN

The application of mixed methods to the formative phase of intervention research is characterized by sequential or concurrent collection of qualitative and quantitative data (see Table A8.1). In SLMHPP, we used a sequential process in which initial qualitative data collection informed theory development and design of psychological measures. These measures were then used to collect quantitative data on a larger and more representative sample and, thus, extend and confirm formative research findings.

As an outgrowth of a project focused on sexual risk among Sri Lankan youth, researchers from the United States developed knowledge of the Sri Lankan youth and educational cultures, identified the need for mental health services, and formed partnerships with professionals and community members. A formative research study was conducted in Sri Lanka in 1995 to examine individual and cultural constructs related to mental health of

Table A8.1

Mixed Methods Designs Applied to Multiyear Research and Development Projects		
PROJECT PHASE	DESIGN	TYPES OF DATA COLLECTED IN SLMHPP
Formative/basic research	Qual →/+ Quan	Focus group interviews Individual in-depth interviews Key-informant interviews Participant observation Archival materials (e.g., school records) Cultural and historical literature Popular mental health literature and popular media Secondary data analysis (qualitative and quantitative data from previous project on sexual risk among older adolescents and young adults from same community)
Theory development or modification and testing	Qual → Quan →/+ Qual → Quan ... Qual → Quan	Development of culture-specific theory and quantitative psychological measures (self- and teacher report) based on formative research data
Instrument development and validation	Qual → Quan	Administration of psychological measures to 600 students and 100 teachers Instrument validation and theory testing through combined factor analysis of quantitative (psychological measure) data and reanalysis of qualitative formative data Further theory development through parallel formative research in India (qualitative interviews)
Program development and evaluation	(a) Qual →/+ Quan →/+ Qual →/+ Quan ... Qual →/+ Quan; or (b) Qual→←Quan	Program development based on formative research data Formative program evaluation (program monitoring): Participant observations Teacher interviews/meetings Session logs (teachers and observers) Teacher session evaluations Student session evaluations Staff field notes Student products (from session activities)
Evaluation research	Qual + Quan	Experimental pre-post control group design (summative program evaluation): Pre-post student and teacher psychological measures Postintervention teacher interviews Final session student evaluation activity Reanalysis of formative evaluation data

Note. Qual = Qualitative methods; Quan = Quantitative methods; → = followed by [sequential design]; + = concurrent with [concurrent design]; →/+ = sequential or concurrent; →← = recursive, interactive; SLMHPP = Sri Lanka Mental Health Promotion Project.

the school-aged population in the country and to assess the need for mental health services in the schools (Nastasi, Varjas, Sarkar, & Jayasena, 1998).

Underlying the work was a conceptual model of mental health based in ecological developmental theory (Bronfenbrenner, 1989). A major assumption of the model is that critical individual and cultural factors influence mental health. That is, mental health status of an individual is influenced by (a) *personal vulnerabilities* due to personal and family history (e.g., early school failure, family alcoholism), (b) *social-cultural stressors* (e.g., community violence), (c) the extent to which the individual possesses *culturally valued competencies* (e.g., academic competence, social skills), (d) culture-specific *socialization practices* (e.g., school discipline practices) and *cultural agents* (e.g., family, teacher, media) responsible for promoting the development of competencies, (e) *personal resources* (e.g., problem-solving skills) for coping with daily stresses and major life changes, and (f) *social-cultural resources* available to youth (e.g., peers, family, mental health facilities) to facilitate coping. This conceptual framework has been applied to the development of mental health programs in schools within the United States (Cowen et al., 1996; Nastasi et al., 1998; Nastasi, Moore et al., 2004; Roberts, 1996).

Formative research data, collected in 18 schools in the Central Province of Sri Lanka, were used to develop an understanding of the individual and cultural factors (described above) that influenced mental health of youth in Sri Lanka. Qualitative data collection methods included 51 focus group interviews with students (33) and teachers (18), individual interviews with school principals and teachers, participant observation in schools, archival materials such as school discipline reports, historical and cultural literature, popular mental health literature, and popular media. In addition, secondary analysis of qualitative (in-depth interviews) and quantitative (ethnographically informed psychological measures) data from the previous sexual risk project (Nastasi et al., 1998–1999) focused on older adolescents and young adults from the same community.

■ FINDINGS

The primary qualitative data provided culture-specific definitions of the major mental health constructs (e.g., stressors, competencies) and the basis for elaboration of the proposed conceptual framework (i.e., identification and definition of factors specific to Sri Lanka; Nastasi et al., 1998). Findings from this formative stage also suggested gender differences and similarities in definition of mental health as described by the adolescent students (Sarkar, 2003).

Competencies. Both male and female adolescent students argued that a socially competent individual is respectful to others, loyal, trustworthy, helpful, and caring. They also suggested that such a person advises or guides others, and is socially responsible (e.g., loves her or his country, works for its development). However, friendliness was viewed as an important quality only by the female students. (Unless otherwise indicated, the qualitative findings presented in this section are drawn from Nastasi et al., 1998; Sarkar, 2003.)

Student definitions of academic competencies were directly associated with high academic achievement and striving for maximum performance in academics. An academically competent person is one who is "good at studies as well as at extracurricular activities." In defining behavioral competence, students identified good behavior, humility, and obedience as the most important qualities of a behaviorally well-adjusted person. Students argued that such an individual follows rules, obeys laws of the land, and does not harm the country. Showing respect to the elders was another critical feature of behavioral competence as indicated by the students irrespective of their gender.

Adjustment Difficulties.   Students recognized several adjustment difficulties among Sri Lankan adolescents. For example, smoking, substance abuse, and suicide were viewed as major adjustment difficulties. Suicide rate was reportedly high among the adolescents in Sri Lanka (Nastasi et al., 1998), and the concern for adolescent suicide was reflected in the interviews with students as well. Female respondents indicated that they suffered from anxiety, whereas male respondents described that they felt restless due to the uncertainty of their future. Students from both genders argued that academic adjustment difficulties were primarily related to poor academic achievement or concerns about performance. These included neglecting studies, academic failure (e.g., failure in the examination), and performance anxiety (e.g., "worry about results in the examination").

Social adjustment difficulties among the Sri Lankan students included aggression, neglecting responsibilities or duties, and being untrustworthy and not helpful to others. Sri Lankan boys also described engagement in criminal activities such as stealing, robbing, and joining gangs as forms of social adjustment problems. Sri Lankan girls suggested that interfering in others' personal affairs and slandering or stigmatizing others were indicative of social adjustment difficulties.

Stressors.   Academic stressors identified by students included academic failure, rigorous examination processes, high level of academic pressure with limited opportunities for recreation or leisurely activities, parental or societal pressure for high academic achievement, high level of competition in academics, and uncertainty about the future due to limited access to higher education and high rate of unemployment. Only about 2% of students are allowed access to university study and economic prospects are limited for the rest.

Major family stressors included alcoholism of parents (mainly fathers), poverty or financial difficulties, domestic violence, parental fights, parental divorce or separation, and separation from parents. Students also considered lack of care and attention from parents and abandonment by parents as stressors. Adolescents discussed parentification of children (e.g., children assume household responsibilities in absence of their parents). This was particularly visible in the families where mothers were working in the Middle East. Adolescents also described the physical and sexual abuse of the children in absence of their mothers. Both Sri Lankan males and females spoke of restrictions on male-female interaction in their culture as problematic.

Students also identified financial problems and poverty as major social stressors. In addition, male students spoke of war, terrorism, and injustices in the society as other social problems. Unemployment was another problem that was cited frequently by male students as social stressors. On the contrary, girls did not mention unemployment as a problem. This may be linked to the societal emphasis on the role of men as the primary providers of the family. Furthermore, girls identified gender inequity (such as lack of freedom for women and differential expectations for men and women) and sexual harassment as social stressors specific to their gender. The male students indicated that the ethnic conflicts within Sri Lanka were a major concern for them. In addition, male students exhibited concern about the political violence and the widespread corruption in the country.

Students suggested death of loved ones, loss of relationships, betrayal, and misunderstandings as relationship stressors. According to them, peer ridicule, fighting with friends, and being ignored or neglected by friends hurt their feelings. In addition, fighting with parents, being pushed by the parents to study without recreation, or the controlling behavior of the parents strained the adolescents' relationships with their parents. Despite these relationship concerns, adolescents viewed peers and parents as potential sources of support in the event of relationship stressors.

Vulnerability.   Students also indicated poverty, lack of family support, alcohol and drug abuse, and academic failure as major personal history factors that made them vulnerable to mental health problems. A striking gender difference was noted in reports of anxiety, nervousness, and health problems, which were restricted to female respondents.

Socialization.   When describing socialization processes and agents, adolescents from Sri Lanka argued that the educational system played an important role in the process of socializing youth. Students discussed the cultural emphasis on high academic achievement and the resultant pressure on adolescents for academic study with limited time for recreation. Students also indicated heavy reliance on tuition classes (private tutoring) for additional academic support that could be related to the prime importance of academic performance. In addition, adolescents indicated the Sri Lankan society valued and underscored the importance of professional jobs (e.g., doctors, engineers). Performance on standardized examinations at Grades 10 (O/L, ordinary level) and 12 (A/L, advanced level) determined admission to government-funded colleges and one's major area of study (those with highest scores were admitted to medicine, then engineering, etc.).

Cultural Norms.   With regard to cultural norms, students suggested that society reinforces high levels of respect for elders in Sri Lanka. This norm influences parent-child relationships and may explain reported social and emotional distancing between adults and children. Students also indicated a restriction on male-female interaction. They talked about parental and societal disapproval of relationships between boys and girls. Respondents, particularly females, described the lack of freedom or independence of girls, in contrast to the boys, who were considerably more independent. Among other prominent cultural norms, Sri Lankan adolescents spoke about arranged marriage (i.e., parents arrange and/or approve marriage) and the practice of dowry.

Data collected at this formative stage not only contributed to development of culture-specific theory but also contributed to development of culture-specific assessment, intervention, and teacher training materials that continued over a period of 5 years. The subsequent steps also reflect mixed methods designs.

■ THEORY DEVELOPMENT/MODIFICATION AND TESTING PHASE: QUAL → QUAN →/+QUAL → QUAN . . . QUAL → QUAN

The process of theory development and testing can be depicted as a sequence of qualitative data collection to inform theory development, followed by testing theory quantitatively and modifying theory through qualitative data collection conducted sequentially or concurrently, followed by quantitative methods to test modified theory, and so on. The repeated application of mixed methods across cultures, contexts, and populations can be used to develop theory that reflects both universal and culturally specific constructs. In the SLMHPP project, we developed a culture-specific framework for conceptualizing the individual and social-cultural factors related to mental health (see previous formative stage). The combined use of qualitative and quantitative data analysis informed theory development. This work is reflected in the next section on instrument development. In addition, subsequent qualitative data collection in Calcutta, India, helped to extend theory development to another Asian country (Sarkar, 2003). Ongoing work will examine the application within posttsunami contexts within Sri Lanka.

■ INSTRUMENT DEVELOPMENT AND VALIDATION PHASE: QUAL → QUAN

A number of sources suggest that assessment of abstract psychological phenomena will differ by culture (see Hitchcock et al., 2005); and this is the case when assessing self-concept (Harter, 1999). Instrument development in the SLMHPP project was predicated on the application of mixed methods to instrument development, using a sequential qualitative-quantitative design to develop culturally relevant measures. Qualitative research methods were used to gather data to inform instrument development. Quantitative methods were subsequently employed to conduct instrument validation. As discussed later, this approach has the potential to yield findings that quantitative or qualitative approaches, by themselves, cannot yield. In the SLMHPP, we employed a sequential qualitative-quantitative design to develop culture-specific instruments designed to assess psychological constructs related to mental health. The process of instrument development and validation illustrated in this section overlaps with the process of theory development and testing, which involves a repeated Qual → Quan design as described in the preceding section.

Psychological instruments were developed based on the aforementioned findings on culturally valued competencies, generated via formative research, and self-concept theory of Harter (1999). Harter suggested that positive adjustment requires congruency between culturally valued expectations and self-rated competencies. For example, a male United States–based researcher would typically be in a culture that values skills with statistical analysis over, say, cross-stitching. If this researcher believed he had adequate skills with statistics, there would be congruency between his perceived competencies and what is valued. Meanwhile, his competency with cross-stitching would likely have no impact on the valence of his self-beliefs.

The investigators entered the context with this general theory of self-concept, believing that Sri Lankan adolescent mental health concerns might be tied to disparities between their perception of their competencies and what is valued in the culture. To clarify, we made limited a priori guesses as to what competencies might be valued but did assume that congruence between values and self-beliefs would indicate positive adjustment and vice versa. An example of an a priori expectation we did make was that an adolescent would be experiencing distress if she did not consider herself to be a strong student. Recall that Sri Lankan society places great expectations on educational achievement; indeed, it was believed that a student can shame family members by not performing well on exams, which are high-stakes in nature because they are a gateway to postsecondary education. Other a priori expectations were that Sri Lankan adolescents would have culturally specific stressors, coping mechanisms, support structures, and ways of expressing emotions related to stress. It also was believed that some of these phenomena would be gender-specific. Qualitative data collected during the formative research phase (see previous section) provided the basis for testing these assumptions and developing culture-specific understanding of key constructs.

Two types of scales were developed via a series of individual studies combining ethno-graphic and factor analytic techniques. The first scale type (a total of five scales were developed) assesses the relationship between culturally specific competencies and values (Nastasi, Jayasena, et al., 1999a). The second scale type (a total of seven scales) includes culturally specific scenarios that adolescents should find stressful (based on formative data) and follow-up items to assess how adolescents might respond to such stress (i.e., emotionally and via active coping, seeking support, or maladjusted behavior; Nastasi, Jayasena, et al., 1999b). Scales in the latter type were used as outcome measures for an exploratory evaluation of an intervention tailored to the needs of Sri Lankan youth (in the forthcoming evaluation design).

The work presented in the *Journal of School Psychology* (Hitchcock et al., 2005) illustrated a mixed method approach for this sort of Qual → Quan instrument development and validation. The article offered a detailed illustration of the approach using the responses 611 Sri Lankan adolescents provided to five ethnographically informed psychological measures. Such instruments offer a key connection between the primary methodologies used (i.e., ethnographic and factor analytic approaches) as they are predicated on qualitative inquiry, can translate these ideas into quantitative data and allow for the application of factor analysis. If the qualitatively derived constructs are comparable to factor analytic results, then triangulation across methods is achieved and a standardized measure can be developed that is sensitive to culturally specific phenomena. The illustration of this approach used data from an ethnographically informed psychological measure of self-concept, which, again, was predicated on Harter's (1999) work.

The scales were back-translated (e.g., English → Sinhala → English to ensure accuracy of meaning), piloted, and refined after obtaining input from local experts with knowledge of the target culture. They were then administered to students ($n = 611$; 315 males, 296 females), Grades 7 to 12, ages 12 to 19, across six schools that represented the range of the student population in terms of ethnicity, religion, and socioeconomic status. A reanalysis of data from focus groups and individual interviews (i.e., with students, parents, and school personnel) and archival information from the culture (e.g., newspapers, school documents, etc.) resulted in the identification of the range of responses to various target questions/issues. Examples of these might be as follows: describe a stressful school scenario, or describe a stressful home scenario, and so on. Qualitative analyses inform the generation of psychological constructs to explain the variation of responses and in turn the development of psychological measures that are highly targeted toward the context of interest.

Secondary analyses of quantitative data were conducted because prior analyses of qualitative data (Sarkar, 2003) indicated that the constructs identified via the factor analyses might be gender specific (Hitchcock et al., 2006). Factors from the first self-concept measure (self-rating of competencies and behaviors) were used to develop subscale scores. MANOVA analyses were performed to test for gender differences. Statistically significant differences were found, as expected, on the Suitable Behavior subscale. Furthermore, structured means analyses demonstrated that the Unsuitable Behavior scale was different for boys and girls. That is, boys and girls appeared to recognize the Unsuitable Behavior construct but report on it in different ways. To summarize, no gender differences were evident on the Personal/Interpersonal Needs construct. Girls reported higher values on the Suitable Behaviors construct, suggesting they engage in suitable behaviors more often than boys. Boys and girls differed on how they answered Unsuitable Behavior items. This last finding is probably due to the fact that the (quantitative) construct/factor is formed by items that deal with joining gangs, carrying weapons, and substance abuse; and the qualitative data indicate that these behaviors are only relevant to males. Meanwhile, female behavior is more rigid and less permissive. Of course, cross-method data triangulation was needed to reach the conclusions and to develop a scale that is sensitive to both gender and culture.

As noted previously, this mixed method approach to scale development yielded insights to Sri Lankan youth culture that could not have been obtained with singular approaches. The formative ethnographic work provided the initial identification of culturally relevant constructs. These constructs in turn generated items that could be administered to hundreds of students (of course, it is generally inefficient to apply qualitative methods when working with larger samples). Analyses of responses provided additional insights into the culturally relevant constructs via cross-method triangulation, clarification of how the constructs appear in quantitative factors, and the opportunity to apply statistical tests of null hypotheses to verify presumed gender differences. One result of SLMHPP is an assessment battery that can be used for future work, and as noted below, this general method also yielded culturally specific outcome measures that can be employed in randomized controlled trials testing culturally specific interventions.

Recall that the second set of scales we developed assessed how Sri Lankan adolescents might respond to culturally specific stressors. Hypothetical stressors were identified via a series of group and individual interviews with stakeholders in the culture, specifically, students, administrators, teachers, and parents (see formative research phase). Three types of stressors emerged from the data: academic, family, and social. Respondents also noted that stressors might be dealt with via emotion-focused coping (or lack thereof), problem-focused strategies, and seeking support from others.

To assess how students might respond to hypothetical culturally specific scenarios, seven scenarios were generated from prior qualitative analyses conducted in the formative research phase (see Table A8.2) and presented as vignettes in the ethnographically informed psychological measures (Nastasi et al., in press). A series of follow-up items were generated, also from prior qualitative analyses of the formative data, to assess how students might respond to these scenarios and the resulting scales were used as outcome measures to evaluate the effects of a culturally specific intervention (more on this below). Each scenario (and follow-up item) was translated into the primary language of the group, using a back translation method (e.g., English → Sinhala → English) to ensure accuracy of meaning.

Table A8.2

Hypothetical Scenarios for Assessing Coping With Stressors

Academic Scenarios Scenario #1
You are currently studying for O/L exams. Your mother is a doctor and your father is an engineer. Your parents want you to be a doctor, so it is important you do well on your O/Ls. You attend tuition 7 days a week and spend all of your free time studying. You have no time to visit with friends or for recreation.

Scenario #2
You have failed A/L exams by a few points and are concerned about your future. You want to be an engineer. Your family cannot afford to send you to private school or to study abroad. You are not sure what you should do.

Scenario #3
You are in a mathematics class with 50 other students and the teacher is explaining a new topic in math. You don't understand but don't ask the teacher because the other students will get at you for using class time.

Relationship Scenario
Scenario #4
You have been having a secret love affair. You and your boy/girlfriend just broke up. You cannot talk to your family or your teacher about it. You have trouble sleeping. Your parents and teachers have asked you what is wrong but you cannot talk to them. You do not know what to do. Meanwhile one of the prefects who searched your school bag found a love letter and gave the letter to the class teacher. The class teacher called your parents. The parents and teacher forbid you to communicate with your lover.

Family Scenarios
Scenario #5
You are living on the street with your family. You have a school uniform but no shoes. You usually feel hungry and sleepy at school, but are a very good student. You like to do handwriting and ask the teacher for her lunch bag to practice writing. After school, you and your sisters and brothers beg on the street.

Scenario #6
Your mother has been working in the Middle East for about a year. She sends money home regularly for the family, but there is little direct communication with the children. You are the eldest child and have been taking care of the four younger children. Your father has brought a stepmother from the village to live with you to help with household tasks. When you object to the stepmother living in the house, your father beats you severely. Because of the severe abuse, you are considering leaving home. Some of your friends have already left home and have formed a gang and invited you to become a member.

Scenario #7
It [is] the day before a big exam in school. You [come] home from school and, when you [enter] your home, your father is yelling at your mother. You father has been drinking arrack. He asks your mother for dinner. She says that dinner is not ready because she had to find money to buy rice. Your parents start arguing about money. When your mother serves dinner, the rice is overcooked. Your father starts yelling and throws the rice on the floor. Your mother says, "I'll cook more," and begins to cry. Your father tells you to clean up the mess he has made. Your mother says that you should study, not to clean up the mess that your father has made. Your father then starts beating your mother.

Source: Reprinted with permission of Sage Publications from Nastasi et al.
Note. O/L = ordinary level; A/L = advanced level.

The instruments were then administered to 120 Sri Lankan students coming from urban and suburban areas, a range of socioeconomic status (SES) levels, and different ethnic groups.

With the exception of the demographic questions, each item utilized a 3-point response format (i.e., *a lot, some, not at all*), and adolescents were asked to rate themselves on a set of culturally defined items capturing perceptions of stress and coping. To assess reactions to each scenario, students were asked to respond to items that assessed their emotional responses; coping strategies; social support (i.e., emotional or instrumental help from others); and behavioral, emotional, or health-related difficulties resulting from stressful experiences such as alcohol abuse, suicidal ideation/attempts, aggression toward peers, and physical symptoms such as headaches or stomach aches.

Qualitative analyses generated the a priori expectation that students would, if faced with the hypothetical stressors, identify with the indicators of adjustment difficulties, coping strategies, and social supports listed in the measure. Note, however, that it was anticipated that factors would likely include a mix of feelings, coping, support, and adjustment difficulty items. To verify these expectations, principal component analyses (PCAs) were conducted (Nastasi et al., in press). Across all scenarios, the analyses yielded the following factors: Adjustment Difficulties—Externalizing, engaging in acting-out behaviors labeled "undesirable/unsuitable" in the culture; Social Support, perceived effectiveness of social resources (family, peer, school/mental health personnel); and Feelings of Distress, affective reactions (e.g., sad, angry, confused) without active coping. The analyses yielded scales that were consistent with qualitative expectations. Furthermore, the factor analyses indicated variation in reactions to stressors as a function of stressful situation and raised questions about the cultural meaning of suicide. Overall, these factors are largely consistent with qualitative findings, providing additional evidence that the three constructs for responding to the scenarios presented above are valid in Sri Lankan youth culture. To assess the reliability of these scales, alpha coefficients computed separately by scenario indicated good to excellent internal consistency (alphas ranging from .70 to .95).

■ PROGRAM DEVELOPMENT AND EVALUATION PHASE: QUAL →/+QUAN →/+ QUAL →/+ QUAN . . . QUAL →/+ QUAN; ALTERNATIVELY, QUAL →/← QUAN

Mixed methods applied to program development and evaluation (see Table A8.1) is characterized by repeated sequential or concurrent use of qualitative and quantitative methods, to design, modify, and evaluate the program. For example, formative qualitative and quantitative data inform program design, and formative evaluation through concurrent or sequential qualitative and quantitative data collection during program implementation informs program modification or adaptation to meet local needs. Alternatively, this process might be characterized as an interactive or recursive process, in which qualitative and quantitative data collected on an ongoing basis inform program design, formative evaluation, and modification/adaptation.

The formative research phase of the SLMHPP provided the basis for designing a mental health promotion program (Nastasi, Varjas, et al., 1999), which was pilot tested in one school in the Central Province of Sri Lanka. The researchers employed a randomized-controlled trial to test the effectiveness of the program, and concurrent and sequential qualitative-quantitative data collection for the purposes of formative evaluation, program monitoring and adaptation, and outcome evaluation. The program consisted of 18 sessions conducted each weekday over a 4-week period with 60 students in Grades 7 through 12. Sessions were cofacilitated by teachers (from participating school) and teacher educators (from participating local university). Students engaged in individual, small group, and large group activities designed to facilitate identification of cultural expectations, stressors, coping mechanisms, and social supports in key ecological contexts (community, family, school, peer group); development and practice of culturally appropriate coping strategies; and participation in peer support activities. An example of the cultural specificity of the program was the sequence of ecological contexts in which students were encouraged to identify stressors and social supports. In contrast to typical social-emotional learning curricula designed for U.S. population, the SLMHPP curriculum focused on the self only in relationship to others (with minimal focus on the self in isolation) and began with an exploration of self within community/societal context and progressing to increasingly more intimate contexts such as school, peer group, and family. Typical programs in the United States begin with focus on self-identity (and self-care), progress to self within interpersonal relationships (caring for others), and conclude with self within society/community (community service).

During program implementation, researchers collected formative evaluation data for each session that focused on examining program acceptability, cultural relevance and social validity, integrity, and immediate impact. The data collection tools included participation observation of curriculum sessions and weekly teacher training meetings; key informant interviews with teachers, students, and school administrators; session evaluation forms completed by students, teachers, and observers; and session products (e.g., student narratives, visual depictions of stressors and supports within ecological contexts; more detailed information about evaluation methods and tools can be obtained from the first author). These data were reviewed after each session and used to inform curricular adaptations and ongoing teacher training and support. Subsequent data collection provided feedback about the success of adaptations and teacher training and support. Thus, an iterative process was reflected in the ongoing integration and application of qualitative and quantitative data to inform decision making during program implementation.

■ EVALUATION RESEARCH PHASE: QUAL →/+ QUAN

Application of mixed methods to evaluation research can be characterized by concurrent use of multiple qualitative and quantitative data collection methods to facilitate data triangulation and evaluate programs in a comprehensive manner. Comprehensive approaches to program evaluation extend beyond traditional notions of evaluating effectiveness to assessment of program acceptability, social validity (application to daily life) and cultural specificity (relevance and appropriateness to cultural background and experiences of participants), integrity or quality of program implementation, immediate and long-term outcomes, and sustainability and institutionalization of program efforts (see Nastasi, Moore et al., 2004).

Furthermore, comprehensive evaluation includes data collection from multiple informants and interpretation from multiple perspectives.

A concurrent qualitative-quantitative design was reflected in the evaluation of the SLMHPP pilot program. As described above, formative evaluation (reflecting an iterative mixed method design) addressed issues of acceptability, social validity and culture specificity, integrity, and immediate program impact. In addition, outcome evaluation was conducted using a pre-post control group design ($N = 120$; 60 experimental, 60 control) with concurrent qualitative and quantitative data collection. Outcome measures included student pre-post self-report measures (culture-specific psychological measures designed from formative data; described in an earlier section), student feedback reflected in final session products (resulting from structured session activity designed for evaluative purposes), and postintervention group interviews with program implementers (teachers and teacher educators).

We used a series of null-hypothesis significance tests and estimates of effects to analyze program impacts, supplemented by analysis of qualitative data collected during program implementation. A 2×2 multivariate analysis of covariance (MANCOVA; controlling for pretest scores) was performed for each of the stressful scenarios (depicted in Table A8.2) to test for intervention effects and gender by intervention group. Tests of the overall MANCOVA were significant for Scenarios 4 (romantic relationship), 5 and 6 (family scenarios); follow-up tests indicated a significant Group $\times$ Gender interaction for those scenarios (Nastasi et al., 2006). (The full presentation of outcome data is beyond the scope of this article. Please contact the first author for more information.)

The quantitative outcomes indicated that the SLMHPP may have heightened the awareness of girls, but not boys, to the potential feelings of distress and limited helpfulness of social support, particularly with regard to situations in which they may have limited control. In addition, exploratory analyses of anticipated responses to complex family stressors (parental alcohol abuse and domestic violence) suggests that the intervention may have heightened girls' awareness of the potential negative impact of such stressors for them personally, that is, internalizing adjustment difficulties. However, the intervention may also have heightened girls' sense of responsibility for resolving complex family problems. The quantitative results were consistent with qualitative data collected during the intervention sessions and during the formative research phase. For example, the heightened sense of responsibility resulting from complex family problems such as absent mother or family alcoholism was evident also in qualitative depictions of stressful situations. These findings have important implications regarding the need for gender specificity in mental health promotion and social-emotional learning programming, and the need for addressing context specificity (e.g., family vs. peer contexts) of coping.

Program acceptability data indicated that students responded positively to activities and opportunities to discuss common stressors and ways of coping. Observations and student reports indicated enjoyment of opportunities to be creative; curriculum activities provided opportunities to express themselves through drawing, writing, role-playing, and discussion. Teachers responded well to on-site support and ongoing skills training. They generally responded favorably to the curriculum; these responses seemed to be influenced by student responses and participation (Bernstein, 2000). For example, teachers reported satisfaction with the program when students showed interest and enjoyment and seemed to benefit from activities. Teachers reported gaining a better understanding of the lives of their students and perceived themselves in a new role as facilitator of students' social-emotional development. These perceptions were consistent with students' favorable reports of emotional support from teachers during the program. Furthermore, in follow-up interviews after program completion, teachers reported that students (both those who had participated in the program and those who were nonparticipants) sought them out for emotional support in the larger school context.

Keep in mind that the initial piloting of the intervention was a small, exploratory study designed to obtain preliminary findings on the effects of a culturally specific intervention. Hence, multiple analyses were conducted using promising outcome measures but nevertheless are still in a development phase. The number of analyses elevate the possibility of making a Type I error, and in all cases the tests were underpowered. In addition, the program was implemented in one school in one community of Sri Lanka and thus the results may not be generalizable to all students and schools within the country. Despite these limitations, the data yield important findings that can be used to guide future intervention work and larger experimental investigations.

As an extension of this work, Nastasi and Jayasena are currently engaged in developing long-term recovery programs for students and parents living in tsunami-affected coastal communities of Sri Lanka. The ongoing data collection using mixed methods designs as described herein is providing information about the applicability of the intervention program to address context-specific stressors such as natural disasters and to extend the program by involving parents as agents for promoting children's mental health. For example, the adapted intervention program included focus on coping with environmental stressors such as natural disasters (Nastasi & Jayasena, 2006). (For more information on this work, contact the first author.)

■ IMPLICATIONS: MIXED METHODS DESIGNS IN INTERVENTION RESEARCH

The work presented in this article illustrates the application of mixed methods designs to the development and evaluation of culturally specific psychological assessment measures and interventions. In this work, formative qualitative data collection was used to identify culturally relevant constructs and develop a culturally specific model of mental health. This model and the qualitative data were then used to develop assessment measures and an intervention program. Mixed methods were used to validate the assessment measure and evaluate the acceptability, integrity, social validity, and outcomes of a pilot intervention. For example, the combination of qualitative analysis of ethnographic data and factor analysis of quantitative data was used to validate scales to measure constructs related to self-concept and coping with stress, which in turn could serve as outcome measures for interventions. Similarly, the evaluation of intervention outcomes was informed by both quantitative indices and qualitative data collected during program implementation. Furthermore, mixed methods were used to monitor and adapt the program to meet context-specific and individual needs of students and teachers. Finally, a new cycle of mixed methods research was instituted to adapt the program model to a new population and context (i.e., students and parents living in tsunami-affected communities).

The repeated application of a recursive research ↔ intervention process using mixed methods can facilitate the development of culture-specific interventions and translation of evidence-based practices to diverse populations and settings. Using a mixed methods approach, researchers can engage local stakeholders (e.g., community members, educators, school administrators) in developing intervention programs that address local cultural, contextual, and population needs (e.g., community violence, drug abuse among middle school students, poor academic performance within a school district); adapting programs across multiple settings (e.g., adapting a sexual risk education program across grade levels and diverse student populations); and translating evidence-based practices to new contexts and populations. The successful application (or translation) of evidence-based interventions developed through randomized-controlled trials to naturalistic settings requires research to identify the conditions necessary for ensuring established program outcomes (see National Institute of Mental Health, 2001). Mixed method designs, as described in this article, are particularly relevant to the comprehensive evaluation of conditions necessary for effective intervention and can thus help to facilitate translational research (e.g., extension of the worked portrayed herein to tsunami-affected areas as described above).

The illustration presented here reflects a multiyear effort to develop and test theory, instruments, and interventions that are specific to culture and context, with the purpose of demonstrating the application of mixed methods designs across the multiple phases of research and development projects. The designs can of course be applied to shorter term and more focused efforts to develop culturally and contextually appropriate interventions. Moreover, as the illustration suggests, the process of ensuring cultural specificity is ongoing through the multiple stages of program design, implementation, evaluation, and translation. Mixed methods designs provide an important mechanism for facilitating development of culturally sensitive interventions and evidence-based practices.

Finally, this article also contributes to the development of multistage program evaluation models. Bamberger, Rugh, and Mabry (2006) and Stufflebeam (2001) noted that mixed methods evaluations are complex and can take the form of multistage projects. However, there appears to be a dearth of examples of such projects in the literature. We have attempted to address this shortcoming here, while advancing mixed methods conceptual frameworks to help others think through how to plan multiphase evaluation projects that use mixed methods.

References

Bamberger, M., Rugh, J., & Mabry, L. (2006). *Realworld evaluation working under budget, time, data, and political constraints.* Thousand Oaks, CA: Sage.

Bernstein, R. (2000). *A demonstration of the acceptability of a mental health project through a participatory culture-specific model of consultation in the country of Sri Lanka.* Unpublished doctoral dissertation, Department of Educational and Counseling Psychology, State University of New York at Albany.

Bronfenbrenner, U. (1989). Ecological systems theory. In R. Vasta (Ed.), *Annals of child development* (Vol. 6, pp. 187–249). Greenwich, CT: JAI.

Cowen, E. L., Hightower, A. D., Pedro-Carroll, J. L., Work, W. C., Wyman, P. A., & Haffey, W. G. (1996). *School-based prevention for children at risk: The Primary Mental Health Project.* Washington, DC: American Psychological Association.

Creswell, J. W. (2003). *Research design: Qualitative, quantitative, and mixed methods approaches.* Thousand Oaks, CA: Sage.

Harter, S. (1999). *The construction of the self: A developmental perspective.* New York, NY: Guilford.

Hitchcock, J. H., Nastasi, B. K., Dai, D. C., Newman, J., Jayasena, A., Bernstein-Moore, R., et al. (2005). Illustrating a mixed-method approach for identifying and validating culturally specific constructs. *Journal of School Psychology, 43*(3), 259–278.

Hitchcock, J. H., Sarkar, S., Nastasi, B. K., Burkholder, G., Varjas, K., & Jayasena, A. (2006). Validating culture-and gender-specific constructs: A mixed-method approach to advance assessment procedures in cross-cultural settings. *Journal of Applied School Psychology, 22*(2), 13–33.

Ingraham, C. L., & Oka, E. R. (2006). Multicultural issues in evidence-based interventions. *Journal of Applied School Psychology, 22*(2), 127–149.

Morse, J. M. (2003). Principles of mixed methods and multimethod research design. In A. Tashakkori & C. Teddlie (Eds.), *Handbook of mixed methods in social & behavioral research* (pp. 189–208). Thousand Oaks, CA: Sage.

Nastasi, B. K., Hitchcock, J. H., Burkholder, G., Varjas, K., Sarkar, S., & Jayasena, A. (in press). Assessing adolescents' understanding of and reactions to stress in different cultures: Results of a mixed-methods approach. *School Psychology International.*

Nastasi, B. K., & Jayasena, A. (2006). *Mental health promotion post-tsunami curriculum.* Minneapolis, MN: Walden University.

Nastasi, B. K., Jayasena, A., Hitchcock, J., Burkholder, G., Varjas, K., & Sarkar, S. (2006, April). *Reactions of female adolescents to a school based mental health program.* Paper presented at the 10th National Convention on Women's Studies, sponsored by Centre for Women's Research, Columbo, Sri Lanka.

Nastasi, B. K., Jayasena, A., Varjas, K., Bernstein, R., Hitchcock, J. H., & Sarkar, S. (1999a). *Student questionnaire: Perceived competencies measure for Sri Lanka Mental Health Promotion Program.* Albany, NY: School Psychology Program, State University of New York at Albany.

Nastasi, B. K., Jayasena, A., Varjas, K., Bernstein, R., Hitchcock, J. H., & Sarkar, S. (1999b). *Student questionnaire: Stress & coping measure for Sri Lanka Mental Health Promotion Program.* Albany, NY: SUNY Press.

Nastasi, B. K., Moore, R. B., & Varjas, K. M. (2004). *School-based mental health services: Creating comprehensive and culturally specific programs.* Washington, DC: American Psychological Association.

Nastasi, B. K., Schensul, J. J., Balkcom, C. T., & Cintrón-Moscoso, F. (2004). Integrating research and practice to facilitate implementation across multiple contexts: Illustration from an urban middle school drug and sexual risk prevention program. In K. E. Robinson (Ed.), *Advances in school-based mental health: Best practices and program models* (chap. 13). Kingston, NJ: Civic Research Institute.

Nastasi, B. K., Schensul, J. J., deSilva, M. W. A., Varjas, K., Silva, K. T., Ratnayake, P., et al. (1998–1999). Community-based sexual risk prevention program for Sri Lankan youth: Influencing sexual-risk decision making. *International Quarterly of Community Health Education, 18*(1), 139–155.

Nastasi, B. K., & Schensul, S. L. (2005). Contributions of qualitative research to the validity of intervention research. *Journal of School Psychology, 43*(3), 177–195.

Nastasi, B. K., Varjas, K., Bernstein, R., Hellendoorn, C., Brewster, M., Hitchcock, J., et al. (1999). *Program for Mental Health Promotion in Sri Lankan Schools: Curriculum manual & instructional guide.* (Developed for implementation in the Central Province Schools, Kandy, Sri Lanka). Albany: School Psychology Program, State University of New York at Albany.

Nastasi, B. K., Varjas, K., Sarkar, S., & Jayasena, A. (1998). Participatory model of mental health programming: Lessons learned from work in a developing country. *School Psychology Review, 27*(2), 260–276.

National Institute of Mental Health. (2001). *Blueprint for change: Research on child and adolescent mental health* (Report of the National Advisory Mental Health Council Workgroup on Child and Adolescent Mental Health Intervention Development and Deployment). Washington, DC: Author.

Roberts, M. C. (Ed.). (1996). *Model programs in child and family mental health.* Mahwah, NJ: Lawrence Erlbaum.

Sarkar, S. (2003). *Gender as a cultural factor influencing mental health among the adolescent students in India and Sri Lanka: A cross-cultural study.* Unpublished doctoral dissertation, State University of New York at Albany.

Schensul, S. L., Mekki-Berrada, A., Nastasi, B. K., & Saggurti, N. (in press). Healing traditions and men's sexual health in Mumbai, India: The realities of practiced medicine in urban poor communities. *Social Sciences and Medicine.*

Schensul, S. L., Nastasi, B. K., & Verma, R. K. (2006). Community-based research in India: A case example of international and interdisciplinary collaboration [Electronic version]. *American Journal of Community Psychology, 38*(1–2), 95–111. Available from http://dx.doi.org/10.1007/s10464-006-9066-z

Schensul, S. L., Verma, R. K., & Nastasi, B. K. (2004). Responding to men's sexual concerns: Research and intervention in slum communities in Mumbai, India. *International Journal of Men's Health, 3,* 197–220.

Stufflebeam, D. L. (2001). Evaluation models. *New Directions for Evaluation, 89,* 7–99.

Tashakkori, A., & Teddlie, C. (2003). *Handbook of mixed methods in social & behavioral research.* Thousand Oaks, CA: Sage.

Aggression Towards Health Care Workers in Spain: A Multi-facility Study to Evaluate the Distribution of Growing Violence Among Professionals, Health Facilities and Departments

Santiago Gascón, PhD; Begoña Martínez-Jarreta, PhD; J. Fabricio González-Andrade, PhD; M. Ángel Santed, PhD; Yolanda Casalod, PhD; M. Ángeles Rueda, PhD

In recent years instances of aggression by patients towards health workers appear to have become more frequent. In Spain, no scientific studies appear to have been performed so far on this question. We analyzed questionnaires on workplace aggression from a stratified sample of 1826 health professionals at 3 hospitals and 22 rural and urban Primary Care facilities located in the Northeast and East of Spain. We found 11% of health workers had been a victim of physical aggression, 5% on more than one occasion, while 64% had been exposed to threatening behaviour, intimidation or insults. About 34% had suffered threats and intimidation on at least one occasion, and 23.8% repeatedly. Over 35% had been subjected to insults on at least one occasion, and 24.3% repeatedly. In general the incidence was higher in large hospitals, with very high levels in services such as Accident and Emergency and Psychiatry.

Keywords: *aggression, violence, healthcare workers, Spain.*

Despite the high quality of care provided in the Spanish National Health System and established systems for handling patient complaints (Gracia, 1989; Osuna Carrillo & Luna Maldonado, 2004), an increase in patient aggression toward health care workers has been observed in recent years. The most severe cases frequently appear in the media and the topic has been the subject of debate both professionally and institutionally. However, scientific studies have not been available in Spain until now. A similar increase has been reported in other highly developed countries (Chappell & Di Martino, 2002; Di Martino, 2002). Studies carried out in Canada (Hesketh, Duncan, & Estrabrooks, 2003), New Zealand (Grenyer, Ilkiw-Lavalle, & Biro, 2004), Australia (Benveniste, Hibbert, & Runciman, 2005), and the United States (Duhart, 2001) have shown that doctors and nurses are at high risk. Their risk has been compared to that faced by police and other law enforcement workers (Hesketh et al., 2003). In the United States, over half the reported instances of aggression at work are towards health workers, who are at a 16 times higher risk compared to other social workers (Duhart, 2001). A variety of measures have been adopted in various European countries to

Source: International Journal of Occupational and Environmental Health, Jan/Mar 2009, Vol. 15, No. 1, 29–35.

Received from the School of Occupational Medicine, Universidad de Zaragoza. This study was carried out with the support of Fondo de Investigación Sanitaria (FIS), Ministerio de Sanidad, Instituto Carlos III.
Disclosures: The authors report no conflict of interest.

protect health care workers against patient aggression (Björkqvist, Österman, & Hjelt-Bäck, 1994; Claix & Pham, 2004; Maljers, 2006; Paoli & Merllié, 2001). For example, in 2002 the United Kingdom set up a "Zero tolerance campaign" in its National Health Service in response to the increasing levels of aggression in this sector (House of Commons, 2003; National Health Service, 2002).

Although this phenomenon has been the subject of research work in recent years, its true scope is still unknown, since all data are based almost exclusively on reported incidents (Benveniste et al., 2005; Di Martino, 2002). Bearing in mind that health workers are likely to report only the most serious cases, the figures do not show the true extent or severity of the problem (Benveniste et al., 2005).

Furthermore, until recently, most relevant studies have been carried out at psychiatric institutions and facilities, and very few studies have dealt with violence in other types of facilities, services and divisions (Henk, Nijman, & Rector, 1999; Stansfeld et al., 1995; Wells & Bowers, 2002). Given the peculiarities and characteristics of the phenomenon of violence in this sector, it is not appropriate to generalize results. The few studies which have taken into account all hospital divisions have all shown that the highest levels of violence occur in Accident and Emergency Departments (A&Es) (Cembrowicz & Shepherd, 1992), although some studies have shown of high rates of violence in other areas as well (Whittington, Shuttleworth, & Hill, 1996; Winstnaley & Whittington, 2004).

Most of the studies have been carried out exclusively on some sub-section of the health care staff, particularly nurses (Anderson & Parish, 2003; Farrell, 1999; Ferns, 2005), even though there is evidence that nurses are not the only health workers affected by violence (Wells & Bowers, 2002; Winstnaley & Whittington, 2004). Since the nursing profession is made up mainly of women, it has also been presumed that female workers are those most affected by violence (Farrell, 1999; Ferns, 2005). Two of the questions this study specifically addresses are whether nurses are more likely to suffer aggressions than other professionals, and if women experience more violent episodes than men.

Finally, many of the studies that have been carried out fail to conceptually delimit the different types of violence, and often do not differentiate between physical aggression, threatening behaviour and verbal aggression (Di Martino, 2002; Winstnaley & Whittington, 2004). For all these reasons, comparisons of studies from different authors and countries are extremely difficult. However, comparisons are desirable for a better characterization of this phenomenon from transcultural, social and economic perspectives.

In Spain, no scientific studies have been performed so far on this question. Nevertheless, it has become a priority to ascertain the main features of its extent and distribution as a prerequisite to designing and assessing the impact of any intervention.

This study aimed to characterize this phenomenon and to address the lack of information in Spain and its consequences for the victims' health.

The study was focused solely on that violence which the California Occupational Safety and Health Administration (CalOSHA) classifies as Type II (exercised by customers, users or patients), excluding other types of aggressions which might coexist in the work environment (California Occupational Safety and Health Administration Cal/OSHA, 1995).

■ METHODS

This was a retrospective study, using self-reporting, for the purpose of researching experiences of aggression and violence over the preceding twelve months. The study was performed in 3 hospitals of different sizes and 22 rural and urban Primary Care facilities located in two regions in the Northeast and East of Spain.

Participant Recruitment

The survey included only permanent staff working continuously in the same post for at least one year. The questionnaires were distributed in informative sessions carried out with groups of between 20 and 30 people, who were provided with information about the study and how to answer study questions. Participants returned surveys to boxes located in each of the healthcare facilities. The surveys were collected over a 1–2 week period. In all 7550 questionnaires were distributed.

Instruments

The health workers completed a booklet containing two questionnaires. A Demographic Data Record asked for with personal, family and workplace information. An Aggression Questionnaire asked participants to rate their experience of various forms of aggression. For each type of aggression, a definition was provided. The definitions, adopted from various international organizations (Di Martino, 2002), had previous been used by other authors. For example, Winstanley and Whittington included definitions for physical aggression, verbal threats, threatening behaviour and verbal abuse (Table A9.1) (Winstnaley & Whittington, 2004). Participants were asked to indicate whether they had experienced each type of violence in the previous 12 months (regardless of the type or the resulting lesion), using a Likert-type scale (0 = never; 1 = never, but has been witness to it happening to others; 2 = on one occasion; 3 = on two or more occasions; 4 = on more than five occasions).

Table A9.1

Violent Behaviors Investigated	
AGGRESSIONS	DEFINITION
Physical aggression	Intentional behavior with the use of physical force, producing physical, sexual, or psychological damage: kicking, slapping, stabbing, pushing and pulling, biting and pinching
Verbal threats or threatening behaviour	The promise of using physical strength or power, which produces the fear of physical, sexual, psychological damage, or other negative consequences
Insults or slander	Verbal behaviour which humiliates, degrades or shows lack of respect

For positive responses, respondents were asked for information on the characteristics of the aggression (punches, kicks, hair-pulling, etc.) and the aggressor (patient, accompanying person), whether the respondent had received specific training with regard to this problem, and whether s/he felt that s/he had the support of the health service administration.

An initial pilot study carried out with 211 health service workers showed no problems with regard to the formulation of the questions or the descriptions of each type of aggression (Martínez-Jarreta & Gascón, 2005).

The questionnaires did not contain any details which could identify the worker and, once collected, were kept in such a manner that only the research team could have access to them, thus ensuring total confidentiality. Informed consent was given by every participant prior to their inclusion in the study and the authorization of the Local Ethics Committee was obtained for every center studied.

■ RESULTS

Of the 7550 questionnaires distributed, 2137 responses were received, and 1826 were used. Forty-three questionnaires were excluded because they were incomplete. An additional 268 were excluded from analysis in order to ensure that the number of responses was proportionate to staff numbers at the various institutions. These exclusions were made based on order of questionnaire submission; the questionnaires submitted latest were excluded first.

Of the 1826 respondents, 1386 worked in a hospital setting. For purposes of analysis, all units of the hospitals were grouped in five categories:

1. Accidents and Emergencies
2. Surgical units
3. Clinical or Medical units
4. Psychiatric
5. Central Services (laboratories, administration and patient attendance, etc.)

Numbers of participants by facility type and position are shown in Table A9.2. Number of hospital-based participants by hospital division and size are shown in Table A9.3.

Table A9.2

Number of Participants and Percent of Workforce Represented, by Facility Type and Post ($n = 1826$)

	NURSES	DOCTORS	MANAGERS	ADMINISTRATION	PATIENT ATTENDANTS	OTHERS	TOTAL PARTICIPANTS
Large hospital	361 (20.0%)	256 (21.5%)	4 (13.0%)	68 (27.4%)	27 (0.6%)	87 (25.7%)	803 (19.9%)
Medium-sized hospital	169 (19.9%)	91 (19.4%)	14 (53.8%)	22 (12.5%)	16 (10.4%)	31 (6.4%)	343 (17.4%)
Small hospital	157 (52.7%)	50 (35.7%)	2 (11.7%)	14 (14.6%)	6 (3.3%)	11 (37.9%)	240 (31.6%)
Rural primary care	41 (7.6%)	56 (11.7%)	3 (33.3%)	10 (22.8%)	0 (0.0%)	0 (0.0%)	110 (8.9%)
Urban primary care	150 (80.2%)	150 (67.3%)	0 (0.0%)	30 (75.0%)	0 (0.0%)	0 (0.0%)	330 (55.4%)
Total	878	603	23	144	49	129	1826 (21.2%)

Table A9.3

Number of Hospital-Based Participants and Percent of Workforce Represented, by Hospital Division ($N = 1386$)					
	A AND E	SURGICAL	MEDICAL	PSYCHIATRY	CENTRAL
Large hospital	123 (29.9%)	169 (26.0%)	361 (32.7%)	73 (32.0%)	87 (25.1%)
Medium-sized hospital	54 (24.4%)	84 (27.2%)	125 (21.5%)	19 (31.1%)	65 (39.9%)
Small hospital	41 (37.9%)	55 (36.9%)	88 (39.8%)	21 (58.3%)	35 (42.6%)

The proportion of respondents by profession was: 33.5% doctors, 47.5% nursing professionals, 7.9% administration staff, 1.7% managers, 2.8% patient attendants, 6.6% technical staff and other professions. The majority of participants were in the ranges of 31–40 and 41–50 years of age. The average age of participants was 41.84 years (SD ± 8.427); 64.2% were women and 35.8% men.

Eleven percent of respondents had been a victim of physical aggression, 5% on more than one occasion, whilst 64% had been exposed to threatening behaviour, intimidation or insults. 34.4% had suffered threats and intimidation on at least one occasion and 23.8% repeatedly, whilst 36.6% had been subjected to insults on at least one occasion and 24.3% repeatedly.

In general the incidence was higher in medium and large hospitals (Table A9.4), with very high levels in services such as A&E and Psychiatry, with the incidences respectively of 48% and 26.9% for aggression, 82.1% and 64.1% for insults, and 87.2% and 58.6% for threats (Table A9.5).

Statistically significant differences were found between large and small hospitals with respect to physical aggression and threats (see Table A9.4). With regard to physical aggression, no statistically significant differences were found between large and medium-sized hospitals and primary care facilities located in urban areas. Neither were there statistically significant differences between small hospitals and rural primary care facilities. Levels of physical aggression were lower at rural primary care centers than urban ones. However, statistically significant differences were found between small hospitals and rural

Table A9.4

Distribution of Incidents of Aggression, by Facility Type ($N = 1826$)							
CENTER	LARGE HOSPITAL	MEDIUM-SIZED HOSPITAL	SMALL HOSPITAL	URBAN RURAL PRIMARY HEALTH	RURAL PRIMARY HEALTH CENTERS	χ^2	SIGNIFICANCE
Physical aggression	21.9%	21.7%	9.5%	17.4%	11.3%	26.435	$p < 0.001$
Insults	58.2%	56.3%	49.7%	59.5%	58.5%	0.087	$p = 0.100$
Threats	55.7%	56.3%	43.2%	57.0%	58.5%	0.120	$p = 0.003$

Table A9.5

Distribution of Incidents of Aggression Against Hospital Workers, by Division ($N = 1386$)

SERVICE	SURGICAL	CENTRAL	MEDICAL	A AND E	PSYCHIATRY	OTHERS	χ^2	SIGNIFICANCE
Physical aggression	6.3%	17.1%	9.2%	48.0%	26.9%	20.0%	45.903	$p < 0.001$
Insults	62.3%	25.0%	47.1%	82.1%	64.6%	25.0%	19.995	$p < 0.001$
Threats	62.3%	24.8%	44.6%	87.2%	58.6%	29.4%	25.825	$p < 0.001$

primary care facilities (9.5% and 11.3%), and between large hospitals and urban primary care facilities (21.9% and 17.4%). Physical violence seems to be associated with the size and complexity of the facility and its location.

No statistically significant differences were found between the different types of care with regard to insults. Statistically significant differences were found only with regard to threats between small hospitals (with a lower incidence of threats: 43.2%) and the other facility types.

Physical Aggression

No statistically significant association was observed between physical aggression and the victim's gender ($\chi^2 = 3.498$; $p = 0.610$), or professional category ($\chi^2 = 8.295$; $p = 0.141$). As has been said, this form of violence was associated more with type of facility and hospital division (see Tables A9.4 and A9.5).

Non-physical Violence

There were differences between facilities in terms of threats, with greater occurrence in large and medium hospitals (Table A9.4). Once again, A&E (87.2% of people threatened) and surgical and psychiatry divisions (62.3% and 58.6% respectively) were shown to have greater levels of occurrence than other services (Table A9.5). Men experienced significantly more threats than women ($\chi^2 = 7.977$; $p = 0.005$), and doctors and people in managerial posts received significantly more threats than other professional workers ($\chi^2 = 22.678$; $p = 0.001$) (Table A9.6).

Table A9.6

Distribution of Incidents of Aggression by Post ($N = 1826$)

POST	ADMIN	POTENTIAL ATTENDANT	MANAGER	NURSE	DOCTOR	OTHERS	χ^2	SIGNIFICANCE
Physical aggression	7.5%	18.2%	10.0%	17.0%	19.4%	11.1%	8.295	$p = 0.141$
Insults	55.0%	50.0%	40.0%	54.6%	61.6%	39.3%	11.614	$p = 0.040$
Threats	42.5%	39.1%	65.0%	49.9%	60.7%	35.7%	22.678	$p < 0.001$

Table A9.7

Percentage of Workers Who Have Suffered More Than One Violent Incident, by Facility Type ($N = 1826$)

CENTER	LARGE HOSPITAL	MEDIUM-SIZED HOSPITAL	SMALL HOSPITAL	URBAN RURAL PRIMARY HEALTH	RURAL PRIMARY HEALTH CENTERS	χ^2	SIGNIFICANCE
Physical aggression	12.9%	8.0%	5.5%	6.7%	2.8%	26.261	$p = 0.001$
Insults	41.7%	39.1%	28.8%	40.0%	35.8%	37.543	$p < 0.001$
Threats	37.9%	35.2%	26.1%	35.6%	29.1%	12.035	$p = 0.150$

A logistic regression analysis confirmed that physical aggression occurred more frequently in the larger facilities, especially in A&E and Psychiatry, while threats were more frequent in surgery and A&E. Working in A&E was predictive of the three types of aggression: physical (OR = 4.734; $p < 0.001$), insults (OR = 3.316; $p < 0.001$) and threats (OR = 3.728; $p < 0.001$).

Working in psychiatry was predictive of physical aggression (OR = 2.881; $p = 0.001$) and of insults (OR = 1.884; $p = 0.001$), while working in the area of surgery was predictive of both forms of verbal violence: threats (OR = 1.586; $p = 0.002$) and insults (OR = 1.732; $p = 0.004$). Gender was predictive only of threats, men being more threatened than women (OR = 1.491; $p = 0.001$).

Repeat Experiences of Violence and Aggression

An important proportion of health workers had been victims of violence on more than one occasion over the past 12 months. The highest levels of repeated violence were once again found in large hospitals (Table A9.7) and in the divisions of A&E and Psychiatry (Table A9.8).

Up to 85% of cases of aggression were perpetrated by the patients themselves (this percentage was lower in A&E, where 27.3% of aggressors were people accompanying patients). In 21% of cases, aggressors were affected by a mental disorder or cognitive deterioration, and 5.7% were under the influence of alcohol or drugs.

Table A9.8

Percentage of Hospital Workers Who Have Suffered More Than One Violent Incident, by Hospital Division ($N = 1386$)

SERVICE	SURGICAL	CENTRAL	MEDICAL	A AND E	PSYCHIATRY	OTHERS	χ^2	SIGNIFICANCE
Physical aggression	3.8%	3.4%	6.9%	21.9%	13.5%	3.3%	45.108	$p < 0.001$
Insults	26.2%	36.6%	43.1%	61.1%	31.7%	18.8%	48.801	$p < 0.001$
Threats	32.9%	34.4%	31.5%	51.9%	23.9%	17.7%	38.216	$p < 0.001$

The most frequent cause of aggression was dissatisfaction with waiting times (58%), followed by anger at not being given a doctor's note for time off work (15%), and disagreement with regard to the prescription of medicine (10%).

Only 8 health care workers in the sample had reported an incident of aggression through formal channels. All these cases involved serious physical attacks, which represents 3.7% of the total number of physical aggressions. None of the episodes of threats or insults had been reported.

■ DISCUSSION

The main limitations of this study come from its retrospective nature. Although it would seem reasonable to assume that those people who had suffered aggression would be more predisposed to answer, we also received anecdoctal information indicating that those who had suffered the most severe episodes did not want to talk about it or to complete the questionnaire. The response rate was low, although typical for Spain (Pariente & Andrés, 2002).

This study is part of a wider research project analyzing the characteristics and consequences of workplace aggression. The overall results show troubling levels of this type of violence in the Spanish health sector. Unfortunately, in our study as has been reported elsewhere, many violent episodes went unreported (House of Commons, 2003; National Health Service, 2002). In this respect, it should be pointed out that future studies should be designed to collect data prospectively, so as to capture the different types of violence conceptually (physical aggression, threatening behaviour and verbal aggression) in such a way that the results can be compared with other research.

As has been seen, not all staff at a facility or all members of a profession are exposed to the same risk of violent incidents. There are differences with regards to the post, to relations with patients and to the work location. Indeed, the use of mean figures for a hospital tends to obscure the high levels of aggression occurring in certain departments and towards certain health workers (Whittington et al., 1996).

The present study shows that the distribution of aggression appears to be related to the size and complexity of the facilities and to different hospital divisions. Facilities in rural and smaller urban areas registered lower levels of physical violence in comparison to larger hospitals.

Certain healthcare institutions suffer the stress of overcrowding and limited time to attend to patients (Al-Sahlawi, Zahid, Shahid, Hatim, & Al-Bader, 1999). The lack of resources, even of space to afford adequate privacy (as in A&E), are problems which lead to the depersonalization of treatment and long waiting times. This may encourage violent behavior.

Owing to the complexity of the system, the particular characteristics of healthcare and the changes occurring in the relationship between healthcare professionals and patients, large hospitals seem to provide a more propitious environment for aggression and violence towards workers by users (Anderson & Parish, 2003; Gracia, 1989). However, further studies are necessary to explain these complex relationships.

It appears that the origin of the problem is to be found in organizational rather than in individual factors (Al-Sahlawi et al., 1999). When professionals have the time and resources to establish rapport with patients, as occurs in rural facilities or in small hospitals, the health-care worker/patient relationship is better, and this may minimize the possibility of aggression (Whittington et al., 1996; Winstnaley & Whittington, 2004).

Regarding the distribution of violence in different departments of the same hospital, various assumptions have been made with regard to the places in which aggression is most frequent and staff most vulnerable. Some studies consider A&E departments have the highest levels of aggression (Cembrowicz & Shepherd, 1992). However, other evidence has shown that violent incidents are also produced outside of the A&E division (Whittington et al., 1996; Winstnaley & Whittington, 2004). This study confirms that A&E is the primary site of physical and non-physical violence but that other areas, especially Surgery and Psychiatry, also show very high indices.

Physical violence is predominately directed towards doctors and nurses. Insults are directly fairly equally towards all staff, while threats vary with hierarchical status, most often being aimed at those who have control or authority and, in consequence, are responsible for making decisions. This appears to be an expression of intentional violence in an attempt to impact decision-making.

Until recently, it had been considered that nursing staff were the most vulnerable to aggression in the health sector, perhaps due to an "a priori" consensus that they were more at risk. Most of the surveys on this problem were carried out exclusively on this group of health workers (Anderson & Parish, 2003; Farrell, 1999; Wells & Bowers, 2002). Our results confirm that nurses are the largest group of health workers affected by violence, as has been pointed out by other authors (Wells & Bowers, 2002; Whittington et al., 1996; Winstnaley & Whittington, 2004). Our results also show, however, that doctors have much violence directed towards them. This suggests that violence and aggression most affects those most in contact with patients.

As this and other studies have shown, only a small fraction of the aggression suffered by health workers is formally reported (House of Commons, 2003). For a variety of reasons, healthcare workers tend to report serious incidents which have required medical intervention, while less serious cases of physical or verbal aggression are rarely reported or followed up.

The incidence and the distribution of physical and non-physical aggression seem very distinct; physical aggression is usually of lower intensity in the healthcare sector, whereas non-physical violence occurs more frequently and, according to Winstanley and Whittington, appears to be associated with the new onset of psychological symptoms among the victims (Winstnaley & Whittington, 2004).

As part of another study, an analysis was performed of the relationship between patients' aggression and psychological symptomatology (depression, anxiety, post-traumatic stress, insomnia, burnout and deteriorated relationships at work). Although no statistically significant association was found between physical aggression and psychological symptomatology, a statistically significant association was found between nonphysical violence and anxiety and symptoms of Post-Traumatic Stress Syndrome. Both physical and non-physical violence had an identical negative impact in terms of burnout, exhaustion, and conflicts of values in health care workers.

To date, little effort has been made to eliminate or minimize this problem (National Health Service, 2002). This may be because, in most countries, studies have not been performed to characterise the problem and allow the effective design of preventive strategies. However, in response to a recent increase in violent incidents, a change of legislation in Spain has meant stronger sanctions for Type II violence, not only in healthcare, but in other settings as well.

Based on the results of this study, we have proposed prevention protocols which include medical and legal counsel as well as psychological support for the victims (Gascón et al., 2008). It should also be the responsibility of the health care center administration to encourage victims to report these incidents, thus sending a clear message that this type of conduct will not be tolerated. Some authors go even further and argue that the health care center administration itself should stand as plaintiff (Yassí, Gilbert, & Cvitkovich, 2005). It is difficult to establish which legal measure would be appropriate to be considered even in the worst cases. This is currently a question of debate in Spain (Alarcón & Ruiz de Adana, 2005).

It would be useful to implement a system which could document and record violence in health centers using a single model, with exhaustive information on the incident, thus facilitating national and international comparative analyses for the whole country.

Data on professionals who repeatedly suffer aggression, and on departments with a high incidence of patient aggression, are of particular interest. We agree with Whittington et al. (1996) that most individuals who have experienced patient aggression have been victims of such aggression more than once. In addition, others have not suffered any aggression at all. This clearly indicates the need to collect information on victims of repeated violence (Whittington et al., 1996). The importance of these variations is clear when we divide the data into areas and professions.

The data from this study help locate the problem and identify the risks, but further research is necessary with regards to the aetiology of the aggression and the vulnerability of certain individuals and groups. Further research is also required with respect to vulnerability to repeated aggression attributable to individual characteristics, workplace role, or working environment. The fact that the healthcare workers are often required to return to work in the same department, and even with the same patient, following an incident may be a factor contributing to recurrence of a similar incident.

In summary, events and patterns shown in our study, many supported by information in the literature, provide evidence for health care administrations to place a high priority on addressing aggression and violence in the workplace and to develop appropriate medical and legal protocols for incidents of aggression and violence, for providing psychological support and medical and legal advice for victims.

References

Alarcón, M. J., & Ruiz de Adana, J. J. (2005). La violencia en el medio sanitario. *Actas del Congreso de la Asociación Española de Derecho Sanitario*, Madrid.

Al-Sahlawi, K. S., Zahid, M. A., Shahid, A. A., Hatim, M., & Al-Bader, M. (1999). Violence against doctors: A study of violence against doctors in accident and emergency departments. *European Journal of Emergency Medicine, 6*(4), 301–304.

Anderson, C., & Parish, M. (2003). Report of workplace violence by Hispanic nurses. *Journal of Transcultural Nursing, 14*, 237–243.

Benveniste, K. A., Hibbert, P. D., & Runciman ,W. D. (2005). Violence in health care: The contribution of the Australian Patient Safety Foundation to incident monitoring and analysis. *The Medical Journal of Australia, 183*(7), 348–351.

Björkqvist, K., Österman, K., & Hjelt-Bäck, M. (1994). Aggression among university employees. *Aggressive Behavior, 20*, 173–184.

California Occupational Safety and Health Administration (Cal/OSHA). (1995). *Guidelines for workplace security.* San Francisco, CA: Department of Industrial Relations, Division of Occupational Safety and Health.

Cembrowicz, S. P., & Shepherd, J. P. (April 1992). Violence in the accident and emergency department. *Medicine Science and the Law, 32*(2), 118–122.

Chappell, D., & Di Martino, V. (2002). *Violence at work* (2nd ed.), Geneva: International Labour Office.

Claix, A., & Pham, T. H. (2004). Evaluation of the HCR-20 violence risk assessment scheme in a Belgian forensic population. *Encephale, 30*(5), 447–453.

Di Martino, V. (2002). *Workplace violence in the health sector—Country case studies (Brazil, Bulgaria, Lebanon, Portugal, South Africa, Thailand, and an additional Australian study): Synthesis report.* Ginebra (SWZ): OIT/OMS/CIE/ISP.

Duhart, D. T. (2001). *Violence in the workplace, 1993–99.* Bureau of Justice Statistics. Special Report. 2001. U.S. Department of Justice.

Farrell, G. A. (1999). Aggression in clinical settings: Nurses' views—A follow-up study. *Journal of Advanced Nursing, 29*, 532–541.

Ferns, T. (2005). Violence in the accident and emergency department. An international perspective. *Accident and Emergency Nursing, 13*, 180–185.

Gascón, S., Martínez-Jarreta, B., López-Verdejo, M. A., Diana, I., López-Torres, J., & Castellano, M. (2008). Respuestas desadaptativas al estrés derivadas de agresiones a profesionales sanitarios [Dis-adaptive responses to stress due to aggression against health professionals]. *Revista de la Sociedad Española de Medicina y Seguridad del Trabajo [Journal of the Spanish Society of Occupational Safety and Medicine], 3*, 113–115 [in Spanish].

Gracia, D. (1989). *Los Cambios en la Relación Médico-Enfermo [Changes in the doctor-patient relation]. Medicina Clinica 93*(3), 100–102 [in Spanish].

Grenyer, B. F. S., Ilkiw-Lavalle, O., & Biro, P. (2004). Safer at work: Development and evaluation of an aggression and violence minimization program. *Australian and New Zealand Journal of Psychiatry, 38*(10), 804–810.

Henk, L., Nijman, M., & Rector, G. (1999). Crowding and aggression on inpatient psychiatric wards. *Psychiatric Services, 5D*, 830–831.

Hesketh, K. L., Duncan, S. M., & Estrabrooks, C. A. (2003). Workplace violence in Alberta and British Columbia Hospitals. *Health Policy, 63*, 311–321.

House of Commons. (2003). *A safer place to work.* Report by the comptroller and auditor general. London.

Maljers, J. (2006). Market forces inevitable in health care. *Nederlands Tijdschrift voor Geneeskunde, 150*(18), 1014.

Martínez-Jarreta, B., & Gascón, S. (2005). Fear of being reported, aggression and pressure. Distinctive aspects of burnout in general practitioners. *Proceedings of Second Mediterranean Academy of Forensic Sciences Congress*, Tunez.

National Health Service. (2002). *Zero tolerance campaign.* http://www.nhs.uk/zerotolerance/intro.htm

Osuna Carrillo, E., & Luna Maldonado, A. (2004). Derechos del enfermo [Rights of the Sick]. In E. Villanueva Cañadas (Ed.), *Medicina legal y toxicología [Legal medicine and toxicology].* Barcelona: Masson.

Paoli, P., & Merllié, D. (2001). *Third European survey on working conditions 2000.* Dublin: European Foundation for the Improvement of Living and Working Conditions.

Pariente, R., & Andrés, R. (2002). Necesidades de orientación de los/as alumnos/as de Magisterio [Guidance needs of education students]. *Educación y futuro: Revista de investigación aplicada y experiencias educativas* [*Education and the Future: Journal of Applied Research and Educational Experience*], no. 6, Madrid [in Spanish].

Stansfeld, S., Feeney, A., Head, J., Canner, R., North, F., & Marmot, M. (1995). Sickness absence for psychiatric illness: The Whitehall II study. *Social Science & Medicine, 40*(2), 189–197.

Wells, J., & Bowers, L. (August 2002). How prevalent is violence towards nurses working in general hospitals in the UK. *Journal of Advance Nursing, 39*(3), 230–240.

Whittington, R., Shuttleworth, S., & Hill, L. (1996). Violence to staff in a general hospital setting. *Journal of Advanced Nursing, 24*, 326–333.

Winstnaley, S., & Whittington, R. (2004). Aggression towards health care staff in a UK general hospital: Variation among professions. *Journal of Clinical Nursing, 13*, 3–10.

Yassí, A., Gilbert, M., & Cvitkovich, Y. (2005). Trends in injuries, illnesses, and policies in Canadian healthcare workplaces. *Canadian Journal of Public Health, 96*(5), 333–339.

Demographic Characteristics as Predictors of Nursing Students' Choice of Type of Clinical Practice

Abstract: *This descriptive study examined predictors of nursing students' choice of field of clinical practice using a convenience sample of 30 baccalaureate students in a Midwestern university. Students voluntarily completed a written questionnaire and responded to a subjective question about experiences influencing their choice of field. Students favored acute settings such as intensive care and emergency rooms over less acute settings, and their age and self-rating of health were related to these choices. Three types of experiences were described as meaningful contributors to choice of field of practice.*

The nursing shortage is of grave concern to the public and to the profession of nursing itself, and nursing workforce planning is a priority. Nursing workforce planning needs to address the number of nurses prepared and the level of nursing preparation at the international level, as well as nationally (Hegyvary, 2006; Peterson, 2005). In considering nursing workforce needs, one needs to consider not just the numbers of nurses but also the choice of clinical practice of those nurses. While declining enrollments in schools of nursing affect the availability of nurses in all settings, settings that are less "popular" among new graduates will be even harder hit by this shortage. This includes long-term health care settings and primary care settings. The needs for nurses in these types of settings vary from country to country. For example, in South Africa, the number of nursing positions in hospitals is much smaller than those in primary health clinics. In contrast, in the United States, the aging population makes needs in long-term care facilities greater than those in primary care.

■ BACKGROUND

In the United States, the general public's image of nursing continues to be the dedicated individual providing bedside nursing for acute health problems. Often the only image nursing students have of the field as they begin their education comes from television shows such as *Scrubs* or *Gray's Anatomy*. These portrayals usually project an image of nurses as either oversexed or always in the midst of life-threatening crises. The impact of such portrayals of nurses is reflected in the common situation when students, who think they may be interested in primary care or public health nursing "someday," often plan to do "real nursing" in a hospital first. As long-term planning for the nursing workforce continues, it will be important to be able to predict which students are more likely to fill gaps in the different and varied fields of nursing practice. This will allow nursing programs to target student recruitment toward those students most likely to move into clinical practice settings with the greatest need. Therefore, this study examined the relationships among nursing students' demographic characteristics and their choice for practice following graduation. Specifically, the study addressed the following three questions:

1. Are age, gender, race, and marital status associated with choice of first clinical practice after graduation?

2. Do older students and those with higher levels of perceived well-being select primary care settings for clinical practice after graduation more often than do younger students and those with lower levels of well-being?
3. What student experiences bring meaning to their choices of field of nursing practice?

■ METHODS

Sample

This study used a convenience sample of undergraduate baccalaureate nursing students in the second semester of their junior year of their program. The students were completing a required research course. The NLN-accredited nursing program located in a large Midwestern university enrolls 120 undergraduate students each year. The university draws students from throughout the Midwest and reports a generally diverse student body, including representative numbers of Latino and black students. Programs to earn a bachelor's degree in nursing include a traditional 4-year program, an RN to BSN program, and an LPN to BSN program. Students in all three of these programs take the research course that provided the sample for this study. Participation in the study was voluntary, and completion of the questionnaire was anonymous. A total of 30 out of 33 students participated.

Procedure

An independent faculty member who was not teaching the course administered the questionnaires, and the subjects placed the questionnaires in a sealed box themselves. Subjects were told that the questionnaire was part of the nursing department's efforts to plan future programs. In order to avoid any overt breach in confidentiality, all students remained in the classroom while the questionnaires were being completed, and all students placed questionnaires in the box, whether or not they had completed the questionnaire.

Measures

The entire questionnaire consisted of three sections. The first section asked about demographic characteristics, the second section asked about postsecondary education, perceived well-being, and planned choice of career, and the last section asked about subjects' preferences of automobiles. The last section was included to be used as a class exercise for the research course itself. Each section is described below.

Demographic characteristics included in this study were age, gender, and marital status. Each of these variables could reflect selected life experiences of students that might influence their choice of practice site after graduation.

The section asking about postsecondary education, well-being, and planned career choice included items asking about completion of previous technical programs, or associate or undergraduate degrees. Subjects were asked whether they were currently licensed to practice as either an LPN or RN and to give the total number of years of postsecondary education they had completed. Well-being was measured on a 4-point scale rating that perceived health as excellent, good, fair, and poor (Kaplan & Camacho, 1983). This single self-report item has been used in a number of studies, including the Human Population Laboratory Studies in Alameda County, CA (Kaplan & Camacho, 1983). The item has demonstrated reliability and validity. It has been shown to be strongly related to a persons' baseline physical health status and to be significantly related to different mortality rates for both men and women of all ages who perceived their health as excellent versus poor (Kaplan & Camacho, 1983).

The last questions in the second section of the questionnaire asked subjects about their anticipated choice of field of nursing immediately post graduation and long-term. Responses were selected from a list of nursing career options, eliminating the need to code individual responses. Subjects also were asked a single open-ended qualitative question, "What experiences in your life have led to your anticipated choice for field of nursing practice?" Subjects were provided with a single page of lined paper for this response.

The third section of the questionnaire regarding automobile preferences included questions about ownership of an automobile, and a rating on a 10-point scale of the condition of that automobile or how much they want an automobile if they do not own one. Subjects were asked to rank their color preferences for automobiles and to answer a series of dichotomous questions about their use of various forms of transportation.

The questionnaire was reviewed for face validity by three undergraduate faculty members of nursing. It was then pilot-tested with a sample of five graduate student nurses in their research course in order to assure clarity and relevancy. Only very minor changes in language resulted from this pilot test.

Analysis

Only the results from the first two sections of the questionnaire are reported here. Objective data from the questionnaires were analyzed using SPSS (Statistical Package for the Social Sciences) software program. Written subjective responses were directly transcribed and were analyzed using common phenomenological methods (Boyd & Munhall, 1993). Analysis included data reduction, identification of common themes, and conclusion drawing and was aided by use of QRS NUD.IST (Non-Numerical Unstructured Data Indexing Searching and Theory-building Multi-Functional) software program.

■ RESULTS

The sample included 30 undergraduate baccalaureate nursing students, 25 female and 5 male. Ninety percent were single ($n = 27$) and the average age of subjects was 23 ($SD = 2$).

The majority of the subjects (60%) were traditional 4-year baccalaureate students; however, subjects did represent all of the different programs offered. Many subjects had completed more than 3 years of postsecondary education ($M = 3.5$, $SD = 1$). Only 20% of subjects rated their own health as "fair or poor." Students' choices of field of nursing immediately post graduation and for a long-term career are reported in Table B.1. In both cases, the majority of students selected acute care settings, with an emphasis on intensive care and emergency department care as their anticipated field of nursing.

Choice of field or setting was dichotomized for acute setting versus nonacute setting for additional analysis. There was a significant difference in age of subjects who

Table B.1

Students' Choices of Field of Nursing

FIELD OF CHOICE	NUMBER (%) SELECTING FIELD IMMEDIATELY POST GRADUATION	NUMBER (%) SELECTING FIELD AS LONG-TERM GOAL
Intensive care (adult)	18 (60%)	9 (30%)
Neonatal or pediatric intensive care	3 (10%)	6 (20%)
Emergency department	3 (10%)	9 (30%)
Obstetrics	1 (3%)	0
Medical/Surgical	0	0
Pediatrics	2 (7%)	2 (7%)
Health department	0	0
Long-term care, nursing home	2 (7%)	0
Primary care clinic or health care provider office	1 (3%)	4 (13%)

selected the two settings ($t = 2.4$, $p < .05$), with younger students selecting acute fields of practice. There also was a significant difference in rating of health ($t = 2.1$, $p < .05$), with subjects who rated their health higher choosing acute care fields of practice more than those with lower levels of self-rated health. Lastly, there was an association between type of nursing program and choice of field of study ($\chi^2_{[10, N = 30]} = 23$, $p < .05$). There was no significant association between race or gender and choice of field of study, and no differences in number of years of postsecondary education and field of study. Logistic regression indicated that only age of subject and rating of health statistically contributed to the odds of selecting a nonacute care field of study when age, health rating, and type of nursing program were entered. One-way analysis of variance indicated that students who were older were more likely to be in the LPN to BSN program or the RN to BSN program.

Analysis of subjective findings yielded three distinct themes that represent the meaning of life experiences related to choice of field of nursing. The themes and selected quotes from subjects are included in Table B.2. The first theme was personal life experiences such as illness or death of a loved one, or their own acute illness. Subjects described experiences with nurses in the emergency room and the hospital and how these gave unique meaning to the health crisis being faced.

The second theme was direct experiences with family or close friends who provided nursing care in the field chosen by the subject. Subjects described love and respect and a desire to follow in the footsteps of these role models who had influenced their plans for the field of nursing.

The last theme was experiences with fictional media including novels, movies, and television shows. These subjects described being moved and excited by descriptions or scenes showing nurses providing care in the fields they expected to choose post graduation.

Table B.2

Definitions of Themes and Examples That Represent Meaning of Experiences in Relation to Choice of Nursing Field

THEMES	EXAMPLES OF EXPERIENCES
Personal life experience: direct interactions with health care providers and the health care system surrounding student's own health or that of others	"Seeing how those nurses took care of my mother as she lay there unconscious with so many tubes and machines hooked to her made me decide right then and there that this was what I wanted to do." "It was the nurse holding my hand as the doctor in the emergency room told me about my brother that made it possible for me to keep going. I want to be like that nurse and help others in such terrible times of life." "After I got home from the hospital a nurse came to visit and change my dressing. She was so caring and kind and gentle. Taking nursing into people's homes is what I want to do."
Experiences with nursing role models: direct interactions with significant others who are nurses	"My aunt was a nurse. She always was so strong and sure of herself—I wanted to be just like her and work in the emergency department." "In our town Mrs. Timms was the person everyone went to with a question or for help. It seemed like her being a nurse just made her able to help everyone. Mrs. Timms worked in the Health Department Clinic so that seems to me to be a good place to practice nursing."
Experiences with fictional media: vicarious experiences of providing nursing care in certain settings as described or depicted in books, television, and the movies	"Watching the nurses in *ER*; they always knew what was going on and were really there for the patients—that is why I want to practice in the emergency room."

■ DISCUSSION

Overall, students in this study identified that their choice of nursing field was intensive care and emergency room care. Maternity care and care of children were the second most commonly identified fields, with public health, primary care, and long-term care being the least frequently chosen. Objectively, the major demographic characteristic that was associated with choice of acute care field of practice was age, with younger nursing students more frequently choosing acute fields compared with older students. Students who were older were more likely to be in the RN to BSN program or the LPN to BSN program, and therefore, the type of baccalaureate program was also related to choice of field. Lastly, self-rating of health was related to choice of field of practice, with students who rated themselves in better health being more likely to choose acute care fields.

Subjectively, students described experiences in their personal lives, with role models and with fictional characters as meaningful in their decisions about choice of field. Age of students may very well relate to these types of experiences, since one would expect that older students would be more likely to have a range of personal life experiences with various fields of nursing. Younger students are more likely to have primarily experienced health care in the acute setting, if at all, and may well depend on role models and fictional characters more than older students. Certainly, the fictional characters available to these students would create an emphasis on acute settings. The differences in self-rating of health further support this idea, since students who are in poor health are more likely to have personal experiences with a variety of health care fields, not just acute care. The subjective transcribed data was not connected to the objective demographic data, so it was not possible to explore these possibilities more completely.

Given the changes in health care in this country and throughout the world and the increased emphasis on primary health care and early discharge from hospitals, it is clear that not all graduates who wish to practice in intensive care and emergency rooms will be able to do so. Nursing programs that are particularly concerned about shortages in nonacute settings may be able to expand this workforce by focusing their recruitment efforts on older students and by further developing or expanding RN to BSN and LPN to BSN programs. In addition, nursing needs to make fields of nursing other than acute care more visible to the public at large in order to widen the number of meaningful experiences nursing students might have that will affect their choice of field of practice.

References

Boyd, C. O., & Munhall, P. L. (1993). Qualitative research proposals and reports. *NLN Publications, 19*(2535), 424–453.

Hegyvary, S. T. (2006). Editorial: Roots of the shortage. *Journal of Nursing Scholarship, 33*(3), 204.

Kaplan, B. A., & Camacho, T. (1983). Perceived health and mortality: A nine-year follow-up of the Human Population Laboratory cohort. *American Journal of Epidemiology, 111*, 292–304.

Peterson, C. A. (2005). In short supply: Around the work, the need for nurses grows. *American Journal of Nursing, 101*(9), 61.

Sample In-Class Data Collection Tool

This questionnaire is for use in this research class only. Completing the questionnaire is entirely voluntary. If you do choose to fill out the questionnaire, please answer each question fully and thoughtfully.

DO NOT PUT YOUR NAME ON THIS FORM

Section One

What is your AGE in years? _____

Are you   MALE   FEMALE (circle one)

What is your MARITAL STATUS? (check one) _____ Single

_____ Married

_____ Divorced or Widowed

_____ Partnered

Section Two

How many YEARS school have you <u>completed</u> since finishing high school? _____

In general, how would you rate your OVERALL HEALTH? (circle one)

Excellent   Good   Fair   Poor

Below, you will find a list of possible fields for nursing practice. Please check which one you want as your FIRST CHOICE for practice when you graduate from this nursing program.

CHECK ONLY ONE!

_____ Emergency Department

_____ Health Department

_____ Intensive Care Unit for Adults

_____ Long-Term Care, Nursing Home

_____ Medical/Surgical Unit

_____ Neonatal or Pediatric Intensive Care

_____ Obstetrics

_____ Pediatric Unit

_____ Primary Care Clinic or Health Care Provider Office

Below, you will find the same list of fields of nursing. This time, please check which one you want as your FIRST CHOICE for practice as a **long-term goal.**

_____ Emergency Department

_____ Health Department

_____ Intensive Care Unit for Adults

_____ Long-Term Care, Nursing Home

_____ Medical/Surgical Unit

_____ Neonatal or Pediatric Intensive Care

_____ Obstetrics

_____ Pediatric Unit

_____ Primary Care Clinic or Health Care Provider Office

On the back of this questionnaire, please describe <u>the one major experience</u> in your life that has led you to select the field of nursing that you indicated above.

Section Three

Do you currently own a car? (check one) _____ YES _____ NO

- IF "YES," please answer the following questions about the car you own.
- If "NO," please answer the following questions for the car you expect to own in the immediate future.

Is the car (check one) _____ NEW _____ USED

Please **rate** the overall condition of the car you own or expect to own in the <u>immediate</u> future by circling ONE rating from the scale below.

1   2   3   4   5   6   7   8   9   10

Terrible   OK   Excellent

Please select your preferences for the CAR OF YOUR DREAMS:

Color (write in your primary color choice) _____

Type (such as SUV, sedan, convertible) _____

Transmission type (check one) _____ Automatic _____ Standard 5 speed

Engine cylinders (check one) _____ 4 cylinder _____ 6 cylinder _____ 8 cylinder _____ Unknown

From a range of 0% to 100%, how often do you wear seat belts while riding or driving in a vehicle? _____ % of the time.

Thank you for completing this questionnaire, which we will use for practice in this class only.

APPENDIX D

In-Class Study Data for Practice Exercise in Chapter 5

CASE NUMBER	MARITAL STATUS	HEALTH RATING
1	Single	4
2	Married	3
3	Divorced/widowed	3
4	Married	2
5	Married	1
6	Single	3
7	Single	1
8	Single	4
9	Single	4
10	Divorced/widowed	3
11	Married	2
12	Single	3
13	Single	3
14	Single	2
15	Married	2
16	Married	3
17	Single	4
18	Single	3
19	Divorced/widowed	3
20	Single	4
21	Married	3
22	Married	2
23	Single	3
24	Single	2
25	Single	3
26	Divorced/widowed	4
27	Single	3
28	Single	3
29	Married	2
30	Married	3

Pacifiers: An Update on Use and Misuse

Abigail Marter and Janyce Cagan Agruss

Abigail Marter, RN, MSN, is a family nurse practitioner and a lieutenant commander in the U.S. Navy, currently practicing at Naval Medical Center Portsmouth, Portsmouth, VA; and Janyce Cagan Agruss, RN, PhD, is a family nurse practitioner, assistant professor of nursing, and coordinator of the family nurse practitioner program at Rush University Medical Center, Chicago, IL.

Purpose.   *The use of pacifiers is a controversial topic; this article looks at the subject from both a historical and cultural perspective, with a review of current research.*

Conclusions.   *The use of pacifiers in infants older than 1 month is currently recommended by multiple researchers to prevent sudden infant death syndrome, and is associated with other benefits for premature infants. However, pacifier use has also been associated with higher risk of otitis media.*

Practice Implications.   *Knowledge of the most recent evidence will enable providers to communicate appropriate guidelines on pacifier use to families.*

Search terms: *breastfeeding, dummy, infants, infant equipment, nonnutritive sucking, otitis media, pacifier, pediatric dental health, premature infants, SIDS, sudden infant death.*

Despite their diminutive size, pacifiers are capable of stirring up a great deal of controversy and heated debate. The purpose of this article is to review the history behind the pacifier, looking at the pacifier's significance over time in different cultures. The article will then discuss benefits and risks associated with pacifier use, as found in recent research literature.

■ HISTORY

"A written word is the choicest of relics…. The symbol of an ancient man's thought becomes a modern man's speech" (Thoreau, 1893, p. 161). This quote from Henry David Thoreau highlights the significance of etymology and the history of language, which we can apply to deepening our understanding of the history of the pacifier. The pacifier, an object that is commonly used to soothe infant cries, has had a long and varied history, and has had many names in different languages over the course of time.

According to the Oxford English Dictionary (1989), use of the widely used current term "pacifier" has only been documented in the English language since the early years of the twentieth century. Alternate names in the past have included some of the following: dummy, sugar rag, binky, soother, sucky, silver spoon, and coral. Continuing to use the etymologic perspective, it is interesting to look at Roget's *New Millennium Thesaurus* for synonyms within the English language for "pacifier." They include the following: peacemaker, placator, appeaser, soother, hypnotic, narcotic, sleeping pill, and tranquillizer. All of these words help to give an appreciation of both the positive and the negative connotations associated with the original word.

Source: Journal for Specialists in Pediatric Nursing, Oct 2007, Vol. 12, No. 4, 278–285.

According to Levin (1971), almost everything written on pacifiers prior to 1900 was in German. Appropriately, the first recorded pictorial representation is in a painting of the Madonna and Child by Albrecht Dürer, a German painter, in 1506 (see Fig. E.1). In the Child's right hand can be found an early form of the pacifier, a "sugar rag" (see Fig. E.2). These were knotted strips of cloths that held different foodstuffs according to the country of origin, which the infant could then suck on without swallowing and choking on the food item. In Europe and Russia, the sugar rags would hold pieces of bread, meat, or fish; Finlanders preferred pieces of fat; while Germans favored poppy seeds or sweetened bread. Sometimes the rag was moistened with brandy or laudanum (a preparation of opium). Not surprisingly, there were occasional observations of babies who became intoxicated from sucking on these sugar rags (unfortunately, we have no reliable rates of intoxication from this era in pacifier history).

A German physician, Christian August Strove, wrote against the sugar rags in 1800 and did not save any sweet words for them.

> One of the most revolting practices is the sucking rag with which one tries to feed or quieten the child. Many a poor mother makes a rag from an old shirt or cloth which was picked up somewhere, possibly in the street, and contained vermin or even the remains of venereal poisons. One dips this rag into lukewarm water, the child throws it on the ground, and it is put back in his mouth in an even dirtier condition. Many flies sit on it, when the child is not observed, flies which a little earlier had been sitting on some poisonous matter in the room. (Levin, 1971, p. 238)

Levin notes that another German observer, Jacob Christian Gottlieb Shaffer, advised that the rag bag should be removed during sleep, to reduce the risk of suffocation.

What were sugar rags to do? They had to change with the times. A very important use for pacifiers of old was to help with teething infants. These devices were called "gum sticks" and were made from animal bone—the bone representing the animal's strength, which would be passed onto the child to help overcome pain. Coral was another substance that gum sticks were made from—coral was believed to be a virtual cure-all, guarding against all kinds of evil and protecting children from spirits as well as from witchcraft and illness. In addition to the use of a coral gum stick, a coral necklace could be added to provide more of the same protection to a baby. According to the Oxford English Dictionary (1989), "coral" was a common reference in the era from the 1600s to the 1800s, and it referred to a baby's teething toy made of coral or bone; both substances felt cool when placed upon the gums. Another alternative often used by wealthy upper-class families in the 1800s was silver—hence, the origin of the expression "to be born with a silver spoon in his mouth" (Oxford English Dictionary, 1989).

In the mid-1800s, rubber became the material of choice for pacifiers, and black, red, or white rubber was used. The "History of the Feeding Bottle" Web site (n.d.) notes that the white rubber of the time period contained a certain amount of lead, which could have contributed to lead poisoning among the infant population of that time. As the rubber pacifier took on the modern shape, the sugar rags, which were still popular until about 1900, rapidly died out. A Sears® Roebuck catalog circa 1908 shows a pacifier shape that is familiar to parents now in the twenty-first century (see Fig. E.3). Interestingly, these 1908 pacifiers had a rattle attached to them on the opposite side from the rubber mouthpiece. This tradition of the teething ring/rattle evolved centuries before, when suckable, cool-feeling coral

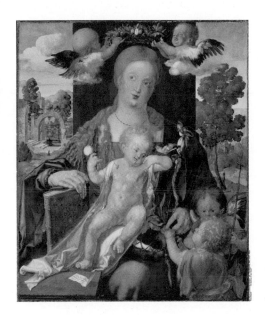

FIGURE E.1 *Madonna with the Siskin:* Albrecht Dürer, 1506. Permission Granted by Art Resource for One-time, Nonexclusive, North American English Language Rights for One Print Edition Only.

on one side was placed in the baby's mouth to rub against sore gums, while bells on the other side would simultaneously rattle and ward off evil spirits.

So, what do parents in the twentieth century think about the pacifier? Levin (1971, p. 240) talked to several mothers, and came up with the following quotes: "little piece of magic," "the most wonderful invention in the world," "worth their weight in gold," "the man

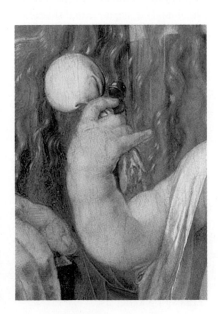

FIGURE E.2 Detail of *Madonna with the Siskin.* Albrecht Dürer, 1506. Permission Granted by Art Resource for One-time, Nonexclusive, North American English Language Rights for One Print Edition Only.

FIGURE E.3. Sears® Roebuck Catalogue Circa 1908, p. 791. Nonexclusive worldwide license to reproduce this figure granted by Sears® Holdings Archives.

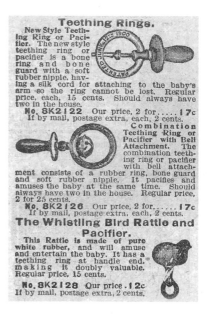

who invented it should be knighted," and "I couldn't have survived without them." On the opposite side, there are parents who are concerned with the sanitary and practical issues involved, in that pacifiers are difficult to keep clean and just plain difficult to keep, with many parents having to buy multiples in the almost inevitable event of loss. Other concerns involve the difficulty inherent in weaning children of the pacifier habit and the negative and shameful parental feelings associated with toddlers who continue to use pacifiers.

Sociocultural context is important in acceptance of a behavior, and attitudes toward pacifiers might predict pacifier use in a population. Thus, it is important within a cultural context to know the attitudes of parents toward their children using pacifiers. Vogel and Mitchell (1997) found predominantly negative parental attitudes to pacifiers in New Zealand, with a national use rate of 9%. Nelson, Yu, Williams, and the International Child Care Practices Study Group Members (2005) did not explore parental attitudes but investigated rates of pacifier use in different countries and found the following: Japan at 12.5%, China at 16%, Italy at 69%, and the Ukraine at 71%.

Levin (1971) noted a predominantly positive attitude toward pacifiers among white South African mothers, but no specific rates were mentioned. In fact, there has been no research on pacifier use within the African continent in the literature, and this could be related to minimal use of mass-produced pacifiers in these countries. In the United States, where recent movies have taken the pacifier, however obliquely, as their subject (e.g., Vin Diesel in *The Pacifier* [2005] and Keanu Reeves in *Thumbsucker* [2005]), rates of pacifier use are on the higher side of the spectrum. According to Hauck, Omojokun, and Siadaty (2005), rates as high as 74% have been reported. Thus, it is apparent that different cultures look at pacifiers from their own unique sociocultural perspectives, which might influence rates of pacifier use.

■ BENEFITS AND RISKS

Research has shown both positive and negative effects of pacifier use in infants. Standley (2003) showed that in preterm infants, nonnutritive sucking (i.e., pacifier use), in combination with lullaby music, increased subsequent feeding rates in previously poor feeders. The author concluded that for premature infants who are neurologically immature, nonnutritive sucking enhances neurological maturity and cognitive growth.

Another study by Li et al. (2006) looked at factors that might be associated with sudden infant death syndrome (SIDS). SIDS is defined as "the sudden unexpected death of an infant under 1 year of age, which remains unexplained after a postmortem examination (autopsy), death scene investigation, and review of the medical history" (Li et al., 2006, p. 18). According to the National Vital Statistics Report from 2003 (Matthews & MacDorman, 2006), SIDS is the third leading cause of infant mortality in the United States, and more than 2,100 deaths are attributed to SIDS each year. Li et al. found that the use of a pacifier was associated with a greater reduction of risk for SIDS with all factors. Thumb sucking was associated with reduced risk of SIDS, but in combination with a pacifier, the risk was even further reduced. Different hypotheses for the correlation (the authors cautioned that the strong association was not proof of a "causal" effect) included the bulky external handle of the pacifier, which might prevent accidental hypoxia as a result of the infant's face being buried in soft bedding, or that sucking on a pacifier could enhance development of neural pathways that control patency of the upper airway.

Hauck et al. (2005, p. 719) conducted a meta-analysis of seven case-control studies and concluded that putting an infant to sleep with a pacifier was a significant factor in protecting the infant from SIDS. Because of the nature of case-control studies, they were not able to attribute a causal effect, but the authors did find that the studies had adjusted for other confounding factors, such as maternal age, infant age, parity, birth weight, socioeconomic status, smoking, and sleep position. The authors discussed potential rationales for their findings based on their review of the literature. A lower arousal threshold has been found in frequent pacifier users (i.e., "light sleepers"—these infants are more likely to wake up out of sleep). Pacifier use may enhance the ability to breathe through the mouth if the nasal airway becomes obstructed. Suffocation and sleep apnea can be caused by retroposition of the tongue, whereas pacifier use "requires forward positioning of the tongue, thus decreasing the risk of oropharyngeal obstruction" (Hauck et al., 2005, p. 720).

One caveat to the Hauck et al. meta-analysis (2005) should be mentioned in that the studies included in the report used a case-control design, where the case group (parents who had SIDS deaths) might be remembering not using a pacifier more than the control group (Stuebe & Lee, 2006). Recall bias is a common problem in case-control studies. However, this problem has been refuted by others, saying that parents would not have known about the research showing pacifiers might reduce risk of SIDS at the time of the interviews in 1996–1997.

Mitchell, Blair, and L'Hoir (2006, p. 1756) noted that studies from New Zealand, the Netherlands, the UK, Ireland, Germany, Scandinavia, and the United States have all shown that routine pacifier use is significant for a reduced risk of SIDS. They also reviewed the literature for possible mechanisms to explain the protective effect of pacifiers on the incidence of SIDS. Proposed rationales included avoidance of the prone sleeping position if the infant is using a pacifier, protection of the oropharyngeal airway, reduction of gastroesophageal reflux through nonnutritive sucking, and lowering of the arousal threshold.

Other studies have been more equivocal regarding pacifier use. Collins et al. (2004) looked at whether pacifier use decreased breastfeeding rates in premature infants. They found that pacifier use was not correlated with lower breastfeeding rates or shorter duration of breastfeeding in preterm infants. The authors concluded that pacifiers should not be withheld from preterm infants less than 34 weeks in a misguided attempt to increase breastfeeding prevalence. Castelo, Gavião, Pereira, and Bonjardim (2005) investigated the effects of pacifier use on temporomandibular dysfunction. They found that nonnutritive sucking (both pacifier use and thumb sucking as defined by the study) was not significantly associated with the presence of signs and symptoms of temporomandibular dysfunction in children ages 3–5 years.

Other research studies show some negative effects in regard to pacifier use. Nelson et al. (2005) found a significant relationship between pacifier use and a lower rate of breastfeeding in different countries, with more pacifier use found in strictly formula-fed groups as well as in those groups where mothers mixed breastfeeding and formula feeding for their infants. However, in this study, countries with both high and low rates of breastfeeding (80% and 4%) showed high pacifier use rates (36% and 42%, respectively). The authors acknowledged that pacifier use could be a marker of breastfeeding difficulties as much as a cause of them. Viggiano, Fasano, Monaco, and Strohmenger (2004) did a retrospective study of children ages 3–5 and concluded that nonnutritive sucking (finger and pacifier use combined as defined by the study) is the main risk factor for dental problems, such as dental occlusion, open bite, and crossbite. They did not address whether spontaneous resolution of the malocclusion occurs when nonnutritive sucking stops.

Howard et al. (2003) were attempting to discover if "nipple confusion," "a breastfeeding problem hypothesized to result from the mechanical differences between suckling at the breast and sucking on a pacifier or bottle nipple" (p. 511), is a significant factor in breastfeeding problems. They found that early pacifier use (within the first month of life) caused a decline in exclusive breast feeding (defined by the infant receiving no other supplementation in addition to breast milk), and was associated with shortened overall exclusive breastfeeding duration. However, pacifier use had no effect on overall breastfeeding (defined as the length of time an infant received any breastfeedings) and no effect on full breastfeeding (defined as breastfeeding combined with less than daily supplementation of water, juice, or other feedings), and no effect on the duration of either type of breastfeeding.

The American Academy of Pediatrics (AAP) (2006) has issued some guidance on the subject of pacifiers. The AAP's policy statement on SIDS notes that the use of pacifiers has been shown to have a protective effect on the incidence of SIDS. Furthermore, the AAP notes that there is a low risk of dental malocclusions related to pacifier use and quotes from the American Academy of Pediatric Dentistry's statement, reinforcing that the use of pacifiers or thumb sucking in children up to the age of 5 is associated with low risk for long-term dental problems (AAP, 2006, p. 332). The AAP also notes that the use of pacifiers has not been shown to decrease breastfeeding duration for both term and preterm infants. The guidelines discuss a 1.2- to 2-fold increased risk of otitis media, which is associated with pacifier use, but quickly remark on this fact by noting that the incidence of otitis media is lower in the first 6–12 months of life, which is the time period of greatest risk for SIDS. As Mitchell et al. (2006) point out, it is important to ask the question in regards to the otitis media findings: are otitis media cases increased because of pacifiers, or are the use of pacifiers an effort to calm an unhappy baby who has ear pain and cannot do anything about it except cry? Several authors (Hauck et al., 2005; Mitchell et al., 2006) approach the otitis media risk by recommending the phasing out of pacifier use by the end of the first year of life, since the highest risk of SIDS is in that first year, and after the first year of life the risk of otitis media increases.

The AAP (2006, p. 332) states that gastrointestinal infections and oral colonization with *Candida* are more common among pacifier users. This last statement by the AAP regarding increased gastrointestinal infections and oral candidal infection does not seem to be supported by recent research. In a review of evidence-based practice on pacifiers by the Joanna Briggs Institute (2006, p. 54), the relationship and evidence that link pacifier use and infection are described as murky at best, due to the limited number of studies available and the variability of results from those studies. The AAP's policy statement on breastfeeding recommends not using pacifiers while mother and baby are initiating breastfeeding and holding off on their use until breastfeeding is well established. However, the AAP notes a distinction for premature infants, in that pacifier use is helpful for nonnutritive sucking and oral training in this population regardless of breastfeeding schedule (Joanna Briggs Institute, 2006, p. 300).

■ HOW DO I APPLY THIS INFORMATION TO NURSING PRACTICE?

In summary, some of the benefits of pacifier use include decreased risk of SIDS, assistance in helping babies to calm down from crying, and assistance for preemies to develop neurological maturity (see Table E.1). Some of the risks of pacifier use include potential for dental misalignment, potential to decrease breastfeeding if initiated within the first month, and a higher risk of otitis media (see Table E.1). Discussion of pacifier use is an important component of a provider's assessment of a family with children. Discussion about pacifier use can begin at the prenatal visit and occur at each visit thereafter, occurring also in the delivery room and postpartum (see Table E.2). The information provided here can serve as the basis for an evidence-based discussion between the healthcare

Table E.1

Potential Benefits and Risk Factors for Pacifier Use	
POTENTIAL BENEFITS	RISK FACTORS
Does not shorten breastfeeding duration when used in preterm infants or in term infants older than 1 month of age	Potential to shorten exclusive breastfeeding duration if initiated within the first month of life in term infants
Lowers the risk of SIDS, especially when used at the time of sleep	Potential for increased incidence of otitis media, especially after the first year of life
Assists in developing neurologic maturity in preterm infants	Potential for dental misalignment, such as open bite or crossbite

Table E.2

Pacifier Education for Parents

- Avoid introducing a pacifier until 4 weeks of age when breastfeeding is more likely to be established (Howard et al., 2003; Mitchell et al., 2006)
- There are risks as well as benefits (Nelson et al., 2005)
- For use only during sleeping periods (Mitchell et al., 2006)
- Do not force a child to use a pacifier (Hauck et al, 2005)
- In a sleeping infant, if the pacifier falls out of the mouth, it should not be reinserted (Hauck et al., 2005)
- At the end of the first year of life, begin to phase out pacifier use (Hauck et al., 2005; Mitchell et al., 2006)

provider and the parents, with the parents making the final decision on the use of pacifiers. With the information contained in this article, all parties will have a better understanding of the risks and current evidence surrounding the use of pacifiers.

■ ACKNOWLEDGMENT

The primary author is a military service member, and this work was prepared as part of said author's official duties. Title 17 U.S.C. 105 provides that "copyright protection under this title is not available for any work of the United States Government." Title 17 U.S.C. 101 defines a U.S. Government work as a work prepared by a military service member or employee of the U.S. Government as part of that person's official duties. The views expressed in this article are those of the author and do not reflect the official policy or position of the Department of the Navy, Department of Defense, nor the U.S. Government.

References

American Academy of Pediatrics. (2006). *Pediatric clinical practice guidelines and policies: A compendium of evidence-based research for pediatric practice* (6th ed.). Elk Grove Village, IL: American Academy of Pediatrics.

Barber, G. (Producer), & Shankman, A. (Director). (2005). *The pacifier* [Motion picture]. Burbank, CA: Buena Vista.

Bregman, A., Stephenson, B. (Producers), & Mills, M. (Director). (2005). *Thumbsucker* [Motion picture]. Culver City, CA: Sony Pictures Classics.

Castelo, P. M., Gavião, M. B., Pereira, L. J., & Bonjardim, L. R. (2005). Relationship between oral parafunctional/nutritive sucking habits and temporomandibular joint dysfunction in primary dentition. *International Journal of Pediatric Dentistry, 15*(1), 29–36.

Collins, C. T., Ryan, P., Crowther, C. A., McPhee, A. J., Paterson, S., & Hiller, J. E. (2004). Effect of bottles, cups, and dummies on breast feeding in preterm infants: A randomized controlled trial. *British Medical Journal, 329*, 193–198.

Hauck, F. R., Omojokun, O. O., & Siadaty, M. S. (2005). Do pacifiers reduce the risk of sudden infant death syndrome? A meta-analysis. *Pediatrics, 116*(5), 716–723.

History of the Feeding Bottle. (n.d.). *Dummies, pacifiers, soothers, what's in a name?* Retrieved July 19, 2006, from http://www.babybottle-museum.co.uk/dummy.htm

Howard, C. R., Howard, F. M., Lanphear, B., Eberly, S., deBlieck, E. A., Oakes, D., et al. (2003). Randomized clinical trial of pacifier use and bottle-feeding or cupfeeding and their effect on breastfeeding. *Pediatrics, 111*(3), 511–518.

Joanna Briggs Institute. (2006). Early childhood pacifier use in relation to breastfeeding, SIDS, infection and dental malocclusion. *Nursing Standard, 20*(38), 52–55.

Levin, S. (1971). Dummies. *South African Medical Journal, 45*(9), 237–240.

Li, D. K., Willinger, M., Petitti, D. B., Odouli, R., Liu, L., & Hoffman, H. J. (2006). Use of a dummy (pacifier) during sleep and risk of sudden infant death syndrome (SIDS): Population based case-control study. *British Medical Journal, 332,* 18–22.

Matthews, T. J., & MacDorman, M. F. (2006). Infant mortality statistics from the 2003 period: Linked birth/infant death data set [Electronic version]. *National Vital Statistics Reports, 54*(16). Hyattsville, MD: National Center for Health Statistics.

Mitchell, E. A., Blair, P. S., & L'Hoir, M. P. (2006). Should pacifiers be recommended to prevent sudden infant death syndrome? *Pediatrics, 117*(5), 1755–1758.

Nelson, E. A., Yu, L. M., Williams, S., & International Child Care Practices Study Group Members. (2005). International Child Care Practices study: Breastfeeding and pacifier use. *Journal of Human Lactation, 21*(3), 289–295.

Oxford English Dictionary (2nd ed.). (1989). Retrieved July 6, 2006, from OED online Web site: http://dictionary.oed.com/cgi/entry/50168989, http://dictionary.oed.com/cgi/entry/50049993, and http://dictionary.oed.com/cgi/entry/50234247

Roget's New Millennium Thesaurus (v 1.3.1). (n.d.). Retrieved July 6, 2006, from Dictionary.com Web site: http://thesaurus.reference.com/browse/pacifier

Sears®, Roebuck & Co. (1908). *Sears® roebuck spring catalogue* [Brochure]. Chicago, IL: Author.

Standley, J. M. (2003). The effect of music-reinforced nonnutritive sucking on feeding rate of premature infants. *Journal of Pediatric Nursing, 18*(3), 169–173.

Stuebe, A., & Lee, K. (2006). The pacifier debate. *Pediatrics, 117*(5), 1848–1849.

Thoreau, H. D. (1893). *Walden, or life in the woods.* Boston, MA: Houghton Mifflin Company.

Viggiano, D., Fasano, D., Monaco, G., & Strohmenger, L. (2004). Breast feeding, bottle feeding, and non-nutritive sucking: Effects on occlusion in deciduous dentition. *Archives of Disease in Childhood, 89*(12), 1121–1123.

Vogel, A., & Mitchell, E. A. (1997). Attitudes to the use of dummies in New Zealand: A qualitative study. *New Zealand Medical Journal, 110*(1054), 395–397.

GLOSSARY

Abstract a summary or condensed version of the research report. Chapter 1, p. 15.

Aggregated data data that are reported for an entire group rather than for individuals in the group. Chapter 11, p. 228.

Analysis of variance (ANOVA) a statistical test for differences in the means in three or more groups. Chapter 5, p. 94.

Anonymous a participant in research is anonymous when no one, including the researcher, can link the study data from a particular individual to that individual. Chapter 7, p. 135.

Assent to agree or concur; in the case of research, assent reflects a lower level of understanding about the meaning of participation in a study than consent. Assent is often sought in studies that involve older children or individuals who have a level of impairment that limits their ability but does not preclude their understanding of some aspects of the study. Chapter 7, p. 140.

Assumptions ideas that are taken for granted or viewed as truth without conscious or explicit testing. Chapter 11, p. 221.

Audit trail written and/or computer notes used in qualitative research that describe the researcher's decisions regarding both the data analysis process and collection process. Chapter 8, p. 153.

Beta (β) value a statistic derived from regression analysis that tells us the relative contribution or connection of each factor to the dependent variable. Chapter 5, p. 96.

Bias some unintended factor that confuses or changes the results of the study in a manner that can lead to incorrect conclusions; bias distorts or confounds the findings in a study, making it difficult to impossible to interpret the results. Chapter 6, p. 111.

Bivariate analysis statistical analysis involving only two variables. Chapter 4, p. 68.

Categorization scheme an orderly combination of carefully defined groups where there is no overlap among the categories. Chapter 4, p. 69.

Central tendency a measure or statistic that indicates the center of a distribution or the center of the spread of the values for the variable. Chapter 4, p. 77.

Clinical trial a study that tests the effectiveness of a clinical treatment; some researchers would say that a clinical trial must be a true experiment. Chapter 9, p. 196.

Cluster sampling a process of sampling in stages, starting with a larger element that relates to the population and moving downward into smaller and smaller elements that identify the population. Chapter 6, p. 114.

Codebook a record of the categorization, labeling, and manipulation of data for the variables in a quantitative study. Chapter 11, p. 226.

Coding reducing a large amount of data to numbers or conceptual groups (see data reduction) in qualitative research; giving individual datum numerical values in quantitative research. Chapter 4, p. 70.

Coercion the involvement of some element that controls or forces someone to do something. In the case of research, coercion occurs if a patient is forced to participate in a study to receive a particular test or service, or to receive or not to receive the best quality of care. Chapter 7, p. 136.

Comparison group a group of subjects that differs on a major independent variable from the study group, allowing comparison of the subjects in the two groups in terms of a dependent variable. Chapter 9, p. 189.

Conceptual framework an underlying structure for building and testing knowledge that is made up of concepts and the relationships among the concepts. Chapter 10, p. 204.

Conceptualization a process of creating a verbal picture of an abstract idea. Chapter 3, p. 55.

Conclusions the end of a research report that identifies the final decisions or determinations regarding the research problem. Chapter 2, p. 25.

Confidentiality assurance that neither the identities of participants in the research will be revealed to anyone else, nor will the information that participants provide individually be publicly divulged. Chapter 7, p. 135.

Confidence intervals the range of values for a variable, which would be found in 95 out of 100 samples; confidence intervals set the boundaries for a variable or test statistic. Chapter 5, p. 88.

Confirmation the verification of results from other studies. Chapter 3, p. 53.

Confirmability the ability to consistently repeat decision making about the data collection and analysis in qualitative research. Chapter 8, p. 153.

Construct validity the extent to which a scale or instrument measures what it is supposed to measure; the broadest type of validity that can encompass both content- and criterion-related validity. Chapter 8, p. 165.

Content analysis the process of understanding, interpreting, and conceptualizing the meanings imbedded in qualitative data. Chapter 4, p. 69.

Content validity validity that establishes that the items or questions on a scale are comprehensive and appropriately reflect the concept they are supposed to measure. Chapter 8, p. 164.

Control group a randomly assigned group of subjects that is not exposed to the independent variable of interest to be able to compare that group to a group that is exposed to the independent variable; inclusion of a control group is a hallmark of an experimental design. Chapter 9, p. 189.

Convenience sample a sample that includes members of the population who can be readily found and recruited. Chapter 6, p. 110.

Correlation the statistical test used to examine how much two variables covary; a measure of the relationship between two variables. Chapter 5, p. 92.

Correlational studies studies that describe inter-relationships among variables as accurately as possible. Chapter 9, p. 189.

Covary when changes in one variable lead to consistent changes in another variable; if two variables covary, then they are connected to each other in some way. Chapter 5, p. 92.

Credibility the confidence that the researcher and user of the research can have in the truth of the findings of the study. Chapter 8, p. 154.

Criteria for participation factors that determine how individuals are selected for a study; they describe the common characteristics that define the target population for a study. Chapter 6, p. 107.

Criterion-related validity the extent to which the results of one measure match those of another measure that is also supposed to reflect the variable under study. Chapter 8, p. 165.

Cross sectional a research design that includes the collection of all data at one point in time. Chapter 9, p. 187.

Data the information collected in a study that is specifically related to the research problem. Chapter 2, p. 27.

Data analysis a process that pulls information together or examines connections between pieces of information to make a clearer picture of all the information collected. Chapter 2, p. 27.

Data reduction organizing large amounts of data, usually in the form of words, so that it is broken down (or reduced) and labeled (or coded) to identify to which category it belongs. Chapter 4, p. 70.

Data saturation the point at which all new information collected is redundant of information already collected. Chapter 4, p. 70.

Deductive knowledge a process of taking a general theory and seeking specific observations or facts to support that theory. Chapter 10, p. 203.

Demographics descriptive information about the characteristics of the people studied. Chapter 4, p. 79.

Dependent variable the outcome variable of interest; it is the variable that depends on other variables in the study. Chapter 4, p. 72.

Descriptive design research design that functions to portray as accurately as possible some phenomenon of interest. Chapter 9, p. 182.

Descriptive results a summary of results from a study without comparing the results with other information. Chapter 2, p. 182.

Directional hypothesis a research hypothesis that predicts both a connection between two or more variables and the nature of that connection. Chapter 10, p. 210.

Discussion the section of a research report that summarizes, compares, and speculates about the results of the study. Chapter 3, p. 52.

Distribution the spread among the values for a variable. Chapter 4, p. 76.

Dissemination the spreading or sharing of knowledge; communication of new knowledge from research so that it is adopted in practice. Chapter 11, p. 227.

Electronic databases categorized lists of articles from a wide range of journals, organized by topic, author, and journal source available on CDs or online. Chapter 1, p. 14.

Error the difference between what is true and the answer we obtained from our data collection. Chapter 8, p. 149.

Ethnography qualitative research methods used to participate or immerse oneself in a culture in order to describe it. Chapter 9, p. 184.

Evidence-based nursing (EBN) the process that nurses use to make clinical decisions and to answer clinical questions about delivery of care to patients. Chapter 1, p. 3.

Exempt a category of research that is free from some of the constraints that are normally imposed upon research involving human subjects (United States Department of Health & Human Services, 2007). Chapter 7, p. 140.

Experimental designs quantitative research designs that include manipulation of an independent variable, a control group, and random assignment to groups. Chapter 9, p. 176.

Experimenter effects a threat to external validity that occurs when some characteristic of the researchers or data collectors themselves influence the results of the study. Chapter 9, p. 182.

External validity the extent to which the results of a study can be applied to other groups or situations; how accurate the study is in providing knowledge that can be applied outside of or external to the study itself. Chapter 9, p. 178.

Factor analysis a statistical procedure to help identify underlying structures or factors in a measure; it identifies discrete groups of statements that are more closely connected to each other than to all the other statements. Chapter 5, p. 96.

Field notes documentation of the participant's tone, expressions, and associated actions, and what is going on in the setting at the same time; they are a record of the researcher's observations about the overall setting and experience of the data collection process while in that setting or field itself; field notes are used to enrich and build a set of data that is thick and dense. Chapter 8, p. 151.

Five human rights in research rights that have been identified by the American Nurses Association guidelines for nurses working with patient information that may require interpretation; they include the right to self-determination, the right to privacy and dignity, the right to anonymity and confidentiality, the right to fair treatment, and the right to protection from discomfort and harm (ANA, 1985). Chapter 7, p. 132.

Frequency distribution a presentation of data that indicates the spread of how often values for a variable occurred. Chapter 4, p. 76.

Generalizability the ability to say that the findings from a particular sample can be applied to a more general population; *see* Generalization. Chapter 6, p. 118.

Generalization the ability to say that the findings from a particular study can be interpreted to apply to a more general population. Chapter 3, p. 56.

Grounded theory a qualitative research method that is used to study interactions to understand and recognize linkages between ideas and concepts, or to put in different words, to develop theory; the term *grounded* refers to the idea that the theory that is developed is based on or grounded in participants' reality. Chapter 9, p. 185.

Group interviews the collection of data by interviewing more than one participant at a time. Chapter 8, p. 152.

Hawthorne effect a threat to external validity that occurs when subjects in a study change simply because they are being studied, no matter what intervention is applied; reactivity and the Hawthorne effect are the same concept. Chapter 9, p. 181.

Historical research method a qualitative research method used to answer questions about linkages in the past to understand the present or plan the future. Chapter 9, p. 185.

History a threat to internal validity that occurs because of some factor outside those examined in a study, affecting the study outcome or dependent variable. Chapter 9, p. 180.

Hypothesis a prediction regarding the relationships or effects of selected factors on other factors under study. Chapter 2, p. 34.

Independent variables those factors in a study that are used to explain or predict the outcome of interest; independent variables also are sometimes called *predictor variables* because they are used to predict the dependent variable. Chapter 4, p. 72.

Inductive knowledge a process of taking specific facts or observations together to create general theory. Chapter 10, p. 203.

Inferential statistics statistics that are most commonly used in quantitative studies allowing the researcher to draw conclusions based on evidence obtained from a sample population. Chapter 4, p. 66.

Inference the reasoning that goes into the process of drawing a conclusion based on evidence. Chapter 4, p. 66.

Informed consent the legal principle that an individual or his or her authorized representative is given all the relevant information needed to make a decision about participation in a research study and is given a reasonable amount of time to consider that decision. Chapter 7, p. 133.

Instrument a term used in research to refer to a device that specifies and objectifies the process of collecting data. Chapter 8, p. 157.

Instrumentation a threat to internal validity that refers to the changing of the measures used in a study from one time point to another. Chapter 9, p. 180.

Institutional review board (IRB) a group of members selected for the explicit purpose of reviewing any proposed research study to be implemented within an institution or by employees of an institution to ensure that the research project includes procedures to protect the rights of its subjects; the IRB is also charged to decide whether or not the research is basically sound in order to ensure potential participants' rights to protection from discomfort or harm. Chapter 7, p. 133.

Internal consistency reliability the extent to which responses to a scale are similar and related. Chapter 8, p. 163.

Internal validity the extent to which we can be sure of the accuracy or correctness of the findings of a study; how accurate the results are within the study itself or internally. Chapter 9, p. 178.

Inter-rater reliability consistency in measurement that is present when two or more independent data collectors agree in the results of their data collection process. Chapter 8, p. 162.

Items the questions or statements included on a scale used to measure a variable of interest. Chapter 8, p. 157.

Key words terms that describe the topic or nature of the information sought when searching a database or the Internet. Chapter 1, p. 15.

Knowledge information that furthers our understanding of a phenomenon or question. Chapter 1, p. 11.

Likert-type scale a response scale that asks for a rating of an item on a continuum that is anchored at either end by opposite responses. Chapter 8, p. 159.

Limitations the aspects of how the study was conducted that create uncertainty concerning the conclusion that can be derived from the study as well as the decisions that can be based on it. Chapter 2, p. 26.

Literature review a synthesis of existing published writings that describes what is known or has been studied regarding the particular research question or purpose. Chapter 2, p. 00; Chapter 10, p. 206.

Longitudinal research design a research design that includes the collection of data over time. Chapter 9, p. 187.

Matched sample the intentful selection of pairs of subjects that share certain important characteristics to prevent those characteristics from confusing what is being explained or understood within the study. Chapter 6, p. 113.

Maturation a threat to internal validity that refers to changes that occur in the dependent variable simply because of the passage of time, rather than because of some independent variable. Chapter 9, p. 185.

Mean the arithmetic average for a set of values. Chapter 4, p. 77.

Measurement effects a threat to external validity because various procedures used to collect data in the study changed the results of that study. Chapter 9, p. 181.

Measure of central tendency a measure that shows the common or typical values within a set of values; central tendency measures reflect the "center" of a distribution, or the center of the spread; the mean, the mode, and the median are the three most commonly used. Chapter 4, p. 77.

Measures the specific method(s) used to assign a number or numbers to an aspect or factor being studied. Chapter 2, p. 32.

Median a measure of central tendency that is the value in a set of numbers that falls in the exact middle of the distribution when the numbers are in order. Chapter 4, p. 77.

Member checks a process in qualitative research where the data and the findings from their analysis are brought back to the original participants to seek their input as to the accuracy, completeness, and interpretation of the data. Chapter 8, p. 154.

Meta-analysis a quantitative approach to knowledge by taking the numbers from different studies that addressed the same research problem and using statistics to summarize those numbers, looking for combined results that would not happen by chance alone. Chapter 2, p. 36.

Metasynthesis a report of a study of a group of single research studies using qualitative methods. Chapter 2, p. 36.

Methods the methods section of a research report describes the overall process of implementing the research study, including who was included in the study, how information was collected, and what interventions, if any, were tested. Chapter 2, p. 29.

Mixed methods some combination of research methods that differ in relation to the function of the design, the use of time in the design, or the control included in the design. Chapter 9, p. 194.

Mode the value for a variable that occurs most frequently. Chapter 4, p. 77.

Model the symbolic framework for a theory or a part of a theory. Chapter 9, p. 190.

Mortality a threat to internal validity that refers to the loss of subjects from a study due to a consistent factor that is related to the dependent variable. Chapter 9, p. 180.

Multifactorial a study that has a number of independent variables that are manipulated. Chapter 9, p. 191.

Multivariate more than two variables; multivariate studies examine three or more factors and the relationships among the different factors. Chapter 2, p. 29.

Nondirectional hypothesis a research hypothesis that predicts a connection between two or more variables but does not predict the nature of that connection. Chapter 10, p. 210.

Nonparametric a group of inferential statistical procedures that are used with numbers that do not have the bell-shaped distribution or that are categorical or ordinal variables. Chapter 5, p. 89.

Nonprobability sampling a sampling approach that does not necessarily assure that everyone in the population has an equal chance of being included in the study. Chapter 6, p. 112.

Normal curve a type of distribution for a variable that is shaped like a bell and is symmetrical. Chapter 4, p. 77.

Novelty effects a threat to external validity that occurs when the knowledge that what is being done is new and under study somehow affects the outcome, either favorably or unfavorably. Chapter 9, p. 181.

Null hypothesis a statistical hypothesis that predicts that there will be no relationship or difference in selected variables in a study. Chapter 5, p. 97.

Operational definition a variable that is defined in specific, concrete terms of measurement. Chapter 8, p. 148.

Outcomes research a type of research that evaluates the impact of health care on the health outcomes of patients and populations, including evaluation of economic impacts linked to health outcomes, such as cost effectiveness and cost utility (NLM, 2008). Chapter 1, p. 5.

Parametric Statistics a group of inferential statistical procedures that can be applied to variables that are (1) normally distributed and (2) interval or ratio numbers such as age or intelligence score. Chapter 5, p. 89.

Participant observation a qualitative method where the researcher intentionally imbeds himself or herself into the environment from which data will be collected and becomes a participant. Chapter 8, p. 151.

Peer review the critique of scholarly work by two or more individuals who have at least equivalent knowledge regarding the topic of the work as the author of that work. Chapter 10, p. 208.

Phenomenology a qualitative method used to increase understanding of experiences as perceived by those living the experience; assumes that lived experience can be interpreted or understood by distilling the essence of that experience. Chapter 9, p. 184.

Pilot study a small research study that is implemented for the purpose of developing and demonstrating the effectiveness of selected measures and methods. Chapter 11, p. 232.

Population the entire group of individuals about whom we are interested in gaining knowledge. Chapter 6, p. 106.

Power analysis a statistical procedure that allows the researcher to compute the size of a sample needed to detect a real relationship or difference, if it exists. Chapter 6, p. 118.

Practice actions that are planned and implemented exclusively for the enhancement of health and the improvement of the well-being of an individual. Chapter 7, p. 131.

Predictor variables those factors in a study that are expected to affect the dependent variable in a specified manner; predictor variables are also called *independent variables*. Chapter 4, p. 72.

Pretest–posttest a research design that includes an observation both before and after the intervention. Chapter 9, p. 191.

Primary sources use of sources of information as they were originally written or communicated. Chapter 10, p. 207.

Printed indexes written lists of professional articles that are organized and categorized by topic and author, covering the time period from 1956 forward. Chapter 1, p. 12.

Probability the percentage of the time that the results found would have happened by chance alone. Chapter 5, p. 88.

Probability sampling strategies to assure that every member of a population has an equal opportunity to be in the study. Chapter 6, p. 113.

Problem section of a research report that describes the gap in knowledge that will be addressed by the research study or a statement of the general gap in knowledge that will be addressed in a study. Chapter 2, p. 33.

Procedures specific actions taken by researchers to gather information about the problem or phenomenon being studied. Chapter 2, p. 31.

Process improvement a management system in which all participants involved strive to improve customer outcomes. Chapter 2, p. 39.

Prospective designs a research design that collects data about events or variables moving forward in time. Chapter 9, p. 187.

Purposive sample inclusion in a study of participants who are intentionally selected because they have certain characteristics that are related to the purpose of the research. Chapter 6, p. 110.

***p* value** a numerical statement of the percentage of the time the results reported would have happened by chance alone. For example, a *p* value of .05 means that in only 5 out of 100 times would one expect to get the results by chance alone. Chapter 2, p. 29.

Qualitative methods approaches to research that focus on understanding the complexity of humans within the context of their lives and tend to focus on building a whole or complete picture of a phenomenon of interest; qualitative methods involve the collection of information as it is expressed naturally by people within the normal context of their lives. Chapter 2, p. 30.

Quality improvement a process of evaluation of health care services to see whether they meet specified standards or outcomes of care. Chapter 2, p. 38.

Quality improvement study a study that evaluates whether or not certain expected clinical care was completed. Chapter 2, p. 38.

Quantitative methods approaches to research that focus on understanding and breaking down the different parts of a picture to see how they do or do not connect; quantitative methods involve the collection of information that is very specific and limited to the particular pieces of information being studied. Chapter 2, p. 30.

Quasi-experimental designs a research design that includes manipulation of an independent variable but will lack either a control group or random assignment. Chapter 9, p. 191.

Questionnaire a written measure that is used to collect specific data, usually offering closed or forced choices for answers to the questions. Chapter 8, p. 157.

Quota sampling selection of individuals from the population who have one or more characteristics that are important to the purpose of the study; these characteristics are used to establish limits or quotas on the number of subjects who will be included in the study. Chapter 6, p. 112.

Random assignment the process ensuring that all subjects in a study have an equal chance of being in any particular group within the study. The sample itself may be one of convenience or purposive, so there may be some bias influencing the results. But, since that

bias is evenly distributed among the different groups to be studied, it will not unduly affect the outcomes of the study. Chapter 6, p. 116.

Random selection the process of creating a random sample; selection of a subset of the population where all the members of the population are identified, listed, and assigned a number and then some device, such as a random number table or a computer program, is used to select who actually will be in the study. Chapter 6, p. 113.

Reactivity effects threats in external validity that refer to subjects' responses to being studied. Chapter 9, p. 181.

Regression a statistical procedure that measures how much one or more independent variables explain the variation in a dependent variable. Chapter 5, p. 96.

Reliability the consistency with which a measure can be counted on to give the same result if the aspect being measured has not changed. Chapter 8, p. 162.

Repeated measures designs that repeat the same measurements at several points in time. Chapter 9, p. 188.

Replication a study that is an exact duplication of an earlier study; the major purpose of a replication study is confirmation. Chapter 3, p. 53.

Research design the overall plan for acquiring new knowledge or confirming existing knowledge; the plan for systematic collection of information in a manner that assures the answer(s) found will be as meaningful and accurate as possible. Chapter 9, p. 175.

Research hypothesis a prediction of the relationships or differences that will be found for selected variables in a study. Chapter 5, p. 97; Chapter 10, p. 210.

Research objectives clear statements of factors that will be measured in order to gain knowledge regarding a research problem; similar to the research purpose, specific aims, or research question. Chapter 10, p. 206.

Research problem a gap in existing knowledge that warrants filling and can be addressed through systematic study. Chapter 10, p. 202.

Research process a set of systematic processes that formalize the development of evidence. Chapter 1, p. 10.

Research purpose a clear statement of factors that are going to be studied in order to shed knowledge on the research problem. Chapter 10, p. 205.

Research questions statements in the form of questions that identify the specific factors that will be measured in a study and the types of relationships that will be examined to gain knowledge regarding a research problem; similar to the research objectives, purposes, and specific aims. Chapter 10, p. 210.

Research utilization the use of research in practice. Chapter 1, p. 3.

Response rate the proportion of individuals who actually participate in a study divided by the number who agreed to be in a study but did not end up participating in it. Chapter 6, p. 123.

Results a summary of the actual findings or information collected in a research study. Chapter 2, p. 27.

Retrospective designs quantitative designs that collect data about events or factors going back in time. Chapter 9, p. 187.

Rigor a strict process of data collection and analysis as well as a term that reflects the overall quality of that process in qualitative research; rigor is reflected in the consistency of data analysis and interpretation, the trustworthiness of the data collected, the transferability of the themes, and the credibility of the data. Chapter 8, p. 153.

Risk-to-benefit ratio a comparison of how much risk is present for human subjects compared with the level of benefit to the study. Chapter 7, p. 134.

Sample a subset of the total group of interest in a research study; the individuals in the sample are actually studied to learn about the total group. Chapter 2, p. 31; Chapter 6, p. 31.

Sampling frame the pool of all potential subjects for a study; that is, the pool of all individuals who meet the criteria for the study and, therefore, could be included in the sample. Chapter 6, p. 112.

Sampling unit the element of the population that will be selected for the study; the unit depends on the population of interest and could be individuals, families, communities, or outpatient prenatal care programs. Chapter 6, p. 118.

Saturation a point in qualitative research where all new information collected is redundant of information already collected; *see* Data saturation. Chapter 4, p. 70; Chapter 6, p. 111.

Scale a set of written questions or statements that in combination are intended to measure a specified variable. Chapter 8, p. 157.

Secondary sources someone else's description or interpretation of a primary source. Chapter 10, p. 208.

Selection bias when subjects have unique characteristics that in some manner relate to the dependent variable, raising a question as to whether the findings from the study were due to the independent variable or to the unique characteristics of the sample. Chapter 9, p. 180.

Selectivity the tendency of certain segments of a population agreeing to be in studies. Chapter 6, p. 122.

Semistructured questions questions asked in order to collect data that specifically targets objective factors of interest. Chapter 8, p. 157.

Simple random sampling a sample in which every member of the population has an equal probability of being included; considered the best type of sample because the only factors that should bias the sample will be present by chance alone, making it highly likely that the sample will be similar to the population of interest. An approach for acquiring the population of interest in which the researcher uses a device such as a random number table or computer program to randomly select subjects for a study. Chapter 6, p. 113.

Significance a statistical term indicating a low likelihood that any differences or relationships found in a study happened by chance alone. Chapter 2, p. 28.

Skew a distribution where the middle of the distribution is not in the exact center; the middle or peak of the distribution is to the left or right of center. Chapter 4, p. 78.

Snowball sampling a strategy for recruiting individuals in a study that starts with one participant or member of the population and then uses that member's contacts to identify other potential participants. Chapter 6, p. 110.

Specific aim clear statements of the factors to be measured and the relationships to be examined in a study to gain new knowledge about a research problem; similar to research purpose, objectives, or questions. Chapter 10, p. 206.

Speculation a process of reflecting on the results of a study and putting forward some explanation for them. Chapter 3, p. 54.

Standard deviation a statistic that is the square root of the variance; it is computed as the average differences in values for a variable from the mean value; a big standard deviation means that there was a wide range of values for the variable; a small standard deviation means that there was a narrow range of values for the variable. Chapter 4, p. 75.

Stratified random sampling an approach to selecting individuals from the population by dividing the population into two or more groups based on characteristics that are considered important to the purpose of the study and then randomly selecting members within each group. Chapter 6, p. 113.

Structured questions questions that establish what data is wanted ahead of the collection and do not allow the respondent flexibility in how to answer. Chapter 8, p. 157.

Study design the overall plan or organization of a study. Chapter 3, p. 58.

Systematic review the product of a process that includes asking clinical questions, doing a structured and organized search for theory-based information and research related to the question, reviewing and synthesizing the results from that search, and reaching conclusions about the implications for practice. Chapter 1, p. 17; Chapter 2, p. 36.

Systematic sampling an approach to the selection of individuals for a study where the members of the population are identified and

listed and then members are selected at a fixed interval (such as every fifth or tenth individual) from the list. Chapter 6, p. 113.

Testing a threat to internal validity where there is a change in a dependent variable simply because it is being measured or due to the measure itself. Chapter 9, p. 180.

Test–retest reliability consistency in the results from a test when individuals fill out a questionnaire or scale at two or more time points that are close enough together that we would not expect the "real" answers to have changed. Chapter 8, p. 162.

Themes results in qualitative research that are ideas or concepts that are implicit in the data and are recurrent throughout the data; abstractions that reflect phrases, words, or ideas that appear repeatedly as a researcher analyzes what people have said about a particular experience, feeling, or situation. A theme summarizes and synthesizes discrete ideas or phrases to create a picture out of the words that were collected in the research study. Chapter 2, p. 27; Chapter 4, p. 70.

Theory an abstract explanation describing how different factors or phenomena relate. Chapter 2, p. 34.

Theoretical definition a conceptual description of a variable. Chapter 8, p. 148.

Theoretical framework an underlying structure that describes how abstract aspects of a research problem interrelate based on developed theories. Chapter 10, p. 204.

Transferability the extent to which the findings of a qualitative study are confirmed or seem applicable for a different group or in a different setting from where the data were collected. Chapter 8, p. 154.

Triangulation a process of using more than one source of data to include different views, or literally to look at the phenomenon from different angles. Chapter 8, p. 155.

Trustworthiness the honesty of the data collected from or about the participants. Chapter 8, p. 153.

***t* test** a statistic that tests for differences in means on a variable between two groups. Chapter 5, p. 90.

Univariate analysis statistical analysis about only one variable. Chapter 4, p. 68.

Unstructured interviews questions asked in an informal open fashion without a previously established set of categories or assumed answers, used to gain understanding about a phenomenon or variable of interest. Chapter 8, p. 151.

Validity how accurately a measure actually yields information about the true or real variable being studied. Chapter 8, p. 163.

Variable some aspect of interest that differs among different people or situations; something that varies: it is not the same for everyone in every situation. Chapter 4, p. 68.

Variance the diversity in data for a single variable; a statistic that is the squared deviations of values from the mean value and reflects the distribution of values for the variable. Chapter 4, p. 74.

Visual analog a response scale that consists of a straight line of a specific length that has extremes of responses at either end but does not have any other responses noted at points along the line. Subjects are asked to mark the line to indicate where they fall between the two extreme points. Chapter 8, p. 160.

Withdrawal a right of human subjects to stop participating in a study at any time without penalty until the study is completed. Chapter 7, p. 136.

INDEX

Note: Page numbers followed by *f* indicate figures; those followed by *t* indicate tables; and those followed by *b* indicate boxed material.